Multiple Choice Questions in Pediatric Dentistry

Multiple Choice Questions in Pediatric Dentistry

Second Edition

MS Muthu, MDS, PHD
Professor and Head
Department of Pediatric Dentistry
Saveetha Dental College and Hospital
Velappanchavadi
Chennai

Director, Pedo Planet
Chennai

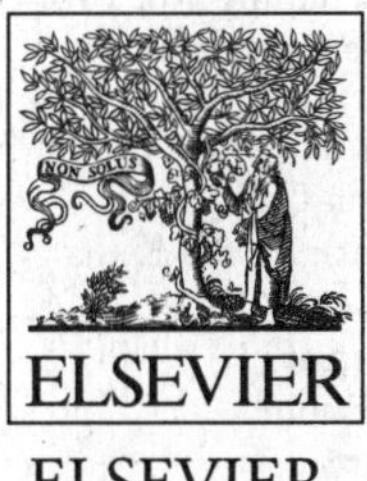

ELSEVIER
A division of
Reed Elsevier India Pvt. Ltd.

Multiple Choice Questions in Pediatric Dentistry, 2/e

Muthu

ELSEVIER
A division of
Reed Elsevier India Private Limited

Mosby, Saunders, Churchill Livingstone, Butterworth Heinemann and Hanley & Belfus are the Health Science imprints of Elsevier.

First Edition 2005
Second Edition 2011

ISBN: 978-81-312-2815-9

Published by Elsevier, a division of Reed Elsevier India Private Limited

Registered Office: 622, Indraprakash Building, 21 Barakhamba Road,
New Delhi-110 001

Corporate Office: 14th Floor, Building No. 10B, DLF Cyber City,
Phase II, Gurgaon-122 002, Haryana, India

Publishing Manager: Ritu Sharma
Commissioning Editor: Nimisha Goswami
Managing Editor (Development): Anand K Jha
Copy Editor: Anu Vig
Manager, Operations: Sunil Kumar
Production Executive: Arvind Booni
Cover Designer: Raman Kumar

Typeset by County Caramels

Printed at Rajkamal Electric Press, Plot No. 2, Phase-IV, Kundli, Haryana.

to

my beloved parents

Mr Murugan (My Dad) and Mrs Balasaraswathi (My Mom)

and

My loving wife K Muthu Prathibha

Foreword

I am delighted to introduce this book written by Dr MS Muthu on Multiple Choice Questions in Pediatric Dentistry.

It is really heartening to know that one of my students has put in tremendous hard work to bring out this book for the benefit of students of dentistry.

Dr Muthu had excelled in pediatric dental practice; both as clinician and academician. Very few books on MCQs in Pediatric Dentistry are available. This book fills the gap. The questions are meticulously selected by the author, which needs appreciation.

I am sure this book will be accepted by undergraduate students as it would encourage them to detect the areas of weakness in their understanding of the subject so that they may return to the text for a more comprehensive review of the topics. Also this book will serve the need and prove extremely useful for students in preparing themselves for competitive exams.

The author deserves to be congratulated for an excellent, well co-ordinated academic venture.

Prof SG Damle
Vice Chancellor
Maharishi Markandeshwar University
Mullana, Ambala (HR)
INDIA-133207

Contributors

Chief Editors

T Chandrapriya BDS
Dental Surgeon
Pedo Planet
Pediatric Dental Centres
2C, AKME Park
Opp S&S Power Ltd
Porur
Chennai

Sharath Asokan
MDS, PHD, MS, MPHIL
Pediatric Dental Surgeon
Reader
Department of Pediatric Dentistry
Meenakshi Ammal Dental College
Maduravoyal, Chennai
Consultant, Pedo Planet
Pediatric Dental Centre

Contributors

Steven Rodrigues MDS
Professor
Department of Pediatric Dentistry
Saveetha Dental College & Hospital
Velappanchavadi
Chennai

SK Jagdish MDS
Junior Resident
Department of Prosthodontics
and Implantology
Mahatma Gandhi Postgraduate
Institute of Dental Sciences
Puducherry

G Deepa MDS
Reader
Department of Pediatric Dentistry
Saveetha Dental College & Hospital
Velappanchavadi
Chennai

Preface to the Second Edition

In the preface to the first edition in 2005, I had mentioned Pediatric Dentistry as a developing field. Six years later, now in 2011, I still believe that the awareness about pediatric dentistry among the doctors, physicians, and pediatricians has not increased in a great way. I still feel that we have a long way to go.

The project of writing a multiple choice questions book was primarily taken up by me with the aim of helping the undergraduate and postgraduate students of Dentistry to strengthen their basics in Pediatric Dentistry.

In the making of the second edition, great efforts have been put forth to synchronize this book with the textbook. A major restructuring of the chapters has also been done. I have included around 21 new chapters and new questions have also been added to the existing chapters. The content of this book has almost been doubled when compared to the first edition. All the questions have been framed with the idea of emphasizing the important facts and points pertaining to each chapter. I have provided clear explanations for most of the questions along with relevant tables, related information and images, which will definitely help the students to understand the subject better. At this stage, I can say that if a student answers these questions and understands the explanations, the basics of the student will definitely be miles ahead of those who have not read this book. Many questions pertaining to applied aspects of clinical pediatric dentistry have also been explained with questions on a variety of clinical situations. Further, each chapter also includes questions which the students usually come across in licensing examinations abroad like National Board Dental Examinations in USA and Canada.

Regarding the effective usage of this book, it is not a book to be read once and considered complete by the students. In this book, many definitions and fundamentals have been framed in the form of questions. In other words, these questions are to be revised many times to reinforce the basics. It may look simple whenever, you see a question with choices as:

a. both the statements are true.

b. both the statements are false, etc.

These questions are framed with the intention of reinforcing some fundamental concepts. Some questions which have the answer as "all of the above" are also framed with the same idea in mind. These questions may seem simple when one answers these questions in isolation. But if the student revises these questions, they may be the key points of a short essay question or a short note question. In a nutshell, this is much more than an MCQ book. In fact, I can confidently say that if a student goes through these questions thoroughly and understands them, he/she will definitely stand apart in their final BDS and MDS examinations as they will be strong with their fundamentals. With many years of experience as an examiner for various universities across the country, I often see students failing in the exams due to their weak basics which upsets the examiners. This book is an answer to such issues.

I have predominantly based the MCQ book on my textbook “Pediatric Dentistry: Principles and Practice”. I personally feel that reading many pages of a theory book can help us to understand the content in general. However, when one goes through MCQs pertaining to the same content, the key points are stressed upon and remembered well. I have always believed that objective questions can evaluate the knowledge of an individual better than any other method. That is probably why many of the competitive examinations worldwide in various fields have objective (MCQs) questions as their method of evaluation. This book will definitely be of great help in efficiently tackling objective competitive examinations.

MS Muthu

Preface to the First Edition

This is an elaborate and penetrating collection of multiple choice questions in the subject of Pediatric Dentistry. This project was primarily taken up by me with the aim of helping the undergraduate and post-graduate students of dentistry to strengthen their basics in this upcoming field.

The competitive examinations of these days demand a sound knowledge of the fundamentals of any subject. Preparation for these entrance exams does not end with merely reading the textbooks. It becomes complete only when the concepts are repeatedly revised by solving the related multiple choice questions.

In this book I have presented about 800 multiple choice questions with relevant explanations. They are organized in a chapterwise manner for the convenience of students. All the questions were framed with the idea of emphasizing the important facts and points pertaining to each chapter. I have provided clear explanations for most of the questions along with relevant tables, related information and images, which will definitely help the students to understand the subject better.

I would sincerely urge the students to repeatedly revise these questions along with their explanations in order to make the most out of this book.

I am sure this book will serve its prime purpose of helping the students to master the fundamentals of Pediatric dentistry.

MS Muthu

Preface to the First Edition

Acknowledgements

First of all I should thank my publisher Elsevier India for publishing the second edition of this book. I would like to thank in particular Mr Rohit Kumar, Managing Director, Ms Ritu Sharma, Publishing Manager, Ms Nimisha Goswami, Commissioning Editor, Mr Anand K Jha, Managing Editor and Ms Anu Vig, Copy Editor for coping with my inconsistencies in delivering the content. However, I have tried my level best to be as efficient as possible.

I should thank Dr Chandrapriya, who has contributed and played a major role in this edition by helping me with the explanations for the newly formed questions and typing it. She has also helped me in integrating the old edition with this edition in a comprehensive and more logical manner.

Dr Sharath Asokan, who has contributed questions for around 10–12 chapters in this edition should be thanked for his voluntary involvement with the book. I have incorporated their names as Chief Editors on the Contributors page of this book. Without their tireless efforts this would not have been possible.

I should also thank Dr Steven Rodrigues, Professor, Department of Pediatric Dentistry, Saveetha Dental College, also my great friend, for checking of all the chapters carefully and giving his valuable inputs. My sincere thanks are due to Dr Deepa G, Reader from the Department of Pediatric Dentistry, Saveetha Dental College for her contribution of MCQs for two chapters in this book and Dr Jagdish, PG student from the Department of Prosthodontics, Mahatma Gandhi Institute of Dental Sciences for his contribution to the chapter on Prosthodontic Considerations.

Mr Saravnan from Print World for delivering me the proofs of the chapters as and when needed. It was a great help getting the printouts delivered at home.

Finally, my better half, Dr Muthu Prathibha, who has really stretched and helped me in going through the proofs and edit the language of all the chapters in a short span of time. This has happened in spite of her pregnancy and the inconsistencies associated with it. Naturally, I have to dedicate this book to her. Without her support and contribution, many of my achievements would not have happened. Undoubtedly, she is the woman behind my success.

I should also thank colleagues of my department Dr Sujatha, and Dr Harini Devi, for effectively managing the department whenever I was unavailable for the department because of this work. I should also thank my PG students who continue to challenge me and help me grow both intellectually and personally, without them I doubt being what I am.

Acknowledgements

Contents

Section V
Dental Caries

Section VI
Restorative Dentistry and Endodontics

Section VII
Injuries to the Teeth—Prevention and its Management

Section VIII
Pediatric Orthodontics

Section IX
Children with Special Health Care Needs and Medical Emergencies

Section X
Interdisciplinary Pediatric Dentistry

Section XI
Miscellaneous

Section I

Fundamentals–Introduction to Pediatric Dentistry

Section 1

Fundamentals–Introduction to Pediatric Dentistry

Chapter 1

Introduction to Pediatric Dentistry

1. Which national society states the following message — "Every child has a fundamental right to his/her total oral health and we have an obligation to fulfill this faith"?

a. European Academy of Pediatric Dentistry
b. Indian Society of Pedodontics and Preventive Dentistry
c. Japanese Society of Pediatric Dentistry
d. American Academy of Pediatric Dentistry

Ans b.

The quote mentioned above is the motto of Indian Society of Pedodontics and Preventive Dentistry (ISPPD).

2. Characteristics of an ideal pedodontist

a. Kindness
b. Patience
c. Empathy
d. All of the above

Ans d.

All of the above-mentioned virtues are characteristics of an ideal pedodontist.

3. Differences between child and adult patient are

a. Physical, emotional and psychological development
b. Dentist to the patient relationship
c. Dentist to the parent relationship
d. Both (a) and (b)

Ans d.

The factors mentioned above in (a) and (b) are significant differences between child and adult patients, which may influence the management of children in the dental office.

Chapter 2

History Taking, Examination, Diagnosis and Treatment Planning in Pediatric Dentistry

1. The carious lesion always appears smaller on the radiograph than it actually is. Likewise, microscopic observation of ground sections of teeth reveal that the progress of the lesion through the enamel and dentin is more extensive than it is evident on the radiograph.

a. Both the statements are false
b. Both the statements are true
c. First statement is true and the second is false
d. First statement is false and the second is true

Ans b.

The answer is self-explanatory.

2. Which of the following is true regarding drug abuse?

a. Symptoms of abuse may include depression, frustration, feeling of inadequacy, helplessness, immaturity, major deficiencies in ego structure and functioning
b. Substances commonly abused are solvents, inhalants, narcotics, stimulants, sedatives, tranquilizers and tobacco
c. Glue sniffing and gasoline sniffing are also different forms of drug abuse
d. All of the above

Ans d.

All the above-mentioned factors are true regarding substance/drug abuse.

3. In extraoral assessment, the height and weight information is recorded for

a. Correlating it to dental disease
b. Establishing the relationship with early childhood caries
c. Comparing with the standard growth curves
d. None of the above

Ans c.

The height and weight information is recorded to compare them with the standard growth curves. If a patient is below the third percentile or above the 97th percentile, referral to a pediatrician may be necessary.

4. All of the following statements are true regarding pain in history taking except

a. Child should be asked whether hot or cold food or drinks have any relation to pain
b. Duration of pain following the exposure to stimulus should be questioned
c. Spontaneous pain indicates reversible pulpitis
d. Pain that is precipitated by pressure indicates periodontal damage

Ans c.

Spontaneous pain indicates irreversible pulpitis. Eliciting an accurate pain history can be very useful in determining the treatment planning for child.

5. (i) Electrical and thermal stimulations are the most common methods of assessing vitality. (ii) Young children are not good candidates for vitality testing as false positive responses are common in primary dentition.

a. Both the statements are true
b. Both the statements are false
c. First statement is true and the second is false
d. First statement is false and the second is true

Ans a.

The answer is self-explanatory.

Chapter 3

Chronology and Morphology of Primary and Permanent Teeth

1. Evidence of development of human tooth can be observed as early as

a. 6th week of embryonic life
b. 11th week of embryonic life
c. 14th week of embryonic life
d. 16th week of embryonic life

Ans a.

Evidence of development of tooth can be observed as early as 6th week of embryonic life. According to Kraus and Jordan, the first macroscopic indication of morphologic development of tooth occurs at approximately 11 weeks in utero. Calcification of the primary maxillary central incisor begins at approximately 14 weeks in utero. Evidence of developing primary canines can be observed between 14 and 16 weeks.

2. Enamel hypoplasia is because of disturbance in _____ stage of tooth development

a. Initiation/proliferation
b. Histodifferentiation
c. Morphodifferentiation
d. Apposition

Ans d.

Refer to the explanation of Q. No. 2.

3. Microdontia or macrodontia of teeth is because of damage in _________ stage of tooth development

a. Initiation/proliferation
b. Histodifferentiation
c. Morphodifferentiation
d. Apposition

Ans c.

Microdontia or macrodontia of teeth is because of damage occurring in the stage of morphodifferentiation. (See Table 3.1 on next page).

Table 3.1

S. No.	Aberration in stage of tooth development	Result
1.	Initiation/proliferation	Supernumerary teeth Partial anodontia Odontoma
2.	Histodifferentiation	Amelogenesis imperfecta Dentinogenesis imperfecta
3.	Morphodifferentiation	Peg teeth Mulberry molars Microdontia Macrodontia Talon cusp
4.	Apposition	Enamel hypoplasia

4. The first macroscopic indication of morphologic development of primary incisors occurs approximately at

a. 11 weeks in utero
b. 14 weeks in utero
c. 16 weeks in utero
d. 6 weeks in utero

Ans a.

Kraus and Jordan have found that the first macroscopic indication of morphologic development occurs at approximately 11 weeks in utero. The maxillary and mandibular central incisor crowns appear identical at this early stage as tiny, hemispheric, mound-like structures.

5. The first evidence of calcification of primary teeth begins approximately at

a. 11 weeks in utero
b. 14 weeks in utero
c. 16 weeks in utero
d. 6 weeks in utero

Ans b.

Calcification of the primary maxillary central incisor begins at approximately 14 weeks in utero, the upper central incisor slightly preceding the lower central.

6. **In primary teeth, cusp of Carabelli is seen in**
   a. Maxillary first molar
   b. Maxillary second molar
   c. Mandibular first molar
   d. Mandibular second molar

Ans b.

Cusp of Carabelli is seen in maxillary second primary molar. Mandibular first primary molar has a central ridge.

7. **Extreme curvature of the buccal side is characteristic of**
   a. Mandibular first primary molar
   b. Mandibular second primary molar
   c. Maxillary first molar
   d. Maxillary second primary molar

Ans a.

Extreme curvature of the buccal side is characteristic of mandibular first primary molar. The buccal curvature of maxillary first primary molar is not as prominent as the mandibular first primary molar.

8. **The primary second molar (mandibular) resembles**
   a. Maxillary first permanent molar
   b. Mandibular first permanent molar
   c. Maxillary second permanent molar
   d. Mandibular second permanent molar

Ans b.

Mandibular second primary molar resembles the mandibular first permanent molar. Maxillary second primary molar resembles the maxillary first permanent molar. Maxillary and mandibular *second* permanent molars do not resemble any primary tooth.

9. **All of the following are true of primary teeth except**
   a. Crowns of the primary teeth are wider in comparison to their crown length than are permanent teeth
   b. Roots of primary molars are long and slender
   c. Primary teeth are usually lighter in color than the permanent teeth
   d. Buccal curvature on primary first molars are not prominent

Ans d.

Extreme curvature of the buccal side is characteristic of mandibular first primary molar. The buccal curvature of maxillary first primary molar is not as prominent as mandibular first primary molar.

10. Clinical emergence of a tooth occurs when

a. One-fourth of the root formation is complete
b. Half of the root formation is complete
c. Three-fourths of the root formation is complete
d. Root formation is complete

Ans c.

According to Gron, tooth emergence appeared to be more closely associated with the stage of root formation than with the chronological or skeletal age of the child. By the time of clinical emergence, approximately three-fourths of root formation would have occurred. Teeth reach occlusion before the root development is complete.

11. According to Moyer, the most favorable sequence of eruption of maxillary permanent teeth is

a. 6,1,2,4,3,5,7
b. 6,1,2,3,4,5,7
c. 6,1,2,4,5,3,7
d. 6,1,2,5,4,3,7

Ans c.

In the maxillary arch, the first premolar ideally should erupt before the second premolar and they should be followed by the canine. The untimely loss of the primary molars in the maxillary arch, allowing the first permanent molar to drift and tip mesially, will result in the permanent canine being blocked out of the arch, usually to the labial side. The position of the developing second molar in the maxillary arch and its relationship to the first permanent molar should be given special attention. Its eruption before the premolars and canine can cause a loss of arch length just as in the mandibular arch.

12. The most favorable eruption sequence for mandibular permanent teeth is

a. 6,1,2,3,4,5,7
b. 6,1,2,4,5,3,7
c. 6,1,3,2,4,5,7
d. 6,1,2,3,7,4,5

Ans a.

The most favorable sequence in mandibular arch is first permanent molar, central incisors, lateral incisors, canines, first and second premolars. It is desirable that the mandibular canine erupts before the first and second premolars. This sequence will aid in maintaining adequate arch length and in preventing lingual tipping of the incisors. Lingual tipping of the incisors not only will cause a loss of arch length but also will allow the development of an increased overbite.

13. Eruption sequestrum is made of

a. A tiny spicule of nonviable bone
b. Dentin and cementum
c. Either osteogenic or odontogenic tissue
d. Any of the above

Ans d.

Eruption sequestrum is defined as a tiny spicule of nonviable bone overlying the crown of an erupting permanent molar just before or immediately after the emergence of the tips of the cusps through the oral mucosa. It can be also composed of dentin, cementum, osteogenic or odontogenic tissue.

14. Among the primary teeth, the problem of ankylosis is most commonly seen with

a. Mandibular molars
b. Mandibular incisors
c. Maxillary incisors
d. Maxillary molars

Ans a.

Ankylosis is most commonly seen in mandibular molars among the primary teeth. Metallic sound on percussion is diagnostic of ankylosed and traumatically intruded tooth. Ankylosed teeth are also called *submerged teeth*.

15. All are features of a Mongoloid child except

a. Bridge of the nose is depressed
b. Mental retardation
c. Delayed eruption of primary teeth
d. Eyes slope downward

Ans d.

All the above-mentioned features are common to Down syndrome children except that the eyes of these children slope upwards.

16. All of the following conditions are associated with delayed eruption of teeth except

a. Hyperthyroidism
b. Hypopituitarism
c. Cleidocranial dysplasia
d. Gardner's syndrome

Ans a.

In hyperthyroidism, premature eruption of teeth is noticed. In hypopituitarism, delayed eruption of teeth is seen. In severe cases, primary teeth do not exfoliate. The underlying permanent teeth also do not erupt. In some cases of cleidocranial dysplasia, primary teeth are retained till 15 years of age. Gardner's syndrome is also associated with delayed eruption of teeth.

17. Maxillary diastema frequently do not close until the eruption of permanent

a. Maxillary lateral incisors
b. Mandibular cuspids
c. Maxillary cuspids
d. Maxillary premolars

Ans c.

In the mixed dentition, physiologic spacing between incisors is normal because of the eruption pattern of permanent teeth. When the canines erupt, all the spaces will close. No treatment should be initiated if there is a possibility of diastema being physiologic or if the canines have not erupted. Abnormal diastema may also result from supernumerary or missing teeth, oral habits, macroglossia or frenula. Hence, an accurate diagnosis is necessary before the treatment is initiated.

18. The crowns of all permanent teeth with the exception of third molars are calcified by the age of

a. 6 years
b. 8 years
c. 12 years
d. 16 years

Ans b.

The enamel formation of all permanent teeth except third molars is complete by the age of 8 years. Hence, drugs like tetracycline which can cause discoloration of teeth should not be given until 8 years of age.

19. The chronological age of a child is

a. Closely related to the physiological age
b. Closely related to the dental age
c. Closely related to the skeletal age
d. Independent of the dental and skeletal ages

Ans d.

Chronological age is not related to dental, physiological or skeletal age. It is the most obvious and easily determined developmental age which is simply figured out from the child's date of birth. The skeletal and the dental ages are based on the skeletal and dental development respectively.

20. In a normal child, the teeth that are generally in the process of calcification at birth are

a. All primary teeth only
b. All primary teeth and first permanent molars
c. Primary anteriors, canines and first primary molars only
d. All primary teeth and all permanent teeth

Ans b.

All the primary teeth and the first permanent molars are in the process of calcification at birth.

21. A radiograph of a 4-year-old child reveals no evidence of calcification of mandibular second premolars. This means that

a. These teeth may develop later
b. The child will probably never develop second premolars
c. It is too early in life to make any predictions concerning the development of any permanent tooth
d. Extraction of primary second molar should be performed to allow the permanent first molars to drift forward

Ans a.

The hard tissue formation of mandibular second premolars begins between 2.25 and 2.5 years. Sometimes it can be delayed and may start after 4 years also. Hence, second primary molar should not be extracted.

22. A disturbance during the calcification stage of tooth development is the cause of

a. Peg teeth
b. Microdontia
c. Oligodontia
d. Interglobular dentin

Ans d.

Disturbance during the calcification stage can result in interglobular dentin formation. Refer to the explanation of Q. No. 2.

23. Tooth buds generally initiated after birth include

a. Entire permanent dentition only
b. All permanent teeth and some primary teeth
c. 1st, 2nd premolars and 2nd and 3rd molars only
d. All primary teeth

Ans c.

All the primary teeth buds are initiated in the intrauterine period itself whereas the tooth buds generally initiated after birth include 1st, 2nd premolars, and 2nd and 3rd molars. Hard tissue formation begins at birth for the first permanent molars and in the intrauterine period itself for all primary teeth.

24. Oblique ridge is formed by union of

a. Mesiobuccal and mesiopalatal cusp
b. Distobuccal and distolingual cusp
c. Mesiopalatal cusp and distobuccal cusp
d. Mesiopalatal and distolingual cusp

Ans c.

The mesiopalatal cusp joins the distobuccal cusp through the oblique ridge which is very characteristic on the occlusal surface of the maxillary primary second molar.

25. The largest cusp on mandibular first primary molar is

a. Mesiobuccal cusp
b. Distobuccal cusp
c. Mesiolingual cusp
d. Distolingual cusp

Ans c.

The largest cusp is mesiolingual cusp. The primary mandibular first molar has four cusps; two on the buccal and two on the lingual. The mesial cusps are larger than the distal ones and the pulp horn of the mesiobuccal cusp may extend high till the DE junction.

26. The largest cusp on mandibular second primary molar is

a. Mesiobuccal cusp
b. Distobuccal cusp
c. Mesiolingual cusp
d. Distolingual cusp

Ans b.

The primary mandibular second molar has five cusps; three on the buccal and two on the lingual. The largest cusp is the distobuccal cusp.

27. The incisal edge of the primary mandibular lateral incisor slopes towards the distal aspect of the tooth. This tooth more closely resembles the maxillary primary lateral incisor than it does the mandibular primary central incisor.

a. Both the statements are true
b. Both the statements are false
c. The first statement is true and the second is false
d. The first statement is false and the second is true

Ans a.

The incisal edge slopes towards the distal aspect of the tooth differentiating it from the central incisor. The distoincisal angle is more rounded.

28. The largest and sharpest cusp of maxillary first primary molar is

a. Mesiobuccal cusp
b. Distobuccal cusp
c. Mesiolingual cusp
d. Distolingual cusp

Ans a.

Mesiobuccal cusp is the largest and sharpest cusp occupying a major portion of the bucco-occlusal surface.

29. All the primary teeth are erupted into the oral cavity by

a. 18 months
b. 24 months
c. 36 months
d. 16 months

Ans c.

All primary teeth are present in the child's mouth by the age of 3 years.

30. What single morphologic characteristic of the permanent first molar necessitates early restorative procedures in most children?

a. Mesial proximal contact
b. Deep grooves and fissures
c. Large pulp chamber
d. Early beginning of calcification
e Presence of an auxiliary cusp

Ans b.

Deep grooves and fissures act like a niche for bacteria and food debris. The manual dexterity in children has to be good enough to remove the retained debris. Children also tend to focus on brushing the anterior teeth rather than the posterior teeth. Pit and fissure sealants are advocated in children with moderate risk of caries.

31. Spacing between primary teeth indicates

a. Bitewings are not needed
b. Greater chance of ectopic eruption
c. An increased likelihood that the larger permanent teeth can be accommodated
d. Increased probability of malalignment later

Ans c.

Spacing between primary anterior teeth is desirable to accommodate the larger permanent teeth.

32. The most frequently impacted permanent tooth is the

a. Mandibular second premolar
b. Maxillary lateral incisor
c. Mandibular canine
d. Maxillary canine

Ans d.

The desired sequence of eruption of permanent teeth is 6,1,2,4,5,3,7. Premature loss of primary molars cause permanent first molar to drift mesially and block out the canines labially or get impacted due to insufficient space. Refer to the explanation of Q. No. 11 also.

33. In females, the permanent maxillary canine usually erupts at age

a. 6 years
b. 9 years
c. 10 years
d. 12 years
e. 14 years

Ans d.

The answer is self-explanatory.

34. The last primary tooth to be replaced by a permanent tooth is usually the

a. Mandibular canine
b. Maxillary canine
c. Maxillary first molar
d. Mandibular second molar

Ans b.

Refer to the explanation of Q. No. 32.

35. After eruption of a permanent tooth, the time required for complete formation of its root is approximately

a. 1/2–1 year
b. 2–3 years
c. 4–5 years
d. None of the above. The time required is unpredictable

Ans b.

In case of primary teeth, root completion occurs 1 year after tooth eruption.

36. Premature exfoliation of a primary canine may indicate

a. An arch length excess
b. An arch length deficiency
c. A skeletal malocclusion
d. An arch length excess more than 10 mm

Ans b.

Arch length reduces on premature exfoliation of primary canines. Loss on one side of the quadrant may cause a midline shift.

37. In examining the primary dentition, if it is observed that a lateral incisor is congenitally missing, it is likely that the

a. Permanent canine will be missing
b. Permanent lateral incisor will also be missing
c. Permanent lateral incisor will be slow in erupting
d. Normal eruption of the permanent lateral incisor is reasonably certain

Ans b.

Congenitally missing primary teeth is a rare entity. When there is a congenitally missing primary tooth, there is a possibility that the successor may also be missing.

38. The color of the primary teeth compared with that of the permanent teeth is

a. Whiter
b. Redder
c. Browner
d. Yellower

Ans a.

The refractive index of primary teeth is close to that of milk and hence called *milk teeth*. They are whiter than their successors.

39. The sum of the widths of primary first and second molars is generally

a. The same as that of the permanent successors
b. 1–2 mm greater than that of the permanent successors
c. 1–2 mm lesser than that of the permanent successors
d. 8 mm lesser than that of the permanent successors

Ans b.

The combined mesiodistal width of C, D, E is greater than 3, 4, 5. The difference is called *leeway space of Nance.*

40. If the eruption sequence of permanent teeth is normal, one can expect

a. Maxillary second premolars to precede maxillary first premolar
b. Maxillary second premolars to precede maxillary canines
c. Maxillary canines to precede mandibular canines
d. Both (a) and (c)
e. Both (b) and (c)

Ans b.

Refer to the explanation of Q. No. 11.

41. The permanent anterior tooth that is most often atypical in size is the

a. Mandibular canine
b. Mandibular central incisors
c. Maxillary canine
d. Maxillary central incisor
e. Maxillary lateral incisor

Ans e.

Every last tooth in the particular sequence has a tendency to have a morphological variation. Lateral incisor, second premolar and third molars show more morphological variations than other teeth. These teeth are last teeth in their corresponding group, namely incisors, premolars and molars.

42. Dental age refers to the

a. State of dental maturation
b. Age at which a given tooth erupts
c. Time periods of an eruption potential
d. Number of years elapsed since a given tooth erupted

Ans a.

Dental age is based on the dental maturation and chronological age is based on the date of birth of the child. Skeletal age is based on the ossification status of certain bones.

43. Which of the following is *least* likely to influence the anteroposterior position of maxillary incisors?

a. Size of the apical base
b. Tongue buccinator mechanism
c. Being a concert clarinetist
d. Congenital absence of third molars

Ans d.

The size of apical base, buccinator mechanism, the tongue posture and the placement of any object or instrument behind the incisors can affect the anteroposterior position of maxillary incisors.

44. If the mandibular second premolars are not radiographically visible by the time a child is 4 years old, the dentist is best advised to

a. Reserve judgment on the presence of the teeth for at least two years
b. Refer the child to a pediatrician to explore the possibility of a systemic condition
c. Assume that the teeth are congenitally missing and extract primary second molars
d. Assume that the teeth are congenitally missing and inform the parents that orthodontic treatment may be necessary when the child is older

Ans a.

Refer to the explanation of Q. No. 21.

45. At what age is a child expected to have 12 erupted primary teeth and 12 erupted permanent teeth?

a. 4.5 years
b. 6.5 years
c. 8.5 years
d. 11.5 years

Ans c.

At 8.5 years, the child has 12 primary teeth (C, D, E in four quadrants) and 12 permanent teeth (all incisors and first molars).

46. The most important morphology or histologic consideration in cavity preparation in primary teeth is the

a. Size of primary molars
b. Thickness of enamel and dentin
c. Direction of the roots below the cementoenamel junction
d. Direction of the enamel rods at the cervical region

Ans b.

Though the size of the tooth, direction of the enamel rods and point of bifurcation of roots vary between primary and permanent teeth, the thickness of enamel is the key factor while considering the tooth for cavity preparation.

47. Which of the following is an abnormal sequence of eruption of permanent mandibular teeth?

a. First molar erupts before central incisor
b. Second molar erupts before second premolar
c. Canine erupts before first premolar
d. First premolar erupts before the second premolar

Ans b.

Refer to the explanation of Q. No. 12.

48. The primary tooth which least resembles any of the permanent tooth is:

a. Maxillary first molar
b. Maxillary second molar
c. Mandibular first molar
d. Mandibular second molar

Ans c.

Mandibular first molar is the tooth which least resembles any permanent tooth. It has a prominent buccal curvature. Maxillary second primary molar resembles the maxillary first permanent molar. Mandibular second primary molar resembles the mandibular second permanent molar.

Chapter 4

Teeth Identification

1. According to the universal system, maxillary left first permanent molar is identified as

a. 16
b. 3
c. 14
d. 26

Ans c.

Universal system uses numbers 1–32 for recording permanent teeth. It starts from maxillary right third molar, which is identified as 1 and progresses around the arch to the maxillary left third molar which is identified as 16. Hence, the left first permanent molar is number 14. Mandibular left third molar is number 17 and progresses around the arch to the mandibular right third molar which is 32.

1	2	3	4	5	6	7	8	9	10	11	12	13	14	15	16
32	31	30	29	28	27	26	25	24	23	22	21	20	19	18	17

Hence 14 denotes maxillary left first permanent molar. Maxillary right third molar is denoted by the number 1. Maxillary right canine and maxillary left third molar are denoted by 6 and 16, respectively.

2. According to the universal system, maxillary left second primary molar is identified as

a. A
b. J
c. K
d. T

Ans b.

In the universal system, the primary teeth are identified by the first 20 letters of the alphabets from A through T. A denotes the maxillary right second primary molar and progresses around the arch to the maxillary left second primary molar which is identified as J. K is mandibular left second primary molar and progresses to T, which is mandibular right second primary molar.

A B C D E	F G H I J
T S R Q P	O N M L K

3. Mamelons are seen in

a. Young permanent incisors
b. Young primary incisors
c. Young primary canines
d. Permanent molars

Ans a.

Mamelons are developmental grooves present on the incisal edges of a newly erupted incisor. These are seen in permanent teeth because the enamel formation in permanent teeth occurs in lobes. These lobes fuse together to form the labial and lingual surfaces of teeth. The lines of fusion which are seen as grooves on the incisal edges of a newly erupted incisor are called *mamelons*. These grooves wear off as the age advances unless the teeth are in crossbite or out of occlusion. Hence, presence of mamelons indicates, that they are young permanent incisors. The mamelons are not seen in primary incisors as the enamel formation takes place from a single lobe and correlating it with the chronology of eruption gives a clue for identification of teeth.

4. In the FDI system of dental recording, which of the following is true?

a. The first digit indicates the quadrant and the second digit the type of tooth within the quadrant
b. Quadrants are allotted the digits 1 to 4 for the permanent teeth and 5 to 8 for the primary teeth in a clockwise sequence, starting from the upper right side
c. Teeth within the same quadrant are allotted the digits 1 to 8 (primary teeth 1 to 5) from the midline backwards
d. This is known as the two-digit system and the digits should be pronounced separately
e. All of the above

Ans e.

All the above mentioned facts are correct.

18 17 16 15 14 13 12 11	21 22 23 24 25 26 27 28
48 47 46 45 44 43 42 41	31 32 33 34 35 36 37 38

55 54 53 52 51	61 62 63 64 65
85 84 83 82 81	71 72 73 74 75

Section II
Growth and Development–Changes in the Dentofacial Structures

Chapter 5

Growth and Development

1. **Which of the following is not a parameter used in growth literature to assess craniofacial increase?**
   a. Magnitude
   b. Velocity
   c. Direction
   d. Increment

Ans d.

The parameters commonly used in growth literature to assess the craniofacial size increase are magnitude, velocity and direction. *Magnitude* refers to the linear dimension overall or that of a part. *Direction* means the vector of size increase as might be described on a three-dimensional coordinate system. *Velocity* is defined as the amount of change per unit of time.

2. **Which of the following is not characteristic of incremental human growth curve?**
   a. Rapid accelerating prenatal growth
   b. Rapid accelerating postnatal growth for the first 2–3 years
   c. Period of slow incremental growth during childhood
   d. Growth acceleration for 2–3 years during pubertal adolescence

Ans b.

Characteristic of an incremental human growth curve is rapid accelerating prenatal growth, rapid decelerating postnatal growth for the first 2–3 years and a period of relatively slow incremental growth during childhood followed by growth acceleration for 2–3 years during pubertal adolescence.

3. **Growth refers to passing from one form (size or shape) to another. Development refers to transition in functional stage or activity.**
   a. Both the statements are false
   b. Both the statements are true
   c. First statement is true and the second is false
   d. First statement is false and the second is true

Ans b.

Growth implies change, a transition from one condition to another. *Conceptual growth* refers to a passing from one anatomic form (i.e. size and shape) to another. Transitions in functional stage or activity refer to *development.* Development also means increased organization or specialization of functioning (physiologic) parts.

4. **Development refers to**
   a. Increased specialization or a higher order of organization
   b. Transition in functional stage or activity
   c. Progression towards maturity
   d. Any of the above

Ans d.

Refer to the explanation of Q. No. 3.

5. **Prenatal period in humans is**
   a. 25 weeks in length
   b. 40 weeks in length
   c. 50 weeks in length
   d. 35 weeks in length

Ans b.

Phases of Growth.

S. No.	Period of growth	Duration of the period
1.	Prenatal period	40 weeks
2.	Infancy	First 2 years after birth
3.	Childhood	2–10 years(Girls) 2–12 years (Boys)
4.	Adolescence	10–18 years (Females) 12–20 years (Males)

6. **The period of infancy usually refers to**
   a. First 2 years after birth
   b. 2–4 years after birth
   c. 3–5 years after birth
   d. First 6 months after birth

Ans a.

Refer to the explanation of Q. No. 5.

7. **The period of adolescence in humans is**

a. 10–20 years
b. 5–10 years
c. 10–14 years
d. 15–20 years

Ans a.

Refer to the explanation of Q. No. 5.

8. **At birth**

a. Neural tissue would have attained 30% of adult stature
b. Neural tissue would have attained 60–70% of adult stature
c. Neural tissue would have attained 90% of adult stature
d. Neural tissue would have attained 15% of adult stature

Ans b.

Neural tissue completes its growth at an early stage whereas the general somatic tissues such as muscle, bone and connective tissue mature at a slower rate.

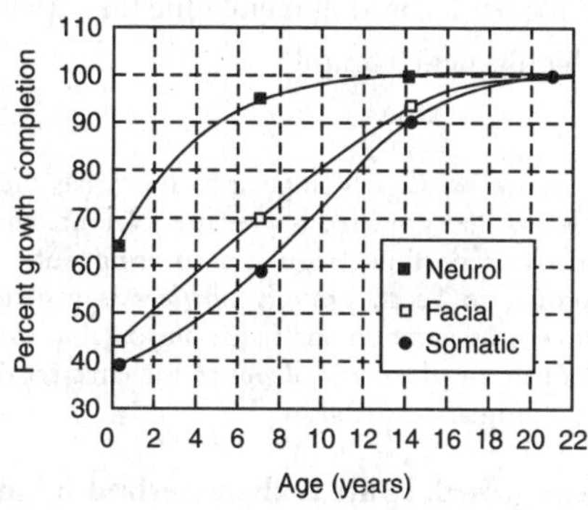

Fig. 5.1 Growth and development of different tissues.

S. No.	Type of tissue	Percentage of growth attained	
		By birth	By middle childhood
1.	Neural tissue	60–70	95
2.	Muscle tissue	40–45	70
3.	Craniofacial lymphoid tissue		125
4.	Craniofacial bone growth	45	70
5.	Craniofacial primary cartilage	75	95

9. The size of craniofacial lymphoid tissue (tonsils and adenoids) is about 125% of adult stature at 5 years of age. Then it decreases gradually to adulthood.

a. Both the statements are false
b. Both the statements are true
c. First statement is true and the second is false
d. First statement is false and the second is true

Ans b.

Refer to the explanation of Q. No. 8.

10. All of the following about primary cartilage is true except

a. Has the capacity for appositional growth
b. Pressure-tolerant
c. Nonvascular
d. Does not require a covering membrane for survival
e. Is under high genetic control

Ans a.

According to Enlow, *cartilage* is singular in form, has the capacity to grow from within (interstitial growth), is pressure-tolerant, noncalcified, flexible and nonvascular and does not require a covering nutrient membrane for survival. According to Scott, *primary cartilage* is genetically predisposed, acts during growth as autonomous tissue and is able to directly influence the craniofacial pattern. *Appositional growth* is characteristic of membranous bones and not of primary cartilage.

11. The adolescent growth spurt is characterized by increased growth velocity at about 10–12 years for females and 12–14 years for males. The maximum velocity or peak height velocity (PHV) of growth is attained approximately 2 years after pubertal onset.

a. Both the statements are false
b. Both the statements are true
c. First statement is true and the second is false
d. First statement is false and the second is true

Ans b.

Maximum velocity of growth is attained approximately 2 years after pubertal onset.

12. During infancy and early childhood, the maxilla will be (most likely) thrusted

a. Backward and downward
b. Forward and downward
c. Forward and upward
d. Backward and upward

Ans b.

Maxilla is thrusted forward and downward.

13. Petrovich's hypothesis of craniofacial growth is

a. Genetic theory
b. Nasal septum theory
c. Functional matrix theory
d. Servo system theory

Ans d.

The theory postulates the influence of somatotrophic hormone—somatomedin complex on the primary and secondary cartilages.

14. An early prepubertal growth spurt indicates

a. A longer treatment time
b. Fast maturing child
c. Slow maturing child
d. An endocrine dysfunction

Ans b.

Early prepubertal growth spurt indicates a fast maturing child. In such situations, growth modification treatment should be started earlier than normal individuals.

15. The downward and forward direction of facial growth results from

a. Upward and backward growth of the maxillary sutures and the mandibular condyle
b. Downward and forward growth of the maxillary sutures and the mandibular condyle
c. Interstitial growth in maxilla and mandible
d. Vertical eruption and mesial drift of dentitions

Ans b.

The downward and forward direction of facial growth results due to the downward and forward growth of maxillary sutures and mandibular condyle.

16. Which of the following is correct in relation to timing of growth spurt?

a. Boys have earlier growth spurt than girls
b. Girls have earlier growth spurt than boys
c. Boys and girls have growth spurts almost at the same time
d. Girls have prolonged growth compared to boys

Ans b.

Puberty and the adolescent growth spurt occur on the average approximately 2 years earlier in girls than in boys. However, early maturing boys will reach puberty ahead of slow maturing girls and it must be remembered that chronologic age has very little to do with where an individual stands developmentally.

17. Period of ovum is between

a. 0–2 weeks
b. 2–8 weeks
c. 8–12 weeks
d. 12–16 weeks

Ans a.

The period of ovum includes the time from fertilization to implantation. This period lasts until the dividing ovum or the blastocyst becomes attached to the wall of the uterus. It usually lasts for 10–14 days.

18. Embryonal period is characterized by

a. Differentiation of tissue and formation of organs
b. Osseous development
c. Formation of mandible
d. Formation of neural tissues

Ans a.

Embryonal period is characterized by differentiation of tissue and it ranges from 2 to 8 weeks. Osseous development occurs in the fetal period between 8 and 40 weeks.

19. The most rapid growth occurs in humans during

a. First year of life
b. 2–5 years
c. 5–8 years
d. Puberty

Ans a.

In the entire human lifespan, maximum growth takes place in the first year of life. After the first year, growth rate tapers but the height–weight increase remains predictable through adolescence.

20. **Sutural dominance theory was given by**
   a. Sicher
   b. Melvin Moss
   c. Scott
   d. Petrovic

Ans a.

Sicher ascribed equal value to all osteogenic tissues, cartilages, sutures and periosteum. But he considered that the suture remains the primary growth center.

21. **Functional matrix theory was given by**
   a. Sicher
   b. Melvin Moss
   c. Scott
   d. Petrovic

Ans b.

Functional matrix theory is the most widely accepted theory of craniofacial growth. It comprises of the skeletal and functional units.

22. **Postnatal development of maxilla occurs entirely by**
   a. Intramembranous ossification
   b. Endochondral ossification
   c. Both endochondral and intramembranous ossification
   d. Displacement only

Ans a.

Postnatal development of maxilla occurs by intramembranous ossification. However, growth occurs in two ways: (a) apposition of bone at the sutures that connect maxilla to the cranium and cranial base and (b) surface remodeling.

23. **Development of mandible is associated with**
   a. Moss's cartilage
   b. Meckel's cartilage
   c. Medullary cartilage
   d. Cartilage of the body of the mandible

Ans b.

Bone begins to develop lateral to Meckel's cartilage during 7th week of intrauterine life and continues until the posterior aspect is covered with bone. Between 10th and 14th weeks, secondary accessory cartilages appear. They are head of condyle, part of coronoid process and mental protuberance. Meckel's cartilage disappears by 24th week of intrauterine life.

24. Meckel's cartilage disappears by

a 12th week of intrauterine life
b. 16th week of intrauterine life
c. 24th week of intrauterine life
d. Two weeks after birth

Ans c.

Refer to the explanation of Q. No.23.

25. Development of mandible takes place by

a. Intramembranous ossification
b. Endochondral ossification
c. Both endochondral and intramembranous ossification
d. Displacement only

Ans c.

Endochondral ossification occurs in the condylar region. All the other areas of the mandible grow by direct surface apposition and remodeling (intramembranous ossification).

26. Endomorphic individuals are

a. Late maturers
b. Early maturers
c. Normal maturers
d. None of the above

Ans b.

Endomorphic individuals are the early maturers. They are stocky having abundant subcutaneous fat and highly developed digestive viscera. Somatic structures are relatively underdeveloped.

27. A boy of chronologic age of 9 years is 125 cm in height. The mean for this age is 133.71 cm with a standard deviation of 5.49 cm. His skeletal age is assessed as 8 years. This boy may be regarded as

a. Somewhat physically retarded but with potential to "catch up"
b. Severely physically retarded with little potential to "catch up"
c. Just at the right level
d. Destined to be a short-statured individual

Ans a.

The child is physically retarded to a small extent based on the standard average for his age. But he can definitely catch up with the mixed dentition growth spurt (8–11 years) and adolescent growth spurt (14–16 years).

28. If a child's teeth do not form, this would primarily affect the growth of the

a. Alveolar bone
b. Whole face
c. Mandible
d. Maxilla

Ans a.

Teeth and the supporting periodontium is the functional matrix and the alveolar bone is the skeletal unit. In the absence of the tooth, the alveolar bone is primarily affected.

29. There is a differential between girls and boys with respect to age at which the growth velocity reaches its peak. The difference is that

a. Boys are six months ahead of girls
b. Girls are six months ahead of boys
c. Girls are one year ahead of boys
d. Girls are two years ahead of boys

Ans d.

The human body does not grow at the same rate throughout life. Different organs grow at different rate to a different amount and at different times. There is a variation in the differential growth between boys and girls as well.

30. The "V" principle of growth is best illustrated by the

a. Nasal septum
b. Mandibular ramus
c. Mandibular symphysis
d. Spheno-occipital synchondrosis

Ans b.

Enlow's expanding "V" principle is best illustrated by growth of mandibular ramus.

31. The greatest period of cranial growth occurs between

a. Birth and 5 years of life
b. 6 and 8 years of age
c. 10 and 12 years of age
d. 14 and 16 years of age

Ans a.

The growth in the cranial vault is because of the growing brain. The rate of bone growth is more during infancy and by fifth year of life more than 90% growth of the cranial vault is achieved.

32. At birth, which of the following structures is nearest to the size it will eventually attain in adulthood?

a. Cranium
b. Mandible
c. Clavicle
d. Middle face

Ans a.

Refer to the explanation of Q. No. 31.

33. What is the relationship between the growth curves for lymphoid tissues and sexual characteristics?

a. Both curves slope upward in parallel form
b. Lymph tissues grow more slowly than genital tissues
c. Lymph tissues stop growing when genital tissues begin growing
d. Lymph tissues regress as genital tissues develop

Ans d.

Scammon divided the tissues into four types: lymphoid, neural, somatic and genital. The growth of lymphoid tissue increases after birth and reaches 100% by 7 years. It is about 200% by 10 years and thereafter it regresses in size. Neural tissue attains 90% growth by 7 years of age. Somatic shows a stable "S" shaped growth with age. Genital tissues growth gets accelerated during puberty.

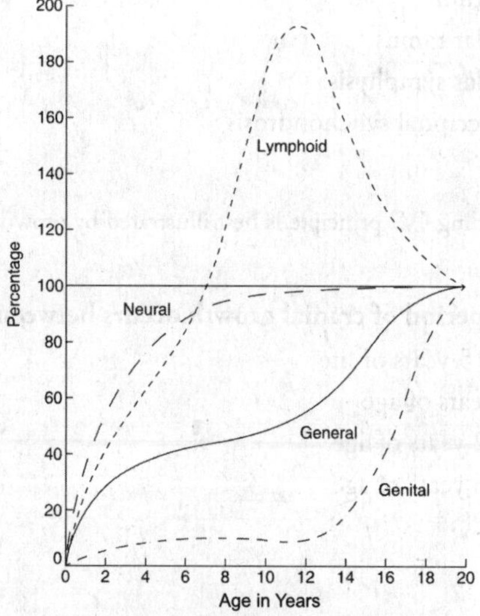

Fig. 5.2 Scammon's growth curve.

34. Which of the following is the basic sex difference in facial growth during puberty?

a. Greater vertical development of the female face
b. Greater vertical development of the male face
c. Greater overall growth in the posterior cranial base in the female
d. Greater horizontal growth of the posterior cranial base in the male

Ans b.

The answer is self-explanatory.

35. The major growth site of mandible is in the

a. Gonial angle
b. Condylar cartilage
d. Posterior border of the ramus
d. Lateral aspect of the body of the mandible

Ans b.

Growth sites are growth fields that have a special significance in the growth of a particular bone, e.g. condyle in the mandible. The growth sites may possess some intrinsic growth potential (debatable).

36. Which of the following tissues grows to 200% of its normal adult mass during ages 6–12 years?

a. Neural
b. Genital
c. Lymphoid
d. General

Ans c.

Refer to the explanation of Q. No. 33.

37. Sexual development in girls occurs two years earlier than in boys because estrogen specifically promotes female sexual development.

a. Both statements and reason are correct and related
b. Both statements and reason are correct and but not related
c. The statement is correct but the reason is not
d. The statement is not correct but the reason is an accurate statement

Ans b.

The answer is self-explanatory. Refer to the explanation of Q. No. 33 also.

38. The second molar of a 6-year-old patient is located in the ramus of the mandible. The body of the mandible increases in length to accommodate the second molar by

a. Apposition of bone in the condyle
b. Apposition of bone on the alveolar margin and the lower surface of the mandible
c. Apposition of bone at the symphysis and the posterior surface of the ramus of the mandible
d. Resorption of bone along the anterior surface of the ramus and apposition of bone on the posterior surface of the ramus

Ans d.

The resorption (anterior surface) and apposition (posterior surface) will accommodate the 2nd molar later.

39. The cranial vault increases rapidly in size the first few years post-natally and completes approximately 90% of its growth by 6 years of age. This growth is typical of which of the following types of tissues?

a. Neural
b. Dental
c. Genital
d. Lymphoid
e. General

Ans a.

Refer to the explanations of Q. Nos. 31 and 33.

Chapter 6

Development of Dentition and Occlusion

1. Ameloblasts are derived from

a. Stomodeal ectoderm
b. Cranial neural crest-derived (ecto) mesenchymal cells
c. Branchial arches
d. Stomodeal arches

Ans a.

Mammalian teeth develop from two types of cells: stomodeal ectoderm, which forms ameloblasts; and cranial neural crest-derived (ecto) mesenchymal cells which form odontoblasts and cementoblasts.

2. Dental lamina formation begins by

a. 1st week of intrauterine life
b. 6th week of intrauterine life
c. 12th week of intrauterine life
d. 24th week of intrauterine life

Ans b.

Dental lamina begins at 6 weeks of intrauterine life and tooth buds arise from the lamina. Initiation of primary teeth is seen from second month in utero.

3. All of the following structures are derived from mesoderm except

a. Enamel
b. Dentin
c. Pulp
d. Periodontal tissues

Ans a.

Enamel is derived from the ectoderm and the mesoderm contributes to the formation of the dentin, pulp and periodontal tissues.

4. In the stages of tooth development, the proliferation of cell ends by

a. Morphodifferentiation
b. Histodifferentiation
c. Apposition
d. Initiation

Ans b.

Histodifferentiation marks the end of proliferation as the cells lose the capacity to multiply. There is differentiation of the cells in the dental papilla into odontoblasts and the cells of the inner epithelium into ameloblasts.

5. Sequence of eruption of primary teeth is

a. A,B,D,C,E
b. A,C,D,E,B
c. A,B,C,D,E
d. A,D,C,B,E

Ans a.

Sequence of eruption is A, B, D, C, E but the sequence of calcification is A, D, B, C, E.

6. In Nolla's stages of tooth development, crown completion occurs by

a. Stage 5
b. Stage 6
c. Stage 4
d. Stage 3

Ans b.

Crown completion occurs by Nolla's stage 6. Stage 8 indicates that two-thirds of roots are completed and tooth is ready for eruption.

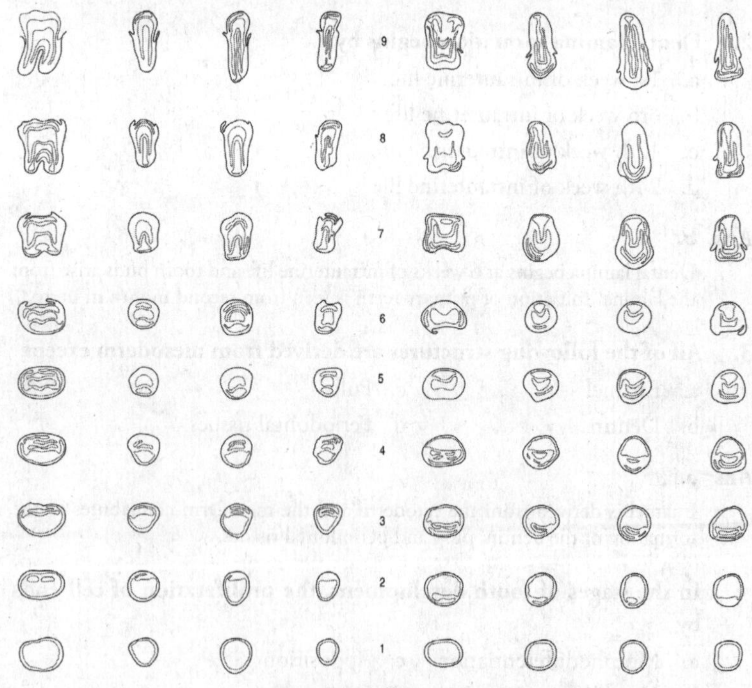

Fig. 6.1 Nolla's stages.

7. **Epstein's pearls are seen in**

a. Attached gingiva
c. Midpalatine raphe
b. Floor of the mouth
d. Tongue

Ans c.

Epstein's pearls are formed along the midpalatine raphe and are considered epithelial remnants of epithelial tissue trapped along the raphe. Dental lamina cysts originate from the remnants of the dental lamina and are found on the crest of the maxillary and mandibular dental ridges.

8. **An 8-year-old patient has maxillary permanent central incisors erupted to the extent that two-thirds of the anatomic crowns may be seen clinically. A 3 mm diastema exists between these teeth. In such cases, the diastema is usually a result of**

a. A failure of fusion of the premaxilla
b. An abnormal labial frenum
c. A supernumerary tooth in the midline
d. The normal eruption pattern of these teeth

Ans d.

The appearance of a midline diastema with flared upper incisors during the eruption of the incisors and canines is called ugly duckling stage or Broadbent phenomenon. It is a self-correcting anomaly which gets corrected when the maxillary canines erupt.

9. **In the average child, teeth generally in the process of calcification at birth are**

a. All primary teeth only
b. All primary teeth and first permanent molars
c. The primary anteriors, canines and first primary molars only
d. All primary teeth and all permanent teeth

Ans b.

Calcification of primary teeth occurs in intrauterine life (4–6 months) and for permanent first molars, it occurs at birth.

10. **Ankylosis of teeth is generally observed after a change in the continuity of the occlusal plane. This change is caused by**

a. Differential eruption sequences
b. Ankylosed teeth sinking into the alveolar bone
c. Localized growth inhibition of the alveolar process
d. Continued eruption of nonankylosed teeth and growth of the alveolar process

Ans d.

Continued eruption of the nonankylosed teeth gives a submerged effect to the ankylosed teeth. In case of a congenitally absent second premolar, the roots of the second primary molar resorbs at a slower rate and may get ankylosed.

11. The eruption of permanent teeth in cases of extremely early loss of primary teeth will result in

a. No change in the time of eruption
b. Early eruption of the permanent teeth
c. Delayed eruption of the permanent teeth
d. None of the above

Ans c.

Loss of primary molar before the age of 7 years will lead to delayed emergence, whereas the loss after 7 years of age leads to an early emergence of succedaneous tooth.

12. Which of the following represents the normal relationship of the primary canine?

a. The distal inclined plane of the maxillary canine articulates with the mesial inclined plane of the mandibular canine
b. The mesial inclined plane of the maxillary canine articulates with the distal inclined plane of the mandibular canine
c. Normal articulation of primary canines is end-to-end
d. Either (a) or (b) depending on age

Ans b.

Class I canine relationship is the most common relationship. The mesial inclined plane of the maxillary canine articulates with the distal inclined plane of the mandibular canine.

13. Prolonged retention of primary teeth may

a. Cause resorption of the roots of adjacent teeth
b. Cause ankylosis of the succeeding permanent tooth buds
c. Disturb the path of eruption of the permanent teeth
d. Cause warping of the alveolar bone in the area

Ans c.

Prolonged retention of primary teeth can cause ectopic eruption of the underlying permanent tooth.

14. In predicting the adult occlusion, a flush terminal plane in the primary dentition

a. Insures good vertical growth probability
b. Insures an angle Class I molar relationship
c. Insures an angle Class II molar relationship
d. Insures a good anteroposterior growth probability
e. Is considered normal, but provides no guarantee for the ultimate molar relationship

Ans e.

A flush terminal plane can result in an end on molar relation with normal growth. With the shift in teeth and normal growth it attains a Class I molar relationship. With continuous downward and forward growth of the mandible it can result in a Class III molar relationship.

15. Eruption of the permanent maxillary second molar before the maxillary second premolar is a sequence that is

a. Usual and desirable
b. Unusual and desirable
c. Usual and undesirable
d. Unusual and undesirable

Ans d.

According to Moyer's, the most favorable sequence of permanent tooth eruption is 6,1,2,4,5,3,7. If the maxillary second molar erupts before the second premolar, the premolar (2nd) can erupt buccally or may get impacted.

16. In the absence of a permanent second premolar, the roots of the primary second molar will most likely

a. Show no resorption as the initial force is absent
b. Resorb more rapidly than normal
c. Resorb more slowly than normal
d. Resorb at a normal rate

Ans c.

Refer to the explanation of Q. No. 10.

17. Ectodermal cells are responsible for

a. Alveolar bone
b. Periodontal tissues
c. Cementum formation
d. Determining crown and root shape

Ans d.

Refer to the explanation of Q. Nos. 1 and 3.

18. Clinical examination of a 15-year-old girl reveals permanent central incisors, permanent canines anterior to premolars. This suggests

a. Thumb sucking habit
b. Ankylosed primary molars
c. Impacted primary canines
d. Congenitally missing permanent lateral incisors

Ans d.

The permanent lateral incisors usually erupt around 8–9 years. The permanent canines and second molars are usually the last teeth to erupt around 11–13 years. The child is 15 years old and the most common scenario could be the congenital absence of permanent maxillary lateral incisors.

19. At birth, jaws are large enough to accommodate

a. Primary incisors
b. All primary teeth, if they are to erupt simultaneously
c. No teeth; the arches are long enough, but the ridges are too narrow
d. None of the above

Ans b.

Ten round or ovoid swellings are seen in each arch during the initiation stage of tooth formation. These swellings occupy the positions due for the primary teeth. The gum pads are the alveolar arches or the edentulous arches of an infant. At birth, jaws are large enough to accommodate all the primary teeth.

20. When is tooth enamel mineralization complete?

a. At the time of eruption
b. At some time following eruption
c. By the time enamel apposition is complete
d. Prior to eruption but after root formation has begun

Ans b.

Enamel mineralization and maturation occurs after eruption of the tooth. Care should be taken to prevent the immature enamel from having dental caries at an early age.

21. In the resorption of roots of a primary tooth, the dental pulp

a. Becomes a nonvital fibrotic mass
b. Functions as a passive participant
c. Initiates resorption from inner surfaces
d. Develops secondary dentin that slows resorption

Ans b.

Resorption of roots (exfoliation) in primary teeth is an apoptotic phenomenon. The pulp can become fibrotic with age but need not become nonvital. Internal resorption occurs when the pulp responds to stimuli like caries and causes the resorption of roots from the pulpal end. But in general, the pulp functions as a passive participant.

22. Supervision of a child's development of occlusion is most critical at ages

a. 3–6 years
b. 7–10 years
c. 11–14 years
d. 14–17 years

Ans b.

The most critical time is the mixed dentition period. The early mixed dentition can help, prevent, intercept or correct a developing occlusal disharmony.

23. Which of the following factors is most frequently responsible for congenital absence of teeth?

a. Heredity
b. Endocrine disturbance
c. Lack of space in the arches
d. Calcium–phosphorus imbalance

Ans a.

Congenital absence of teeth is mostly seen as a hereditary defect.

24. How will extraction of a primary maxillary central incisor in a 5-year-old child with incisal spacing affect the size of the intercanine space?

a. The intercanine space will increase in size
b. The intercanine space will decrease in size
c. There will be no change in the size of the intercanine space
d. None of the above

Ans c.

Extraction of primary maxillary incisor at 5 years of age does not interfere with the establishment of intercanine width and does not cause a space problem.

25. Which of the following dental sequelae is likely in a child with a history of generalized growth failure ("failure to thrive") in the first 6 months of life?

a. Retrusive maxilla
b. Enamel hypoplasia
c. Retrusive mandible

d. Small permanent teeth
e. Dentinogenesis imperfecta

Ans b.

Enamel hypoplasia is seen in children who have a generalized growth failure. It occurs due to environmental factors (nutritional deficiencies, neurological defects, birth defects, fluorides) and local factors (infection, trauma and iatrogenic surgery).

26. Before eruption, the position of permanent mandibular incisor buds relative to primary incisors is

a. Superior and facial
b. Superior and lingual
c. Inferior and facial
d. Inferior and lingual

Ans d.

Permanent mandibular incisors are usually inferior and lingual to their primary predecessors. They erupt lingually and tongue pressure guides them to their correct position.

27. If a 7-year-old patient loses a primary mandibular canine about the same time the adjacent lateral incisor is erupting or shortly thereafter, the dentist should be alert to the possibility of

a. A tongue habit
b. A developing crossbite
c. Early eruption of the permanent canine
d. Lingual collapse of mandibular anterior teeth

Ans d.

Exfoliation of lower primary canine occurs around 9–10 years. If the lateral incisor is erupting around the same time, the eruption could have caused the early exfoliation of the canines due to reduced space. The lingual collapse of mandibular anteriors causes arch length reduction.

28. Calcification of teeth begins during which stage of pregnancy?

a. First trimester
b. Second trimester
c. Third trimester
d. First two weeks of first trimester

Ans b.

Calcification of primary teeth occurs between 4 months (central incisor) and 6 months (canines and second molars) intrauterine life.

29. The average age at which calcification of crowns of permanent central incisors is completed is

a. At birth
b. 2–3 years of age
c. 4–5 years of age
d. 6–7 years of age

Ans c.

Crown completion in permanent central and lateral incisors occur at 4–5 years of age. First molars: 3 years; first premolars: 5–6 years; canines and second premolars: 6–7 years; second molars: 7–8 years.

30. After premature loss of a primary mandibular canine, the space closes most rapidly from

a. Mesial migration of molars on the affected side
b. Lateral and lingual migration of mandibular incisors
c. Neither of the above; canine spaces do not actually close

Ans b.

Refer to the explanation of Q. No. 27.

31. Radiographs of a 5-year-old patient show permanent maxillary first molar inclined mesially with resulting resorption of the distal portions of the roots of primary second molars. The condition described is

a. Ankylosis
b. Ectopic eruption
c. Premature eruption
d. Internal resorption

Ans b.

The permanent first molar positioned too far mesially in its eruption can result in the resorption of the distal roots of the second primary molar.

32. Tooth buds generally initiated after birth are

a. Entire permanent dentition only
b. All permanent teeth and some primary teeth
c. First and second premolars and second and third molars
d. All premolars only

Ans c.

Refer Table 6.1 on next page.

Table 6.1 Chronology of human dentition by Lunt and Law (1974)

Tooth	Hard tissue formation begins	Amount of enamel at birth	Enamel completed	Eruption	Root completed
PRIMARY					
Maxillary					
Central incisor	14 (13-16) week in utero	five-sixths	1.5 months	10 (8-12) months	1.5 years
Lateral incisor	16(14.7-16.5) week in utero	two-thirds	2.5 months	11(9-13) months	2 years
Canine	17(15-18) week in utero	one-third	9 months	19(16-22) months	3.25 years
First molar	15.5(14.5-17) week in utero	cusps united	6 months	16(13-19) months (↗)	2.5 years
				16(14-18) months (↙)	
Second molar	19(16-23.5) week in utero	cusps united	11 months	29(25-33) months	3 years
Mandibular					
Central incisor	14 (13-16) week in utero	three-fifths	2.5 months	8(6-10) months	1.5 years
Lateral incisor	16 (14.75-) week in utero	three-fifths	3 months	13(10-16) months	1.5 years
Canine	17(16-) week in utero	one-third	9 months	20(17-23) months	3.25 years
First molar	15.5(14.5-17) week in utero	cusps united	5.5 months	16(14-18) months	2.25 years
Second molar	18(17-19.5) week in utero	cusps united	10 months	27(23-31) months (↗)	3 years
				27(24-30) months (↙)	

33. A 10-year-old patient has cusp-to-cusp molar relationship in the mixed dentition. This will probably become a Class I molar relationship by

a. The maxillary molar drifting 0.9 mm posteriorly
b. The mandibular molar drifting 3.4 mm forward
c. Both molars drifting forward with the mandibular molar drifting about twice as far as the maxillary molar
d. Orthodontic intervention only

Ans c.

Refer to the explanation of Q. No. 14.

34. The terminal plane relationship of primary second molars determines the

a. Bimolar dimensions of permanent first molars
b. Future anteroposterior positions of permanent first molars
c. Vertical dimensions of the mandible upon eruption of permanent first molars
d. Amount of leeway space that is available for permanent premolars and canines

Ans b.

The answer is self-explanatory.

35. Variations in the time of eruption of primary teeth and in the time of exfoliation are frequently observed in pediatric patients. How much of variation in time in exfoliation of primary teeth is considered normal?

a. 6 months
b. 18 months
c. 36 months
d. 48 months

Ans b.

A variation of 18 months in the exfoliation time of primary teeth may be considered normal. Exfoliation of teeth in the absence of trauma in children younger than 5 years of age merits special attention because it can be related to pathologic conditions of local and systemic region.

36. Local or systemic factors that interfere with the normal matrix formation cause enamel hypocalcification. Factors that interfere with calcification and maturation produces enamel hypoplasia.

a. Both the statements are false
b. Both the statements are true
c. First statement is true and the second is false
d. First statement is false and the second is true

Ans a.

Interference during matrix formation results in hypoplasia and interference with calcification results in hypocalcification.

37. Which of the following statements regarding primary enamel hypoplasia is/are true?

a. Hypoplasia of primary enamel that forms before birth is rare
b. It is common in prematurely born, very low birth weight children
c. If ameloblastic activity is disrupted for a long time, gross areas of irregular enamel occur; if disrupted for a short period of time, it manifests as a thin line or a pit
d. All of the above

Ans d.

The answer is self-explanatory.

38. All of the following can result in enamel hypoplasia except

a. Deficiency of vitamins C and D
b. Brain injury and neurologic defects
c. Nephrotic syndrome
d. Deficiency of vitamin K

Ans d.

Vitamin K does not have any role in epithelial differentiation or calcification of teeth.

39. All of the following are true regarding Turner's hypoplasia except

a. It is usually due to local infection
b. It manifests as hypoplastic or hypocalcified areas on the crown of permanent teeth
c. It can be seen in primary teeth also
d. Inflammatory processes of primary teeth extend toward the buds of the permanent teeth and affect them during the prefunctional stage of eruption
e. It can be seen in second mandibular premolar

Ans c.

Turner's hypoplasia occurs usually because of trauma to primary teeth or infection of primary teeth affecting the permanent tooth germ. Hence, it cannot be seen in the primary teeth.

40. Which of the following can be a method of managing enamel hypoplasia?

a. Topical fluoride application
b. Restoration with glass ionomers
c. Enamel color modification by controlled hydrochloric acid-pumice abrasion
d. Enamel microabrasion
e. Any of the above

Ans e.

Topical fluoride application and glass ionomers are the commonly used strategies. *Enamel microabrasion* (Croll) is a technique in which a specially prepared abrasive compound (Prema) is applied to the discolored enamel areas, similar to prophylaxis paste, using a synthetic rubber applicator in a 10:1 gear-reduction handpiece. Frequent water rinsing and re-evaluation of the tooth for color correction are required. In the hydrochloric acid technique, slurry of fine pumice and 18% HCl is applied under pressure and abrasion with a wooden stick. The slurry is rinsed away after each 5-second application until the desired color change has occurred.

41. Apart from the permanent third molars, the most commonly missing permanent tooth is

a. Mandibular second premolars
b. Maxillary lateral incisors
c. Maxillary second premolars
d. Mandibular central incisor

Ans a.

The most commonly missing permanent teeth are the mandibular second premolars, maxillary lateral incisors and maxillary second premolars. Glenn and Grahnen confirm this order of frequency in their studies.

42. Which of the following can cause midline diastema?

a. Oral habits
b. Supernumerary tooth
c. Macroglossia
d. Peg lateral and congenital absence of permanent lateral incisors
e. Abnormal labial frenum
f. Any of the above

Ans f.

The answer is self-explanatory.

43. The labial frenum is composed of two layers of epithelium enclosing a loose vascular connective tissue. Muscle fibers if present are derived from the zygomaticus major muscle.

a. Both the statements are false
b. Both the statements are true
c. First statement is true and the second is false
d. First statement is false and the second is true

Ans c.

Muscle fibers for the labial frenum are derived from the orbicularis oris muscle.

44. An abnormal labial frenum can cause

a. Interference with tooth brushing
b. Stripping of tissue from neck of tooth
c. Accumulation of food particles which leads to pocket formation
d. Interference with speech
e. Any of the above

Ans e.

The answer is self-explanatory.

45. The interval between crown completion and the beginning of eruption until the tooth is in full occlusion (for permanent teeth) is approximately

a. 2 years
b. 12 months
c. 3 years
d. 5 years

Ans d.

Once the crown formation is complete, the tooth moves through the bone at the rate of 1 mm every 4–6 months. To reach the antagonistic tooth and stabilize itself in occlusion, it takes approximately 5 years.

46. Extraction of primary molars at 4 or 5 years of age delays the eruption of premolars. Extraction of primary molars at 9 or 10 years of age also delays the eruption of premolars.

a. Both the statements are false
b. Both the statements are true
c. First statement is true and the second is false
d. First statement is false and the second is true

Ans c.

According to Posen, extraction of primary molars at 4 or 5 years of age delays the eruption of the premolars whereas extraction at 9 or 10 years of age accelerates the eruption of the premolars.

47. Eruption of mandibular second permanent molar before second premolar can cause arch length deficiency. It is desirable that the mandibular canines erupt before the first and second premolars.

a. Both the statements are false
b. Both the statements are true
c. First statement is true and the second is false
d. First statement is false and the second is true

Ans b.

Eruption of mandibular second permanent molar before second premolar will push the first permanent molar mesially and cause arch length deficiency. In the mandibular arch if the premolar erupts ahead of the canines it can lead to labial positioning of the canines.

48. Which of the following regarding teething is/are true?

a. It is associated with increased salivation
b. The child puts the hand and fingers into the mouth
c. Diarrhea and fever are incorrectly attributed to teething
d. All of the above

Ans d.

As teething is a physiological process, its association with fever and systemic disturbances is not justified. Fever or respiratory tract infection at this time should be considered coincidental with the eruption process rather than relating to it. Observations like increased salivation and the child putting the hand and fingers into the mouth may be the only indications that the teeth will soon erupt.

49. Which of the following is/are true regarding ankylosis of primary molars?

a. It follows a familial pattern
b. It occurs because of missing permanent successors
c. It occurs because of solid union developing between the bone and the primary teeth during reparative process of resorption
d. Any of the above

Ans d.

The answer is self-explanatory.

50. All of the following are true regarding ankylosed teeth except

a. Ankylosis usually occurs in the primary molar region
b. Ankylosed teeth are otherwise called submerged teeth
c. If ankylosis occurs early, the involved tooth may lie below the plane of occlusion
d. Ankylosis always occurs after the eruption of tooth into the oral cavity

Ans d.

Ankylosis can occasionally occur even before the eruption and complete root formation of primary tooth.

51. Diagnosis of ankylosed tooth can be made by the

a. Presence of tooth out of occlusion
b. Break in continuity of the periodontal ligament in a radiograph
c. Metallic sound while percussing the suspected tooth
d. Any of the above

Ans d.

Because eruption has not occurred and the alveolar process has not developed in normal occlusion, the opposing molars in the area seem to be out of occlusion. The *ankylosed tooth* will have a metallic sound on percussion whereas the normal tooth will have a cushioned sound because it has an intact periodontal membrane that absorbs some of the shock of the blow. A break in the continuity of the periodontal membrane on a radiograph indicates ankylosis.

Section III

Psychology, Behavior and Behavior Management

Chapter 7

Child Psychology

1. **A child aged 4 would be classified developmentally according to Stone and Church as a**
   a. Toddler
   b. Preschooler
   c. Middle year child
   d. Adolescent

Ans b.

Stone and Church's classification:

Infant	–	Till 15 months
Toddler	–	5 months to 2 years of age
Preschooler	–	2 to 6 years of age
Middle year child	–	6 to 12 years of age
Adolescent	–	12 years till maturity

2. **A 2-year-old preschooler shows active happy hustle-bustle type of reception room behavior. His most likely response for oral examination will be**
   a. Definitely negative
   b. Negative
   c. Positive to modeling
   d. Positive to effective communication

Ans b.

A 2-year-old child is classified by Wright as too young to cooperate. Hence the response for oral examination may invariably be negative.

3. **When a patient is exposed step by step in a hierarchy from the least to the most stressful procedures repeatedly until there is no evidence of stress, the procedure is known as**
   a. Modeling
   b. Restraining
   c. Desensitization
   d. Reinforcement

Ans c.

This procedure is known as *desensitization*. Systematic desensitization as a behavior modification procedure uses two important elements:

i. Gradational exposure of the child to his or her fear.

ii. Induced state of incompatibility with his or her own fear.

4. Appraising the child's positive behavior in front of parent verbally is known as ___________ reinforcer.

a. Social
b. Material
c. Activity
d. None of the above

Ans a.

Praise, positive facial expressions, nearness and physical contact come under social reinforcers and they represent the majority of all reinforcing events.

	Reinforcers
Social	In the form of a pat on the back of shoulder, shaking hands, hugging the child or verbal praise in the presence of parent for which the child will be happy.
Material	In the form of gifts like toothbrush kits, drawing kits, favorite cartoon stickers or toys appropriate for their age.
Activity	In the form of allowing the child to perform his/her choice of activity like watching a favorite TV show or movie or playing his favorite instrument for some time or games of interest.

5. Which of the following is not a part of Erikson's model for personality development?

a. Trust versus mistrust
b. Initiative versus guilt
c. Autonomy versus doubt
d. None of the above

Ans d.

All the above-mentioned concepts are a part of Erikson's psychosocial theory (see Table 7.1 on next page).

Table 7.1

Ages	Freud's Stages	Erikson's Stages
Birth to 1 year	*Oral Stage* A child's primary source of pleasure is through the mouth, via sucking, eating and tasting	*Trust vs. Mistrust* Children learn to either trust or mistrust their caregivers
1–3 years	*Anal Stage* Children gain a sense of mastery and competence by controlling bladder and bowel movements	*Autonomy vs. Doubt* Children develop self-sufficiency by controlling activities such as eating, toilet training and talking
3–6 years	*Phallic Stage* The libido's energy is focused on the genitals. Children begin to identify with their same sex parent	*Initiative vs. Guilt* Children begin to take more control over their environment
7–11 years	*Latent Period* The libido's energy is suppressed and children are focused on other activities such as school, friends and hobbies	*Industry vs. Inferiority* Children develop a sense of competence by mastering new skills
Adolescence	*Genital Stage* Children begin to explore romantic relationships	*Identity vs. Role Confusion* Children develop a personal identify and sense of self
Adulthood	According to Freud, the genital stage lasts throughout adulthood. He believed the goal is to develop a balance between all areas of life	*Intimacy vs. Isolation* Young adults seek out romantic love and companionship *Generativity vs. Stagnation* Middle-aged adults nurture others and contribute to society *Integrity vs. Despair* Older adults reflect on their lives, looking back with a sense of fulfillment or bitterness

6. When a child is complemented or rewarded in some manner for his or her cooperative behaviors, it is known as

a. Punishment
b. Restrainment
c. Positive reinforcement
d. Negative reinforcement

Ans c.

If a pleasant consequence follows a response, the response has been positively reinforced and the behavior that led to this pleasant consequence becomes more likely in the future dental visits.

7. A child's behavior problem in the dental office can be handled by familiarization if the basis of the problem is

a. The parents
b. Pain
c. Emotional
d. Fear

Ans d.

Once the child is familiar with the things around, he/she becomes comfortable and the fear diminishes.

8. Preventive desensitization means

a. Behavior shaping
b. Tell, show and do procedures
c. Graded introduction of child to dentistry
d. All of the above

Ans d.

All these techniques are effective methods of managing child behavior during initial and subsequent dental visits which can be categorized as preventive desensitization.

9. Id, ego and superego are part of

a. Freud's psychoanalytical theory
b. Erikson's model of personality development
c. Piaget's theory
d. Skinner's theory

Ans a.

Id, ego and superego are components of Sigmund Freud's psychoanalytical theory (see Table 7.2 on next page).

Table 7.2

S. No.	Components	Description	Principle
1.	Id	*Id* is defined as the inherited reservoir of unorganized drives, it is mostly unconscious, is governed by the pleasure–pain principle, aims at immediate satisfaction of libidinal urges, is immoral, illogical and lacks unity of purpose.	Pleasure–pain principle
2.	Ego	*Ego* is defined as the integrating or mediating part of personality, which develops out of interaction of id and environment. It has perception of both the internal and the external world.	Reality principle
3.	Superego	*Superego* is defined as the latest development of the mind embodying the code of society and including concepts of right and wrong, the value system and the ideals.	Moral principle

10. The basic fear of most children under 2 years of age is concerned with

a. Separation from the parent
b. Injection of local anesthetics
c. The reason for dental treatment
d. The instruments to perform dental treatment

Ans a.

The basic fear of most children under the age of 2 years is separation anxiety.

11. The id is based on

a. Reality principle
b. Egoistic principle
c. Pleasure–pain principle
d. Moral principle

Ans c.

Id is the portion of the mind that contains the unconscious drives for pleasure and destruction. It is one of the three hypothetical structures of personality as explained by Sigmund Freud. Id works on pleasure–pain principle and ego is based on the reality principle (also refer to the table and explanation of Q. No. 7).

12. Among the psychic triad, the executive of personality is

a. Id
b. Ego
c. Superego
d. Ego ideal

Ans b.

The psychic triad includes the id, ego and superego. The ego works on a reality principle. It is the mediating part of personality, which develops out of interaction of id and the environment. The superego here is termed as the policeman, monitoring the "right" and "wrong" (also refer to the explanation and table of Q. No. 7).

13. Oedipus and Electra complexes are seen in ________stage of psychosexual theory.

a. Oral
b. Anal
c. Phallic
d. Latency

Ans c.

Children in phallic stage develop a feeling of attraction to the opposite sex parent. This is called *Oedipus complex* in the boys and the *Electra complex* in the girls. They sometimes wish to eliminate the same sex parent whom they envy and fear as a rival for the affection.

14. Oedipus or Electra complex is resolved by a process called

a. Sublimation
b. Identification
c. Fixation
d. Repression

Ans b.

The boy child tries to imitate the father and the girl child tries to imitate the mother to win the love and affection of the opposite sex parent. This specific aspect of identification with parents is adopting their values and morals. Sublimation and repression are other ego defense mechanisms. Freud believed that there are erogenous zones (zones of extreme tension) in different stages of childhood. Concept of fixation is the failure of development in which the individual continues to seek a particular kind of gratification even after he has passed through the stage in which that kind of pleasure is normally is sought.

15. The basic fear of oral sensory stage according to Erikson is

a. Fear of abandonment
b. Fear of bodily injury
c. Fear of loss of love
d. Fear of sudden movements

Ans a.

The conflict in the oral sensory stage is basic trust versus mistrust. The tight bond between the parent and the child is reflected in a strong sense of "separation anxiety" in the child when separated from the parent. They have the fear of abandonment when tried to separate from the parent in the dental office.

16. Mastery of skills is characteristic of ________stage of psychosocial theory.

a. Adolescence
b. Latency
c. Locomotor genital
d. Muscular anal

Ans b.

Children in this stage go to school, learn about people, culture, values, skills, their capacities and interests. They like to participate and compete to improve their skills. Erogenous zone is absent in this stage of Freud's theory.

17. Object permanence is seen around _____ months according to Jean Piaget.

a. 2–3 months
b. 4–6 months
c. 6–8 months
d. 8–12 months

Ans d.

Object permanence is the notion that an object continues to exist even after it disappears from view. It is seen in the end of the preverbal sensorimotor period. Till this comes into existence, peak-a-boo game works magic with these children.

18. Adolescent girls feeling constantly onstage is called

a. Imaginary audience c. Personal fable

b. Centration d. Egocentrism

Ans a.

Imaginary audience makes young adolescents self-conscious and particularly susceptible to peer influence. They feel they are the center of attraction and are very conscious of their appearance. This phenomenon was proposed by David Elkind. The notion that "others care about my appearance and feelings as much as I do" leads adolescents to think that they are unique, special individuals. As a result of this, a second phenomenon called "personal fable" emerges. This concept holds good that because I am unique, I am not subject to consequences others will experience. The personal fable is a powerful motivator that allows us to cope in a dangerous World. Both these factors can also result in dysfunctional behavior and fool hardy risk taking.

19. Match the following:

A. Sigmund Freud - 1. Cognitive theory

B. Erik Erikson - 2. Operant conditioning

C. Jean Piaget - 3. Hierarchy of Needs

D. Ivan Pavlov - 4. Psychosexual theory

E. Skinner - 5. Observational Learning

F. Abraham Maslow - 6. Psychosocial theory

G. Albert Bandura - 7. Classical conditioning

Ans

A-4, B-6, C-1, D-7, E-2, F-3, G-5

20. Negative reinforcement is

a. Presenting unpleasant stimulus

b. Removing unpleasant stimulus

c. Presenting pleasant stimulus

d. Removing pleasant stimulus

Ans b.

Rescheduling an extraction appointment based on the child's wish and decision, substituting a high speed handpiece with a slow speed handpiece or spoon excavator are classical examples of negative reinforcement.

21. Which of the following processes is not a part of classical conditioning?

a. Acquisition d. Discrimination

b. Generalization c. Equilibration

Ans c.

Acquisition, generalization, discrimination, spontaneous recovery and extinction are the five processes associated with classical conditioning. Equilibration is a part of the cognitive theory put forward by Jean Piaget (see Table 7.3).

S. No.	Name of the process	Explanation
1.	Acquisition	Acquiring/learning a new experience (fear of dentist, fear of white coat, drilling, needles)
2.	Generalization	Generalizing all similar stimuli (all white coat people can be dangerous and can cause pain)
3.	Discrimination	Differentiating individual stimuli (not all dentists or not all dental procedures are painful)
4.	Extinction	Disappearance of the acquired knowledge (loss of fear of dentist and dental procedures)
5.	Spontaneous recovery	Reappearance of the extinguished response (in the subsequent dental visits, if the dentist takes it for granted the child knows the procedure very well and fails to use adequate behavior management strategies, fear of dental procedure reappears)

22. Intuitive stage in Piaget's theory is

a. Less than 2 years
b. 2 to 4 years
c. 4 to 7 years
d. More than 7 years

Ans c.

The preoperational period of Jean Piaget's theory is divided into preconceptual period (2 to 4 years) and intuitive period (4 to 7 years).

23. Withdrawal of pleasant stimulus is

a. Escape
b. Time-out
c. Punishment
d. Reward

Ans b.

The best example for time-out or omission is sending the mother out of the dental operatory when the child does not cooperate for the dental treatment. The child is first explained what he is expected to do in the dental office. But on repeated attempts if the child fails to cooperate, the child is informed that the mother will be sent outside if the child does not cooperate. In spite of instructions if the child fails to cooperate the mother is asked to wait outside.

24. Characteristic of a preschooler is

a. Stranger anxiety
b. Role playing
c. Time of loose tooth
d. Peer group influence

Ans b.

Role playing is very characteristic in preschoolers (2 to 6 years). They tend to imitate or model-like parents, siblings and teachers. The best behavior management technique used to manage these children is modeling (imitation).

Chapter 8

Behavior Management

1. **Pedodontic treatment triangle was given by**
   a. G.Z. Wright
   b. Henry Kempe
   c. Evangeline Jordan
   d. Addleston

Ans a.

G.Z. Wright introduced the pedodontic treatment triangle. Henry Kempe introduced the term *battered-child syndrome*. Evangeline Jordan introduced hand-over-mouth exercise. Addleston introduced TSD (tell, show and do) technique.

2. **Which of the following about pedodontic treatment triangle is correct?**
   a. Child is at the apex of the triangle
   b. The arrows placed on the lines of triangle indicate that the communication is reciprocal
   c. This triangle illustrates the 1:2 relationship in Pediatric Dentistry
   d. All of the above

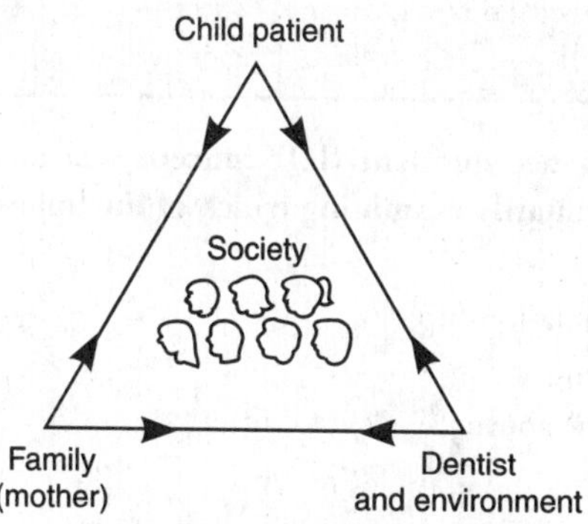

Fig. 8.1 Pedodontic treatment triangle.

Ans d.

As the child is the primary focus in Pediatric Dentistry, he or she is placed at the apex of the triangle. The communication is between child and dentist, dentist and parent, and parent and child, which is indicated by arrows on the triangle. As the dentist communicates with both the child and the parents, it is a 1:2 relationship. On the other hand, in adult dentistry the dentist communicates only with the patient (1:1 relationship).

3. The average age range by which a child stands alone is

a. 3–4 months
b. 9–18 months
c. 20–24 months
d. 1–2 months

Ans b.

Average age range of selected physical developmental milestones

S. No.	Developmental task	Average age	Normal range
1.	Focuses on light	2 weeks	1–4 weeks
2.	Lies on stomach, lifts chin	3 weeks	1–10 weeks
3.	Birth weight doubles	6 months	5–7 months
4.	Rolls from back to stomach	7 months	5½–11 months
5.	Sits alone	7 months	6–11 months
6.	Stands with support	10 months	7½–14 months
7.	**Stands alone**	**13½ months**	**9–18 months**
8.	Walks alone	14 months	10–20 months
9.	Attains bowel control	18 months	1–2½ years
10.	First menstruation (in girls)	12 years 9 months	10–17 years

4. The intelligence quotient (IQ) concept was measured by Alfred Binet by primarily examining which of the following tasks?

a. Memory
b. Spatial relationship
c. Reasoning
d. All of the above

Ans d.

The IQ is measured by evaluating memory, reasoning and spatial relationship.

5. **The IQ formula used by Binet was**

a. $IQ = \frac{\text{Mental age}}{\text{Chronologic age}} \times 100$

b. $IQ = \frac{\text{Chronologic age}}{\text{Mental age}} \times 100$

c. $IQ = \frac{\text{Mental age}}{\text{Dental age}} \times 100$

d. $IQ = \frac{\text{Skeletal age}}{\text{Chronologic age}} \times 100$

Ans a.

The formula gives a numerical value which is quoted as IQ.

6. **According to American Association of Mental Deficiency classification, which of the following descriptions describe "mild" mental retardation?**

a. Can be educated in special classes to gain elementary school level academic skills
b. Can be trained to perform self-help skills and to achieve sheltered workshop employment
c. Abilities typically limited to simple language usage and the mastery of basic self-help skills
d. Consistent custodial care required

Ans a.

Refer the American Association of Mental Deficiency classification, given below.

S. No.	IQ range	Description	Practical description
1.	**52–68**	**Mild**	**Can be educated in special classes to gain elementary school-level academic skills**
2.	36–51	Moderate	Can be trained to perform self-help skills and to achieve sheltered workshop employment
3.	20–35	Severe	Abilities typically limited to simple language usage and the mastery of basic self-help skills
4.	19 and below	Profound	Consistent custodial care required

7. **A child visits the dental clinic, has a good rapport with the dentist, is interested in the dental procedures, is laughing and enjoying the treatment. According to Frankl, what is the rating given for this behavior?**

   a. Rating 1
   b. Rating 2
   c. Rating 3
   d. Rating 4

Ans d.

Frankl behavior rating scale:

Rating 1—Definitely negative—Refusal of treatment, crying forcefully, fearful or any other avert evidence of extreme negativism.

Rating 2—Negative—Reluctant to accept treatment, uncooperative, some evidence of negative attitude but not pronounced (sullen, withdrawn).

Rating 3—Positive—Acceptance of treatment, at times cautious, willingness to comply with the dentist, at times with reservation, but patient follows the dentist's directions cooperatively.

Rating 4—Definitely positive—Good rapport with the dentist, interested in dental procedures, laughing and enjoying.

8. **A child aged 2 years reports to the dental office with her parents and resists examination by the dentist. According to Wright's classification of child's behavior, which category will the child fall in?**

   a. Cooperative.
   b. Lacking cooperative ability
   c. Potentially cooperative
   d. Timid behavior

Ans b.

Refer the classification below.

Wright's classification of child behavior

A. **Cooperative**—Most children in the dental office cooperate

B. **Lacking cooperative ability**

   1. Children with whom communication cannot be established and comprehension cannot be expected (children less than 3 years of age).

   2. Those children who lack cooperative ability because of debilitating or disabling condition.

C. **Potentially cooperative**—In this category, the child's behavior can be modified and the child can become cooperative. This is further classified into uncontrolled, defiant, timid, tense cooperative, whining and stoic behavior.

9. Which of the following statements is true?

a. Preappointment behavior modification refers to anything that is said or done to positively influence the child's behavior before the child enters the operatory.
b. In recent years, preappointment behavior modification is done with audiovisual aids for modeling and preappointment mailings.
c. This strategy prepares the pediatric patient in advance and makes the first dental visit pleasant.
d. All the above statements are true.

Ans d.

All of the above-mentioned statements are true regarding preappointment behavior modification.

10. Behavior shaping is a form of behavior modification. It is based on the established principles of social learning.

a. Both the statements are true
b. Both the statements are false
c. First statement is true and the second is false
d. First statement is false and the second is true

Ans a.

Behavior shaping is that procedure which very slowly develops behavior by reinforcing successive approximations of the desired behavior, until the desired behavior comes to be.

11. TSD was introduced by

a. Levitas
b. Wright
c. Addleston
d. Gesell

Ans c.

Addleston in 1959 first described the *TSD* (tell, show and do) *technique*. This technique addresses the anxiety of the child and provides acceptable means to cope with it by making the "unknown" known to the child (by telling, showing and doing).

12. HOME was introduced by

a. Levitas
b. Evangeline Jordan
c. Addleston
d. Gesell

Ans b.

This technique was first described by Dr Evangeline Jordan in 1920 and she named it hand-over-mouth technique. Levitas renamed this technique *HOME* (hand-over-mouth exercise).

13. The primary objective of HOME and voice control is

a. To gain the attention of a highly oppositional child so that communication can be established

b. To do filling in the same appointment

c. To make the child understand that improper behavior will lead to punishment

d. To prepare the child for eventual extraction

Ans a.

HOME and voice control are used to manage children showing disruptive behavior. When a child is crying uncontrollably, these methods are used to muffle the noise so that the dentist can convey whatever has to be conveyed.

14. Aversive Conditioning (HOME) is not used routinely but as a method of last resort, in children having appropriate communicative abilities in the age group of

a. 2–3 years

b. 3–6 years

c. 9–12 years

d. 12–15 years

Ans b.

A child less than 3 years of age may cry even more forcefully when voice control is used. Hence, these techniques are used only in children in 3–6 years age group.

15. A bribe is promised to induce the behavior. A reward is recognition of good behavior after the completion of the operation, without previously implied promise (by FINN).

a. Both the statements are true

b. Both the statements are false

c. First statement is true and the second is false

d. First statement is false and the second is true

Ans a.

The question explains the difference between a bribe and a reward.

16. Modeling is based on

a. Observational learning
b. Classical conditioning
c. Operant conditioning
d. Instrumental conditioning

Ans a.

Observational learning has two components: acquisition and actual performance. Children are capable of acquiring most behavior which they observe very closely. *Modeling* is learning by imitation of the models.

17. According to Wright, precooperative children are classified under

a. Cooperative
b. Lacking cooperative
c. Potentially cooperative
d. Uncooperative

Ans b.

Precooperative is the term used to describe very young children (2½ years) who are emotionally immature and who lack the cooperative ability. Lacking cooperative category also includes the special children. Potentially cooperative category includes uncontrolled, defiant, timid, tense cooperative and whining children (also refer classification given in Q. No. 8).

18. The borderline behavior seen in children who are classified as potentially cooperative is

a. Defiant
b. Timid
c. Tense cooperative
d. Whining

Ans c.

Tense cooperative children accept and cooperate for the dental treatment but are extremely tensed. They may speak with a tremor in their voice. Their eyes might follow every movement of the dentist and the assistant. These children are easily *mismanaged* because they accept treatment. Defiant children are the "stubborn" or "spoilt" children. Timid children are shy and tend to hide behind parents. Whining children allow the dentist to perform dental treatment but whine throughout the procedure (also refer classification given in Q. No. 8).

19. Bell termed the parent–child relationship as

a. One-tailed
b. Two-tailed
c. Three-tailed
d. Multi-tailed

Ans a.

Many of the child's characteristics like his or her personality, behavior and the reaction to stressful situations are the direct product of parental—especially maternal—characteristics. Most of the mother's attitude coincides with their children's attitude.

20. The overindulgent overprotective mother is associated with _______ child.

a. An aggressive and demanding
b. A shy and anxious
c. A timid and fearful
d. An overactive and disobedient

Ans a.

These children expect constant attention and service even from the dentist. They may not be anxious in a dental setting, but denying their wishes may result in temper tantrums and/or physical assault. Dominant overprotective mothers are associated with shy and anxious children. Children of overanxious parents may be shy, timid and fearful.

21. The term protective stabilization denotes

a. Retraining
b. Sedation
c. General anesthesia
d. Physical restraints

Ans d.

Protective stabilization is defined as the restriction of patient's freedom of movement, with or without the patient's permission, to decrease risk of injury while allowing safe completion of treatment. It is otherwise termed as *medical immobilization.*

22. Retraining does not include

a. Avoidance
b. Substitution
c. Distraction
d. Reinforcers

Ans d.

Avoidance—avoid what the child does not want or cannot take now (postponing extraction for subsequent visits).

De-emphasis or *substitution*—substituting a particular stimulus with another less threatening one (slow-speed hand piece substituted for high-speed hand piece).

Distraction—diverting the child's attention (story-telling, counting numbers).

Reinforcers are a part of contingency management. Reinforcers are pleasant or unpleasant stimulus which on presentation or withdrawal alters the behavior.

23. Match the following:

a. HOME – 1. Lampshire
b. Emotional surprise therapy – 2. Kramer
c. Aversive conditioning – 3. Evangeline Jordan

Ans A-3, B-1, C-2

24. In managing a 7-year-old child, the dentist should keep in mind that a child of this age is

a. Frequently negative
b. Susceptible to praise
c. Generally uncooperative
d. Prone to separation anxiety and extremely afraid of strangers

Ans b.

School-going children like to compete and they constantly try to improve their skills. The conflict in this stage is industry versus inferiority. Every praise from their environment is going to make them perform better.

25. A broad understanding of the "development" of human behavior requires knowledge of the basic concepts of

a. Maturation and learning
b. Masculinity and femininity
c. Dependence and independence
d. Generalization and facilitation

Ans a.

Development is the act or process of growing. Development of human behavior requires knowledge of learning and maturation.

26. A young child's fear of dentistry is primarily

a. Objective in nature
b. Subjective in nature
c. Equally subjective and objective
d. Introspective in nature

Ans b.

Fear based on the feelings and attitudes described to the child by others is called *subjective fear*. The child actually does not have the personal experience regarding the fear factor.

27. Fears produced in a child by direct, physical stimulation of sense organs are ____________ type of fears.

a. Wholesome
b. Objective
c. Subjective
d. Inordinate

Ans b.

Fears produced by direct, physical stimulation are objective fears.

28. While dealing with a frightened child, the dentist should

a. Reprimand the child.
b. Delay the appointment
c. Reason with the child
d. Ask about the child's fears

Ans d.

Identifying the child's fear is the key to behavior management. Allowing the child to express and own his/her feelings is important rather than to just deny it saying "there is nothing to be scared of".

29. During what stage of development is peer group identity the strongest?

a. Toddler
b. Latency
c. Pre-puberty
d. Teenager
e. Adult

Ans d.

Adolescents feel they are very unique and are very self-conscious of themselves. They go through a strong peer pressure. Parental influences keep reducing particularly in this stage.

30. An attempt to alter human behavior and emotion in a beneficial way and in accordance with the laws of learning is

a Behavior management
b. Behavior shaping
c Behavior guidance
d. Behavior modification

Ans d.

The answer is self-explanatory.

31. A child crying forcefully and showing extreme negativism is categorized according to Frankl as

a. Rating 4
b. Rating 3
c. Rating 2
d. Rating 1

Ans d.

Refusal of treatment, crying forcefully and extreme negativism are features of Frankl 1. Refer classification given in Q. No. 7.

32. Which of the following does not belong to potentially cooperative category of Wright's classification of cooperative behavior?

a. Defiant
b. Timid
c. Whining
d. Stoic

Ans d.

Stoic person is one who has great self-control and bears great pain and discomfort. This behavior is commonly seen in children who have been physically or emotionally abused (also refer to the classification provided in Q. No. 8).

33. Uncontrolled behavior is also known as

a. Timid
b. Incorrigible
c. Defiant
d. Stubborn

Ans b.

Uncontrolled behavior is seen in young children between 3 and 6 years. These children throw temper tantrums, cry out loud and lash out the extremities (also refer to the classification provided in Q. No. 8).

34. Appointment time for children in general should not exceed

a. 30 minutes
b. 45 minutes
c. 60 minutes
d. 90 minutes

Ans a.

Children tend to be comfortable with short duration of appointments. Hence, 30 minutes is optimal for most children.

35. Which of the reinforcers should not be given to children?

a. Toys
b. Watching favorite TV show
c. Bribe
d. Reward

Ans c.

Refer to the explanation of Q. No. 15.

36. Protective stabilization is a type of

a. Positive reinforcement
b. Negative reinforcement
c. Time-out
d. Punishment

Ans d.

Protective stabilization is a type of punishment under contingency management. It is the presentation of an unpleasant stimulus (like a restraining device) (also refer explanation of Q. No. 21).

Chapter

9 Pharmacological Behavior Management

1. Which of the following statements will you take into account when a child patient is posted for dental treatment under general anesthesia?

a. Narrow airways in children
b. Children have reduced tolerance to airway obstruction
c. Cardiovascular parameters are different for a child
d. All of the above

Ans d.

In a pediatric patient, narrow nasal passages and glottis combined with hypertrophic tonsils and adenoids, enlarged tongue and greater secretions produce a greater risk of airway obstruction. Because of their reduced tolerance to respiratory obstruction, sudden apnea is a greater concern. The heart rate is faster and the blood pressure is lower than the adult patient.

2. Which of the following is not true of conscious sedation?

a. A pharmacologically induced controlled state
b. Minimally depressed level of consciousness
c. Ability to maintain airway independently and continuously
d. Inability to respond to physical stimuli and verbal command

Ans d.

Conscious sedation is defined as a controlled, pharmacologically induced, minimally depressed level of consciousness, in which the patient retains the ability to maintain airway independently and continuously and respond to physical stimuli and verbal command.

3. All of the following are true regarding deep sedation except

a. Controlled state, induced pharmacologically
b. Patient not easily aroused
c. Partial loss of protective reflexes
d. Minimally depressed consciousness

Ans d.

Deep sedation is defined as controlled, pharmacologically induced, deeply depressed level of conscious state in which there is partial loss of protective reflexes from which the patient is not easily aroused.

4. Which of the following is true regarding general anesthesia?

a. Pharmacologically induced state
b. State of unconsciousness
c. Partial or complete loss of reflexes
d. All of the above

Ans d.

General anesthesia is a pharmacologically induced state of unconsciousness where there is partial or complete loss of reflexes.

5. Which of the following is an indication for conscious sedation?

a. Patient who cannot understand or cooperate
b. Patient who cannot cooperate because of lack of psychological maturity
c. Patient who cannot cooperate because of cognitive, physical or medical disability
d. All of the above

Ans d.

All the above situations are indications of conscious sedation.

6. Which of the following is a requisite for sedation procedures?

a. Informed consent
b. Careful patient evaluation and availability of emergency services
c. Knowledge of agents used
d. All of the above

Ans d.

All of the above-mentioned factors are requisites for sedation procedures.

7. The most commonly used routes for sedation are

a. Inhalational, oral and intravenous
b. Inhalational, oral and submucosal
c. Intramuscular, intravenous and oral
d. Intravenous, oral and rectal

Ans a.

Sedative drugs may be administered by inhalational, oral, rectal, submucosal, intramuscular or intravenous routes. But the most commonly used routes are inhalational, oral and intravenous.

8. Which of the following is not an objective of conscious sedation?

a. Patient's mood should be altered
b. Child should remain unconscious
c. All vital signs should be stable
d. Pain threshold should be elevated

Ans b.

In conscious sedation, the patient should be conscious. Refer to the explanation of Q. No. 2.

9. Which of the following is an objective of conscious sedation?

a. Amnesia should occur
b. To provide most efficient high quality dental care
c. To provide positive psychologic attitude
d. All of the above

Ans d.

The primary objective of these techniques is to produce a quiescent patient to ensure the best quality of care and to help train a child to willingly accept, future dental care.

10. The most commonly used agent for inhalational conscious sedation is

a. Nitrous oxide–oxygen
b. Halothane
c. Ether
d. Fluorothane

Ans a.

Nitrous oxide–oxygen is the most commonly used inhalational sedating agent. All the other above-mentioned agents are general anesthesia agents.

11. One of the primary advantages of inhalational route in conscious sedation is

a. Sedation can be reversed at any moment
b. Drug absorption is less
c. Postoperative complications are less
d. Patient tolerance is good

Ans a.

Sedation can be reversed at any moment by withdrawing the mask and thereby introducing nitrous oxide–oxygen into the system.

12. Nitrous oxide is

a. Colorless
b. Slightly sweet smelling
c. Heavier than air
d. All of the above

Ans d.

Nitrous oxide is slightly heavier than air with a specific gravity of 1.53. It has a blood-gas partition coefficient of 0.47. Because of its low solubility in blood it has a very rapid onset and recovery time.

13. Which of the following statements is false regarding nitrous oxide administration for conscious sedation?

a. It is physically dissolved in the serum fraction of the blood
b. Nitrous oxide has a minimum alveolar concentration of 105
c. It has chemical combination with the blood components
d. When the concentration gradient is reversed, the gas is rapidly excreted by the lungs

Ans c.

Nitrous oxide is physically dissolved in blood but has no chemical combination with any of the blood components. Also, it does not undergo any biotransformation.

14. Nitrous oxide–oxygen anesthesia can cause

a. Hypoxic hypoxia
b. Diffusion hypoxia
c. Nitrous hypoxia
d. Hypoxia with cyanosis

Ans b.

A phenomenon termed *diffusion hypoxia* may occur as the sedation is reversed at the termination of the procedure. Nitrous oxide rapidly escapes into the alveoli so that the oxygen present in the alveoli becomes diluted. The oxygen–carbon dioxide exchange is disrupted and a period of hypoxia is created. This is termed as diffusion hypoxia, which can be minimized by oxygenation for about 5 minutes after the sedation procedure.

15. When does diffusion hypoxia occur during the conscious sedation procedure?

a. At the beginning of the procedure
b. At the end of the procedure
c. In between the procedure
d. Five minutes after starting the procedure

Ans b.

Diffusion hypoxia may occur as the sedation is reversed at the termination of the procedure. However, this phenomenon is reported not to occur in healthy pediatric patients.

16. The side effects of nitrous oxide exposure for prolonged periods include

a. High rates of spontaneous abortion
b. Neurotoxicity
c. Hepatotoxicity
d. All of the above

Ans d.

Chronic exposure to nitrous oxide can produce recreational abuse, neurotoxicity, impotence, renal and liver toxicity, higher rate of spontaneous abortions and decrease in fertility.

17. Which of the following is true of nitrous oxide–oxygen sedation?

a. It causes an altered sense of consciousness
b. It is a CNS depressant
c. It produces limited analgesia state of awareness
d. All of the above

Ans d.

All of the above-mentioned factors are true regarding nitrous oxide–oxygen sedation.

18. First step after placing the mask in nitrous oxide sedation procedure is

a. Administering 30% nitrous oxide and 70% oxygen
b. Administering 50% nitrous oxide and 50% oxygen
c. Administering 100% oxygen
d. Administering 70% nitrous oxide and 30% oxygen

Ans c.

First, the bag is filled with 100% oxygen and delivered to the patient for 2–3 minutes at an appropriate slow rate typically between 4 and 6 liters per minute. Then, nitrous oxide can be introduced in slowly increasing concentrations (at increments of 10%–20%) to achieve the desired level.

19. Maintenance dose of nitrous oxide–oxygen for conscious sedation is

a. Nitrous oxide 70% and oxygen 30%
b. Nitrous oxide 30% and oxygen 70%
c. Nitrous oxide 50% and oxygen 50%
d. Nitrous oxide 80% and oxygen 20%

Ans b.

The patient can be maintained at 30% nitrous oxide and 70% oxygen or lower and monitored and the contemplated procedure can be carried out.

20. To prevent diffusion hypoxia after nitrous oxide–oxygen sedation

a. 100% oxygen is administered for 5 minutes
b. 100% oxygen is administered for 30 minutes
c. Nitrous oxide–oxygen concentration is reduced gradually
d. 70% oxygen is administered for 5 minutes

Ans a.

To minimize the effect of diffusion hypoxia, the patient should be oxygenated with 100% oxygen for 5 minutes after the sedation procedure.

21. Which of the following is an indication that the patient is adequately sedated?

a. Floating sensation and giddy feeling
b. Tingling sensation of digits
c. Distant gaze or sagging eyelids
d. Any of the above

Ans d.

All the above-mentioned features indicate that the patient is adequately sedated.

22. The dentist who used nitrous oxide for the first time is

a. Colton
b. Horace Wells
c. Long
d. Priestley

Ans b.

The answer is self-explanatory.

23. Whose demonstration of properties of nitrous oxide instigated Horace Wells to use nitrous oxide for tooth extraction?

a. Colton
b. Horace Wells
c. Long
d. Priestley

Ans a.

Colton's (a physicist) demonstration of properties of nitrous oxide instigated Horace Wells to use nitrous oxide for tooth extraction.

24. All of the following antihistamine drugs are used for conscious sedation except

a. Hydroxyzine
b. Promethazine
c. Chlorpromazine
d. Meperidine

Ans d.

Meperidine being a narcotic drug cannot be used for conscious sedation.

25. Which of the following agents is used for sedation only by inhalational route?

a. Halothane
b. Nitrous oxide–oxygen
c. Promethazine
d. Isoflurane

Ans b.

Nitrous oxide–oxygen is used for sedation only by inhalational route. Halothane and isoflurane are general anesthetic agents. Promethazine is a phenothiazine with sedative and antihistaminic properties.

26. Which of the following benzodiazepines is frequently used nowadays for conscious sedation?

a. Diazepam
b. Midazolam
c. Hydroxyzine
d. Fentanyl

Ans b.

Midazolam is used as an intravenous sedative agent. It is a benzodiazepine group of drug. After intravenous administration, sedation occurs in 3–5 minutes.

27. Which of the following conditions in a 6-year-old patient is a contraindication to the usage of nitrous oxide–oxygen analgesia?

a. The child has cold

b. The child is mentally retarded

c. The child has a history of diabetes

d. The child is allergic to local anesthesia

Ans a.

The answer is self-explanatory.

28. Which of the following intravenous agents is commonly used as an induction agent?

a. Diazepam

b. Ketamine

c. Thiopental

d. Phenobarbitone

Ans c.

Thiopental and methohexital are ultrashort acting barbiturates commonly used as induction agents.

29. Commonly used drug combination for oral sedation is

a. Chloralhydrate + hydroxyzine

b. Chloralhydrate + hydroxyzine + meperidine

c. Meperidine + hydroxyzine

d. Any of the above

Ans d.

All of the above-mentioned drug combinations are used for oral sedation.

30. Which of the following routes are titrable?

a. IV and inhalational

b. IV and IM

c. IV and oral

d. Oral and subcutaneous

Ans a.

IV and inhalational routes are titrable. Titration refers to the incremental administration of small amounts of a drug until a desired clinical effect is observed. This is possible in inhalational sedation and it allows the dentist to administer the correct dose of the drug to the patient.

31. Which of the following is a contraindication for conscious sedation?

a. If medical history reveals him or her to be a high risk patient
b. Pregnancy
c. ASA III and IV group patients
d. All of the above

Ans d.

The answer is self-explanatory. Refer the table below.

American Society of Anesthesiologists Classification

S. No.	Class	Description
1.	Class I	There is no organic, physiologic, biochemical or psychiatric disturbance. The pathologic process for which operation is to be performed is localized and is not a systemic disturbance.
2.	Class II	Mild-to-moderate systemic disturbance caused either by the condition to be treated surgically or by other pathophysiologic processes.
3.	Class III	Severe systemic disturbance or disease.
4.	Class IV	Indicative of the patient with severe systemic disorders that are already life threatening.
5.	Class V	The moribund patient who has little chance of survival without the planned procedure.

32. Which drug should be available if meperidine is used for premedication?

a. Atropine
b. Naloxone
c. Promethazine
d. Lactamine

Ans b.

Meperidine is a narcotic agent. When it is used for premedication, narcotic antagonist. Naloxone should be available.

33. The nitrous oxide administered for conscious sedation in a patient

a. Gets excreted by the kidneys
b. Is detoxified in the liver

c. Is exhaled by lungs
d. Is metabolized to NO and oxygen

Ans c.

Nitrous oxide does not combine chemically with blood components. Hence, it is just exhaled by the lungs.

34. A child who has been given a sedative dose of barbiturate (short acting) is active and excited. This indicates

a. A normal response to the drug
b. An excessive dose of drug
c. Insufficient dose of drug
d. Unexpected reaction

Ans c.

If the dose is insufficient, barbiturates can cause excitement in children instead of sedation.

35. The combined use of nitrous oxide and oxygen was introduced by

a. Colton
b. Horace Wells
c. Andrews
d. Jorgenson

Ans c.

In 1863, Andrews, an American physician introduced the combined use of nitrous oxide and oxygen inhalation. Refer also to Q. No. 23.

36. The first successful intravenous anesthetic agent is

a. Methohexital
b. Hexobarbital
c. Midazolam
d. Diazepam

Ans b.

Hexobarbital was introduced by Weese in Germany in 1932.

37. Thiopental was first used in medicine by

a. Colton
b. Jorgenson
c. Lundy
d. Leffingwell

Ans c.

Thiopental was synthesized in 1932 but Lundy used it in medicine in 1934.

38. Who is called the father of intravenous conscious sedation?

a. Jorgenson
b. Horace Wells
c. Colton
d. Lundy

Ans a.

Jorgenson is called the father of intravenous conscious sedation. Jorgenson and Leffingwell from Loma Linda University developed a technique using multiple agents like pentobarbital, meperidine and scopolamine. They called it the Jorgensen or Loma Linda technique.

39. Which of the following is incorrect regarding pediatric patients?

a. BMR is high in children leading to greater oxygen consumption
b. Apnea or hypoxia develops faster in children
c. Airways are smaller and shaped in a tubular form with the narrowest part lying above the vocal cords
d. Oxygen reserve is limited in children

Ans c.

In children, the airways are smaller and shaped in a funnel form, with the narrowest part of the trachea lying below the vocal cords. In adults, the airway is in a tubular form. The cardiac output and oxygen demand is also high in children.

40. The dosage of midazolam is

a. 0.5 mg/kg
b. 0.02 mg/kg
c. 1 mg/kg
d. 0.004 mg/kg

Ans a.

Refer also to Q. No. 26.

41. Diffusion hypoxia is observed in

a. Ketamine sedation procedure
b. Nitrous oxide–oxygen sedation procedure
c. Mask induction with halothane
d. Intravenous midazolam sedation procedure

Ans b.

Refer to the explanation of Q. No. 14 and 15.

42. One of the difficulties with premedication is "paradoxical excitement", which occurs most frequently with

a. Narcotics
b. Barbiturates
c. Nitrous oxide
d. Comedication

Ans b.

Barbiturates are nonselective central nervous system depressants, capable of producing all degrees of depression from mild sedation and hypnosis to general anesthesia, deep coma and death. In some patients, especially children and the elderly, drowsiness may be paradoxically preceded by transient euphoria, elation, excitement and confusion.

Section IV

Preventive Dentistry

Chapter 10

First Dental Visit

1. The first dental visit of a child should be carried out by

a. The time early changes of dental caries is seen on primary teeth
b. One year of age or as soon as the first primary tooth erupts into the mouth
c. Five years of age
d. Three years of age

Ans b.

Increased prevalence of early childhood caries lead to the need for an early first dental visit as soon as the first primary tooth erupts into the mouth.

2. All of the following should be avoided during a first dental visit in a 3-year-old child except

a. Deep caries excavation
b. Extraction of a tooth
c. Minor surgical procedures
d. Fluoride application

Ans d.

Any procedure which can cause pain and discomfort can be avoided in the first dental visit. Procedures like fluoride application are nonthreatening and carried out without any pain or discomfort.

3. Separation anxiety is a common phenomenon in which of the following age group?

a. 1–3 years
b. 5–8 years
c. 4–8 years
d. 8–12 years

Ans a.

Children in the age group most likely have separation anxiety. Hence separating them from their parents should be avoided.

Chapter 11

Principles of Preventive Dentistry

1. **All of the following are primary preventive measures except**
    a. Primordial prevention
    b. Health promotion
    c. Specific protection
    d. Disability limitation

Ans d.

Disability limitation is a tertiary preventive measure. Refer the Figure 11.1 given below:

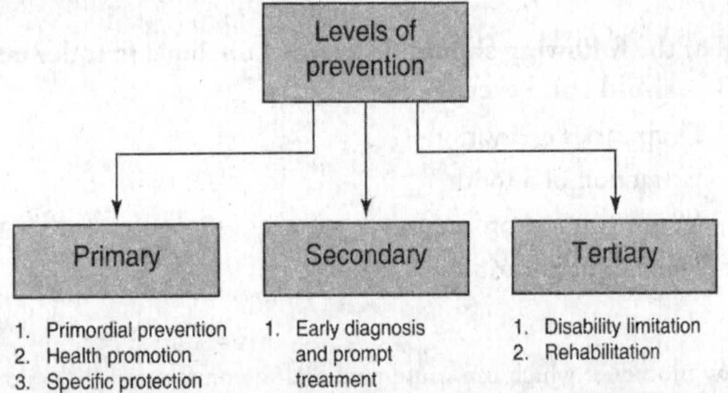

Fig. 11.1 Schematic diagram showing levels of prevention.

2. **Disability limitation and rehabilitation are forms of**
    a. Primary preventive measure
    b. Secondary preventive measure
    c. Tertiary preventive measure
    d. Not a type of preventive measure but a measure of rehabilitating an individual

Ans c.

Refer explanation and diagram of Q. No.1 above.

3. Immunization is a type of primary preventive measure categorized under

a. Health promotion
b. Specific protection
c. Primordial prevention
d. Health services

Ans b.

Immunization, mouth guards, car seat restraints, chlorination of drinking water, water fluoridation, pit and fissure sealants are various forms of primary preventive measures categorized under specific protection.

4. The action which halts the progress of the disease at its incipient stage and prevent complications is

a. Primary prevention
b. Secondary prevention
c. Tertiary prevention
d. Final prevention

Ans b.

Primary preventive measures include procedures that prevent occurrence of oral disease and oral abnormalities. The question is the definition of secondary prevention. Tertiary preventive measures are to reduce or limit disabilities and minimize suffering.

Chapter 12

Infant Oral Health and Anticipatory Guidance

1. **The concept of anticipatory guidance was proposed by**
   a. Nowak c. McDonald
   b. Tinanoff d. Pinkham

Ans a.

Anticipatory guidance is defined as proactive counseling of parents and patients about developmental changes that will occur in the interval between health supervision visits that includes information about daily care taking specific to that upcoming interval. This guidance has a defined protocol for every age group in it, starting from 6 to 12 months to adolescence.

Anticipatory guidance protocol

Major area	Topics to be discussed
Oral development	Eruption of the first tooth Eruption schedule Teething problems
Oral hygiene	Mouth cleaning Brushing position Consequence of inadequate cleaning
Fluoride adequacy	Water evaluation and supplementation Breastfeeding Formula milk Safety of fluoride Topical fluoride agents
Nutrition and diet	Role of carbohydrates Weaning Role of plaque Early childhood caries
Habits	Nonnutritive sucking Pacifiers

Continue...

Injury prevention	Child abuse Accidents Car safety Electric cord safety Emergency instructions

2. The concept of dental home is derived from

a. Hand-over-mouth exercise described by Evangeline Jordan
b. Medical home by American Academy of Pediatrics
c. Preventive measures taken at home
d. Ancient philosophy of dental care

Ans b.

The concept of *dental home* is derived from the American Academy of Pediatrics definition of medical home. The essential concept of medical home as described by American Academy of Pediatrics states that medical care of children of all ages is best managed when there is an established relationship between the practitioner who is familiar with the child and the child's family. Medical home becomes the place where a child receives preventive instructions, immunizations, counseling and anticipatory guidance.

3. Which of the following is true about infant examination?

a. Lift the lip examination is performed
b. Presence of plaque is recorded
c. Carried out in a "knee-to-knee position" with proper illumination
d. All of the above

Ans d.

The answer is self-explanatory.

4. Caries Assessment Tool (CAT) helps to assess

a. The risk of a child for developing caries
b. The treatment needed for children in the age group of 3–5 years
c. The pattern of caries (smooth surface or pit and fissure) observed in children
d. Salivary mutans levels of infants

Ans a.

Using CAT, children can be categorized to be in high, moderate or low risk for caries and the preventive measures can be planned accordingly.

Chapter 13

Fluorides

1. **Which of the following is the mechanism by which fluoride exerts the cariostatic action?**
   a. Incorporation of fluoride into dentin and enamel of unerupted teeth
   b. Secretion of fluoride in saliva, which decreases acid production in plaque and enhances remineralization of enamel
   c. Fluoride in saliva helps in the maturation of enamel of newly erupted teeth which decreases caries susceptibility
   d. All of the above

Ans d.

All the above-mentioned factors are true regarding cariostatic action of fluoride.

2. **The first fluoride containing dentifrice (CREST) had**
   a. Stannous fluoride
   b. Sodium fluoride
   c. Acidulated phosphate fluoride
   d. Sodium monofluorophosphate

Ans a.

The dentifrice CREST contained stannous fluoride in combination with calcium pyrophosphate as the cleaning and polishing system and was accepted as the first therapeutic dentifrice by the Council on Dental Therapeutics of the American Dental Association in 1964.

3. **The concentration of sodium fluoride used for professional topical fluoride application is**
   a. 0.2%
   b. 2%
   c. 0.02%
   d. 0.002%

Ans b.

Four applications of 2% sodium fluoride solution during a 2 week period, with the series of applications at 2–3 year intervals, has shown to decrease the caries incidence by 40%.

4. The concentration of stannous fluoride and acidulated phosphate fluoride used for professional topical fluoride application are

a. 8% and 12.3%
b. 0.8% and 1.23%
c. 0.8% and 12.3%
d. 8% and 1.23%

Ans d.

Stannous fluoride is available in powder form, in either bulk containers or preweighed capsules. The recommended concentration is 8%. Acidulated phosphate fluoride (APF—1.23%) is available as either a solution or a gel or a foam all of which are stable and ready to use.

5. All of the following are true regarding stannous fluoride except

a. 8% stannous fluoride solution is obtained by dissolving 0.8 g of powder in 100 mL of distilled water
b. Stannous fluoride solution is acidic with a pH of 2.4 to 2.8
c. Stannous fluoride solution is not stable, hence it has to be prepared immediately before use
d. Stannous fluoride is available in powder form in either bulk containers or preweighed capsules

Ans a.

Stannous fluoride (8%) is obtained by dissolving 0.8 g of powder in 10 mL of distilled water.

6. APF gel or solution contains all except

a. Sodium fluoride
b. Hydrofluoric acid
c. Phosphoric acid
d. Hydrochloric acid

Ans d.

APF system consists essentially of a mixture of sodium fluoride, hydrofluoric acid and phosphoric acid, with concentrations of 1.23% fluoride and 0.98% phosphoric acid with a pH of 3 to 3.5.

7. APF gels can be usually stored for

a. 1 year
b. 2 years
c. 5 years
d. 4.5 years

Ans b.

The APF systems are chemically stable for at least 2 years when stored in plastic containers, but there may be a decrease in the viscosity of the gels after several months of storage.

8. The usual time recommended for topical fluoride application is

a. 4 minutes
b. 8 minutes
c. 2 minutes
d. 6 minutes

Ans a.

A 4 minute treatment time is recommended for either solution or gel. Topical application of APF gel, solution or foam should be repeated at least every 6 months.

9. Which of the following is/are true about carrying out a topical fluoride application for a child patient?

a. Both trays can be inserted at once
b. Patient sits in an upright position with head tipped slightly forward to allow excess saliva and gel to flow towards the lips
c. The trays are in place for 4 minutes
d. Patient may need assistance or positive reinforcement during the procedure
e. All of the above

Ans e.

The choices describe the technique of application.

10. Patients are encouraged not to drink, eat or rinse after fluoride application for

a. 1 hour
b. 15 minutes
c. 30 minutes
d. 90 minutes

Ans c.

Patients are encouraged not to drink, eat or rinse after fluoride application for 30 minutes to maximize the fluoride uptake into the enamel.

11. The concentration of fluoride used for mouth rinse is

a. 0.2% NaF rinse once weekly
b. 0.05% NaF rinse once daily
c. 0.02% NaF rinse once daily and 0.05% NaF rinse once weekly
d. Both (a) and (b)

Ans d.

The answer is self-explanatory.

12. Transfer of fluoride does occur from the mother to the fetus through placenta. The benefit of caries prevention is more for the primary teeth than the permanent teeth because of this transmission from mother to fetus.

a. Both the statements are false
b. Both the statements are true
c. First statement is true and the second is false
d. First statement is false and the second is true

Ans b.

Transfer of fluorides does occur from mother to fetus. Those who support prenatal fluorides usage agree to this point. However, how much fluoride is transferred from the mother's blood remains uncertain. Researchers generally agree that some benefits accrue to the primary teeth but considerable doubt exists about the benefits to the permanent teeth.

13. The administration of fluoride supplements should commence shortly after birth and should continue through the time of eruption of second permanent molars. If the natural fluoride content of water is 0.7 ppm or more, supplements should not be recommended.

a. Both the statements are false
b. Both the statements are true
c. First statement is true and the second is false
d. First statement is false and the second is true

Ans b.

The answer is self-explanatory.

14. One of the following is not a disadvantage of stannous fluoride topical application

a. Bad taste
b. Etch porcelain restoration
c. Stain silicate restoration
d. Pigmentation of arrested lesions

Ans b.

Stannous fluoride solutions do not etch porcelain restorations like APF gels or solutions. Hence, this is an advantage of stannous fluoride solutions.

15. All of the following are advantages of APF gel except

a. It has a better taste than stannous fluoride
b. It has no staining or pigmentation
c. It can be applied to both arches simultaneously
d. It damages porcelain restorations

Ans d.

APF gel can be detrimental to porcelain resorations.

16. The quantity of stannous fluoride solution required for treating a patient is approximately

a. 10 mL
b. 20 mL
c. 30 mL
d 40 mL

Ans a.

The answer is self-explanatory.

17. In tray application of APF gel, the quantity of gel taken for one application is

a. 2/3 of the trough area of the tray
b. 1/3 of the trough area of the tray
c. Fill the tray completely
d. Less than 1/3 of the trough area of the tray

Ans b.

APF gel or foam is placed to fill one-third of the trough area so that they properly fit over each dental arch. Avoid overloading the tray; this could lead to excessive ingestion.

18. Sodium fluoride solution is a

a. Neutral solution
b. Acidic solution

c. Alkaline solution

d. None of the above

Ans a.

Sodium fluoride solutions are of neutral pH and have a more acceptable taste than stannous fluoride.

19. The fluoridated dentifrice has fluoride in the following concentration

a. 450–1500 ppm

b. 200–300 ppm

c. 2000–2500 ppm

d. 1800–2200 ppm

Ans a.

The answer is self-explanatory. A 25 to 35% caries reduction can be expected with the use of fluoride dentifrices. Increased benefit is observed with two or three brushings per day when compared to one brushing.

20. Gel-Kam has

a. 0.4% NaF

b. 0.4% APF

c. 0.4% stannous fluoride

d. 0.6% NaF

Ans c.

Gel-Kam has 0.4% stannous fluoride (1000 ppm F).

21. The fluoride concentration in school water fluoridation is

a. 2 times the city water supply

b. 4.5 times the city water supply

c. 8 times the city water supply

d. Equal as the city water supply

Ans b.

The answer is self-explanatory. School water fluoridation shows 35% caries reduction with supervised daily or weekly rinses. Refer explanation of Q. No. 28.

22. Denti di chiaie was reported by

a. McKay

b. J.M. Eager

c. Trendley Dean

d. G.V. Black

Ans b.

In 1902, Dr J.M. Eager reported that in Italy certain people have ugly brown stains on teeth (*dent di chiaie*), teeth with writing (*denti scritti*) or black teeth (*denti neri*).

23. Fluoride was identified excessively in water through spectrometric analysis by

a. McKay
b. JM Eager
c. Trendley Dean
d. HV Churchill

Ans d.

In 1931, H.V. Churchill did a thorough spectrometric analysis of a sample of bauxite water and found that it showed a high fluoride content.

24. Shoe leather survey was carried out by

a. McKay
b. JM Eager
c. Trendley Dean
d. HV Churchill

Ans c.

Shoe leather survey was done to study the relationship between fluoride concentration in drinking water, mottled enamel and dental caries. In 1931, Dr Trendley H Dean was appointed to find the extent and geographical distribution of mottled enamel in USA.

25. Formula to calculate the appropriate fluoride level in community water based on the temperature is

a. F = 0.34/E
b. F = E/0.34
c. F = E + 0.34/t
d. F = E + 0.34 + t

Ans a.

The formula was given by Galagan and Vermillion in 1957. In the formula E= 0.038 + 0.0062t (where E is the estimated daily water intake for children in ounces per pound of body weight, t is yearly mean of the daily maximum temperature in Fahrenheit).

26. The appropriate fluoride level for caries prevention in community water fluoridation is

a. 0.5 ppm

b. 0.7–1.2 ppm
c. 0.2–0.5 ppm
d. 2–3 ppm

Ans b.

The optimal level of fluoride in water is 1 ppm. But usually it ranges between 0.7 and 1.2 ppm depending on mean temperature of a particular area. Because people in cold climates consume less water, water in those areas has higher fluoride levels. But people in warmer areas consume more water and so the water in those areas has lower fluoride content.

27. Nalgonda technique is a technique for

a. Adding fluoride to community water fluoridation
b. Defluoridation
c. School water fluoridation
d. School topical fluoride application

Ans b.

This is a more economical method of defluoridation. In this method, the fluoridated water is defluoridated by addition of lime and aluminium sulfate. This technique was introduced in the town of Kadiri in Andhra Pradesh in 1980.

28. The recommended concentration of fluoride in school water fluoridation is

a. 4.5–6.3 ppm
b. 1.5–3.5 ppm
c. 1.5–4.5 ppm
d. 6–8 ppm

Ans a.

School water fluoridation is a suitable alternative where community water fluoridation is not feasible, because school children would consume it in school. However, high concentration of 4.5–6.3 ppm fluoride is added in school water supply since children would only be exposed to the fluoridated water for a limited period (during school hours). Also there would be no exposure to fluoridated water during the vacations.

29. The concentration of stannous fluoride used for topical application is

a. 2%
b. 1.23%
c. 8%
d. 4%

Ans c.

Stannous fluoride (8%) solution has a pH of 2.1–2.3. The concentration of fluoride in 8% stannous fluoride is 19360 ppm. Sodium fluoride is used in 2% concentration and APF gel is used in 1.23% concentration.

30. Knutson technique is application of

a. Sodium fluoride
b. Stannous fluoride
c. APF gel
d. APF solution

Ans a.

Sodium fluoride was developed by Knutson et al. in 1947. It has a neutral pH of 7 and available fluoride is 9040 ppm. Application of stannous fluoride is known as *Muhler technique.*

31. Certainly lethal dose of fluoride is

a. 12–24 mg/kg
b. 32–64 mg/kg
c. 1 mg/kg
d. 5 mg/kg

Ans b.

Certainly lethal dose of fluoride for a 70 kg adult is 5000 to 10000 mg of sodium fluoride or 32–64 mg F/kg body weight. Survival after consuming this amount of fluoride is unlikely.

32. Which of the following is the most effective way to combat dental disease?

a. Establishing a milk and salt fluoridation Program
b. Careful dietary control emphasizing elimination of sweets
c. Incremental dental care coupled with community water fluoridation
d. Use of a Program composed of community water fluoridation and additional topical fluoridation

Ans c.

Fluoridation of public water supplies is the most effective of many fluoride therapies that has been proved repeatedly. Fluoridation benefits children and adults and the benefits continue for a lifetime if consumption continues.

33. Topical application of fluoride for patients who have had the benefits of water fluoridation since birth is desirable because

a. Benefits are additive

b. It has been a state law for 2 years
c. Two different types of fluorides are used
d. None of the above. The premise is false

Ans a.

Topical fluorides are applied to the tooth surfaces in regular intervals in order to prevent the development of caries. They exert an anticaries effect by increasing the concentration of fluorides on the outer most surface of the enamel. Benefits of topical application of fluorides along with community water fluoridation are additive.

34. If a child lived for only the first month of his life in a fluoridated community, one would expect to find the fluoride in a fully developed permanent first molar deposited in the

a. Cervical enamel
b. Enamel near the dentinoenamel junction only
c. Cusp tip enamel and dentinal layers near the dentinoenamel junction
d. Enamel occlusal surface and the dentinal layers adjacent to the pulp chambers

Ans c.

The mineralization of the permanent teeth is initiated around the time of birth on average, beginning with the first permanent molar. Hence, if a child has lived in a fluoridated area for only the first month of his life, this will benefit the first permanent molars cusp tips.

35. A child is born and lives his first 8 years in a community in a temperate zone, the water supply of which contains 2.5 ppm of fluoride. It can be expected that some mottling will develop in

a. All teeth
b. All permanent teeth, except third molars
c. Lateral incisors, canines, premolars and third molars
d. None of the above. This concentration is not sufficient to cause mottling

Ans b.

The calcification of all permanent teeth ends before the age of 8, except third molars. A concentration of 2.5 ppm is higher than the optimal level of water fluoridation which can cause mottling in all permanent teeth if the child lives in the community for the first 8 years.

36. The most effective immediate action for a child who has accidently swallowed 10 cc of a 10% fluoride solution is to

a. Have the child drink copious quantities of water to dilute the solution
b. Have the child drink a 10% sodium bicarbonate solution
c. Have the child drink milk or some other calcium-containing liquid
d. Send the child immediately to the emergency room of a hospital

Ans c.

Give calcium orally (milk) to relieve gastrointestinal symptoms and observe for a few hours. Induced vomiting is not necessary. Please refer the following table:

Table 13.1 Emergency treatment for fluoride toxicity

Amount of fluoride ingested	Treatment
Less than 5 mg/kg body weight	Give calcium orally (milk) to relieve gastrointestinal symptoms and observe for few hours. Induced vomiting is not necessary. Empty the stomach by inducing vomiting with an emetic. For example, Ipecacuanha emetic mixture (Ipecac syrup) can be given-Dose: 6–18 month old child — 10 mL Older children — 15 mL Adults — 30 mL
5–15 mg/kg body weight	Give orally soluble calcium in any form (milk, 5% calcium gluconate or calcium lactate solution) Epsom salts or aluminium hydroxide antacid can also be given to slow down the absorption of any remaining fluoride Admit in a hospital and observe for a few hours
More than 15 mg/kg body weight	Admit in a hospital immediately Induce vomiting Begin cardiac monitoring and be prepared for cardiac arrhythmias. Electrolytes, especially calcium and potassium should be monitored and corrected as necessary Slowly administer intravenously 10 mL of 10% calcium gluconate solution Adequate urine output should be maintained using diuretics if necessary General supportive measures for shock

37. Which of the following statements best describes the relationship with the fluorides and dental caries?

a. Children living in areas of endemic mottling tend to show higher DMF index than those living in areas where mottling is rare
b. Children living in areas of endemic mottling tend to show a lower DMF index than those living in areas where mottling is rare
c. Children drinking optimal quantities of fluoridated water have about the same number of interproximal carious lesions but significantly fewer pit and fissure caries than the children who bring the same quantities of nonfluoridated water
d. Optimal effects of fluorides can be achieved only at levels where mottled enamel also occurs

Ans b.

The answer is self-explanatory.

38. Using a topical fluoride rinse before acid etch direct bonding of orthodontic bracket is contraindicated because fluoride

a. Decreases the solubility of the enamel
b. Increases the pH of the etching agent
c. Causes copious amounts of saliva
d. Directly reacts chemically with the bonding agent

Ans a.

Primarily etching is done to demineralize enamel to a depth of 20–30 nm and render it porous. During remineralization, if fluoride is present in the oral environment due to topical application, these fluoride ions get incorporated into the tooth surface thereby forming fluorapatite crystals which are more stable and resistant to demineralization.

39. A 5-year-old patient who lives in an area where the fluoride content of the drinking water averages 0.75 ppm should be supplemented with how much fluoride per day?

a. 0 mg
b. 0.25 mg
c. 0.5 mg
d. 1.0 mg

Ans a.

Please refer the following Tan;e 13.2 on next page.

Table 13.2 Dietary fluoride supplementation as recommended by AAPD

Age of Child	Water fluoride concentration		
	<0.3 ppm	0.3–0.7 ppm	>0.7 ppm
Birth to 6 months	Not recommended	Not recommended	Not recommended
6 months to 3 years	0.25 mg	Not recommended	Not recommended
3 to 6 years	0.5 mg	0.25 mg	Not recommended
6 to 16 years	1 mg	0.5 mg	Not recommended

40. When determining the dosage of systemic fluoride supplements for a child, it is most important to consider which of the following?

a. Age and weight of the child
b. Age of the child and mean annual temperature
c. Age of the child and fluoride content of drinking water
d. Weight of the child and fluoride content of drinking water

Ans c.

The dietary fluoride supplementation schedule is recommended by American Academy of Pediatric Dentistry (AAPD) in 2002 according to the age of the child and the amount of fluoride present in the drinking water where the child resides.

41. The water supply of a community has 0.28 ppm fluoride. Which of the following supplemental procedure is appropriate for a 3-year-old child?

a. Prescribe a fluoride rinse
b. Prescribe 0.5 mg fluoride per day
c. Place the child on 3 month recall and apply fluoride topically each visit
d. Fluoride supplement is unnecessary because the crowns of most permanent teeth have already formed

Ans b.

Please refer the Table of Q. No. 39.

Chapter 14

Plaque Control Measures in Pediatric Dentistry

1. **The length of bristles in most of the toothbrushes is**
   a. 5–8 mm
   b. 11 mm
   c. 15 mm
   d. 18 mm

Ans b.

The length of bristles in most of the toothbrushes is 11 mm. Brushes are classified as soft, medium or hard based on the width of the bristles. The diameter ranges from 0.16 to 0.22 mm for soft, 0.23 to 0.29 mm for medium and 0.30 mm and greater for hard toothbrushes.

2. **Which of the following bristle ends cause the least amount of gingival irritation?**
   a. Coarse cut
   b. Enlarged bulbous
   c. Round end
   d. None of the above

Ans c.

The three types of bristle ends are coarse cut, enlarged bulbous and round end. Of the three types of bristle ends, the round end is the type of choice for bristle because of its decreased incidence of gingival-tissue irritation. However, even the coarse-cut bristles round off eventually with normal use.

3. **Which of the following is true regarding the powered toothbrush —Interplak?**
   a. It uses the movement of individual tufts of bristles rather than the head of the brush
   b. Interplak has 10 independently driven tufts that rotate approximately 4200 times per minute
   c. Each soft bristled tuft alternatively rotates 11/2 revolutions in one direction and then reverses to rotate 11/2 revolutions in

the opposite direction with adjacent tufts rotating in opposite direction

d. All of the above

Ans d.

All the above-mentioned facts are true regarding the powered tooth brush—Interplak.

4. The novelty of the powered toothbrushes causes an initial increase in use and therefore control of plaque and gingivitis. Any change or experimental manipulation similar to the above situation may induce an improvement in behavior, which is known as the Hawthorne effect.

a. Both the statements are false
b. Both the statements are true
c. First statement is true and the second is false
d. First statement is false and the second is true

Ans b.

A few studies have confirmed that powered toothbrushes are not proved to be more effective than manual brushes in plaque removal for the typical patient over a protracted period. Kerlinger attributes the initial increase in use and initial improvement in plaque and gingivitis control to the novelty of the powered toothbrush. However, with time, the results become comparable to manual brushing.

5. The soft brush is preferable for most uses in pediatric dentistry because of

a. Decreased incidence of gingival tissue trauma
b. Increased interproximal cleaning ability
c. The bristle type is usually round end
d. All of the above

Ans d.

The answer is self-explanatory.

6. The advantage of the new floss made up of Teflon material is

a. It has lower coefficient of friction than nylon
b. It slides easily between tight contacts and minimizes snapping of the floss
c. It does not shred
d. All of the above

Ans d.

Several different types of floss are available—flavored and unflavored; waxed and unwaxed; thin, tape and meshwork. Almost all commercially available floss is made up of nylon. The newly introduced floss made up of Teflon material has the above advantages.

7. Which of the following dye is used in disclosing agents?

a. Gentian violet
b. Erythrosin
c. Fluorescein
d. Basic fuchsin
e. Any of the above

Ans e.

Disclosing agents include iodine, gentian violet, erythrosin, basic fuchsin, fast green, food dyes, fluorescein, etc.

8. The brushing technique naturally adopted by children is

a. Roll method
b. Horizontal scrub method
c. Charters method
d. Modified Stillman method

Ans b.

The horizontal scrub technique removes as much plaque or more plaque than other techniques, regardless of the child's age or if the parent performs the brushing. In addition, it is the technique most naturally adopted by children.

9. Lap-to-lap position is a recommended position for performing oral hygiene procedures in

a. Infants (0–1 year old)
b. Toddlers (1–3 years old)
c. Preschool child (3–6 years old)
d. School age (6–12 years old)

Ans b.

Two adults sit with knees touching using their laps as a table to rest the child. One adult holds the child's legs and arms while the other adult performs the oral hygiene procedures.

10. The oldest antiplaque agent is

a. Listerine
b. Chlorhexidine

c. Cetylpyridinium chloride

d. Sanguinarine

Ans a.

The most widely known noncharged phenolic antiseptic agent is Listerine. It has demonstrated a long history of efficacy and was among the original antiseptic agents studied by W.D. Miller in 1890.

11. Dentifrices

a. Act as plaque- and stain-removing agents

b. Have pleasant colors and flavors which encourage their use

c. Have tartar control properties

d. Have anticaries and desensitizing properties

e. All the statements are true

Ans e.

Dentifrices serve multiple functions in oral hygiene through the use of a variety of agents. They act as plaque- and stain-removing agents through the use of abrasives and surfactants. They have tartar control properties by the addition of pyrophosphates. They have anticaries and desensitization properties through the action of fluoride and other agents.

12. All the following statements are true except

a. More time was spent brushing the upper than lower teeth by the children

b. The contralateral side was brushed more than the ipsilateral side in children

c. Less than 10% of the time was spent in brushing the lingual areas

d. Most popular brushing stroke was the horizontal scrub method in children

Ans a.

More time was spent brushing the lower teeth than the upper teeth.

13. Which of the following mouth rinse has the highest alcohol content?

a. Listerine

b. Chlorhexidine

c. Cetylpyridinium chloride

d. Sanguinarine

Ans a.

Listerine has one of the highest alcohol contents of mouthwashes, approximately 25%.

14. Disclosing agents are available in all of the following forms except

a. Tablets

b. Wafers

c. Gels

d. Capsules

Ans c.

Disclosing gels are not available. These agents are highly desirable for effective plaque removal and patient motivation. A good disclosing agent stains the teeth only very faintly by staining the pellicle in a faint pink color but stains the dental plaque deeply and vividly.

15. The first commercial dental floss was probably introduced in

a. 1782

b. 1882

c. 1970

d. 1910

Ans b.

The first commercial dental floss was introduced in 1882 in Massachusetts and the first patent on dental floss dates back to 1876. The Johnson & Johnson Company manufactured silk dental flosses as early as 1898.

16. All of the following statements regarding floss is/are true except

a. No difference in effectiveness of plaque removal exists between waxed and unwaxed floss

b. Waxed floss tends to fray more than unwaxed floss

c. Each dental floss depending on its thickness is made with 4–18 ends of filaments twisted in a predetermined number of twists per inch

d Waxed floss is used much more in dental offices than unwaxed floss

Ans b.

Bass was a strong proponent of the unwaxed floss because of fear of wax being left on the interproximal surfaces from waxed floss; also unwaxed floss is usually thinner and splays more on use.

17. Which of the following is/are undesirable side effects of chlorhexidine?

a. Brown diffuse discoloration of teeth
b. Unpleasant bitter taste
c. Dryness of the mouth
d. Burning sensation of the tongue
e. All of the above

Ans e.

All the side effects mentioned above are undesirable effects of chlorhexidine.

18. An ideal chemotherapeutic plaque control agent should have

a. Specificity only for pathogenic bacteria
b. Substantivity and chemical stability
c. Toxicologic and ecologic safety
d. Ease of use
e. All of the above

Ans e.

Substantivity is the ability to attach and to be retained by oral surfaces and then be released overtime without loss of potency. Though no agent has yet been developed that has all the above features, chemotherapeutic agents still play a role in maintaining oral health.

19. One of the following agent is not used as or component of disclosing agent

a. Basic fuchsin
b. Erythrocin
c. Fast green
d. Acidic fuchsin

Ans d.

Various agents used as disclosing agents are basic fuchsin, erythrocin, fast green and vegetable and fruit coloring dyes. Refer Q.No. 7 and its explanation.

20. Any change or experimental manipulation will induce an improvement in behavior, apparently because of a novelty effect. The introduction of powered toothbrushes caused an initial increase in use and therefore plaque and gingivitis were controlled. After some time, the results became comparable to those with manual brushes. This is called

a. Bass effect
b. Charter's effect

c. Hawthorne effect
d. Kerlinger effect

Ans c.

Studies on plaque removal effectiveness failed to demonstrate greater efficacy for powered than for manual tooth brushes. Although improvement was seen initially, over the time, the level of cleaning achieved with powered toothbrushes declined to the same level obtained using manual toothbrushes. This is called *Hawthorne effect* by Kerlinger.

21. All of the following are true regarding electric toothbrushes except

a. They have oscillating or rotating motions
b. They are generally useful in children who lack manual dexterity
c. Their cleaning efficiency is always better than manual brushes
d. Some brushes uses low-frequency acoustic energy to enhance cleaning

Ans c.

Refer to the explanation of Q. No. 20.

22. The usual concentration of chlorhexidine used for mouth rinses is

a. 0.12%
b. 0.5%
c. 0.6%
d. 0.002%

Ans a.

The usual concentration of chlorhexidine used in mouth rinses is between 0.1 and 0.2%. It has a broad spectrum of antimicrobial activity against gram-positive bacteria, gram-negative bacteria, yeast and *Streptococcus mutans.*

23. One of the following is not an interdental cleaning aid

a. Toothette
b. Single tuft brushes
c. Interdental tips
d. Toothpick in holder

Ans a.

Toothette is a swab of sponge attached to a stick. It is used in oral cleansing in hospitals and in patients having extremely fragile tender gingiva or mucosal lesions.

24. Based on the work of Bass, which type of floss is considered better?

a. Teflon waxed
b. Teflon unwaxed
c. Nylon waxed
d. Nylon unwaxed

Ans d.

Based on the work of Bass, it is said that the nylon unwaxed floss is generally considered the floss of choice because of the ease of use.

25. Parental brushing is recommended up to the age of_____.

a. 6 years
b. 4 years
c. 10 years
d. 12 years

Ans a.

During this period all the primary teeth are present. Spaces that were visible earlier may begin to close. Cleaning the mouth includes brushing the teeth and cleaning the areas where the gingiva touch the teeth. This is a fine motor activity that most 3- to 6-year olds cannot perform completely without assistance. In addition, the lingual surfaces of the mandibular posterior teeth and the buccal surfaces of the maxillary posterior teeth are the most difficult to reach and to see if all the plaque has been removed.

26. All of the following are components of a powder dentifrice except

a. Abrasives
b. Detergents
c. Flavoring agents
d. Binders

Ans d.

The powder dentifrice contains the following components—abrasives, detergents, flavoring agents and sweeteners. Binders are component of gel and paste form dentifrice.

27. The use of which of the following adjunctive aids is necessary to check on the efficacy of an oral prophylaxis for a young patient?

a. Disclosing agent
b. Sandpaper strip
c. Synder test
d. Unwaxed floss

Ans a.

For minimal amounts of plaque, the disclosing solutions were found to be the most sensitive assessment techniques. The clinical significance of these data is that, in measuring a patient's oral hygiene abilities, one must assess plaque deposits immediately after the patient has cleaned his or her tooth.

28. An 11-year-old patient who is wearing a full-banded orthodontic appliance has inflamed gingiva. The dentist should

a. Encourage better oral hygiene
b. Perform deep scaling and curettage
c. Perform gingivoplasty after the bands are removed
d. Ask the orthodontist to remove the bands so healing can occur

Ans a.

If orthodontic treatment is being considered, oral hygiene instructions should be given before the orthodontic treatment is started and should be consistently reinforced during the treatment to maintain good oral hygiene.

Chapter 15

Dental Health Education and School Dental Health Programs

1. The definition of health encompasses all except

a. Physical well being
b. Mental well being
c. Economical well being
d. Social well being

Ans c.

Health is defined as "a state of physical, mental and social well being and not merely an absence of disease or infirmity".

2. Which of the following components are inherent components of health education

a. Information
b. Motivation
c. Maintenance of healthy practices
d. All of the above

Ans d.

Health education is defined as "a process that informs, motivates and helps persons to adopt and maintain healthy practices and lifestyles; advocates environmental changes as needed to facilitate this goal; and conducts professional training research to the same end".

3. Which of the following are well known health education programs?

a. ASKOV dental demonstration
b. Tattle tooth program
c. ABCD — Access to Baby and Child Dentistry
d. All of the above

Ans d.

All the above-mentioned programs are health education programs.

Section V

Dental Caries

Chapter 16

Caries Risk Assessment and Caries Activity Tests

1. Which was the first microbiologic caries activity test that was extensively used by the practitioners?

a. Snyder's test

b. Alban's test

c. Lactobacillus count test

d. Caries risk test

Ans c.

This was the first microbiologic caries activity test that was extensively used by the practitioners. Saliva obtained from the individuals with active caries usually has high numbers of *Lactobacillus acidophilus* organisms.

2. Which of the following caries risk assessment test uses an algorithm to assess the caries risk?

a. DIAGNOdent

b. Quantitative light- induced fluorescence

c. Cariostat

d. Cariogram

Ans d.

Cariogram is a graphical model which summarizes the complex picture of various interrelated caries risk factors, so that it can be used by the dental professional routinely in the clinic. This Program contains an algorithm that presents a weighted analysis of the input data, mainly biological factors. Furthermore, it expresses the extent to which different etiological factors of caries affect the caries risk for a particular individual and provides targeted strategies for those individuals.

3. Which of the following technologies uses infrared fluorescence for diagnosing caries lesions?

a. DIAGNOdent

b. Quantitative light-induced fluorescence

c. Digital imaging fiberoptic trans-illumination

d. Cariostat

Ans a.

DIAGNOdent helps to identify and quantify dental caries of occlusal and smooth surfaces. It uses a diode laser light source and a fiberoptic cable that transmits the light to a handheld probe with a fiberoptic eye in the tip. The light is absorbed and induces infrared fluorescence by organic and inorganic materials. The emitted fluorescence is collected by the probe tip and transmitted through ascending fibers, and processed and presented on a digital display as an integer between 0 and 99.

4. **Which of the following is a colorimetric test?**
   a. Cariogram
   b. Quantitative light fluorescence
   c. Digital imaging fiberoptic transillumination
   d. Cariostat

Ans d.

Cariostat method is an abridged term for caries status. It was formulated by Tsutomu Shimona. As a colorimetric test, it determines the ability of the acid-producing bacteria in dental plaque to change the color of the supplied medium from dark blue to varying shades of blue, green and yellow.

5. **The best method for detection of risk in younger age group children (2–3 years) is**
   a. Cariogram
   b. Quantitative light-induced fluorescence
   c. Digital imaging fiberoptic transillumination
   d. Cariostat

Ans d.

The cariostat test has reliably predicted caries experience in the short term in toddlers, and in the long term by sampling as early as age 3 and predicting of outcomes as long term as age 10 (refer to explanation of Q. No. 4).

6. **The purpose of the Snyder's test is to**
   a. Predict the nature of the combined acidogenic organisms in the oral cavity
   b. Determine the exact nature of a specific organism related to caries prevalence
   c. Predict the rate of salivary flow
   d. Estimate the salivary dissolving capacity of enamel

Ans a.

Snyder's test was based on the fact that lactobacilli are acidogenic and aciduric. Since the amount of acids produced is directly proportional to the number of lactobacilli, the amount of acid produced was kept as a determinant of the risk. The Snyder's medium changes its color based on the amount of acids produced.

7. **The value of caries activity tests is their use in**
   a. Gaining the child's confidence
   b. Predicting the number of new lesions in a specified time
   c. Checking on the patient's cooperation in preventive measures
   d. Determining whether a fixed appliance is better than a removable one

Ans c.

Repeating caries activity tests at the first and subsequent appointments can help the practitioner identify the patient's cooperation in preventive measures. If the patient has not taken any effort to practice preventive measures, the scoring in caries activity test may increase or may not show any significant reduction in the risk.

Chapter 17

Dental Caries

1. The most widely accepted theory of the cause of dental caries is

a. Proteolysis-chelation theory
b. Proteolysis theory
c. Acidogenic theory or chemicoparasitic theory
d. Hypoplastic theory

Ans c.

The most popular and probably the most widely accepted theory is Miller's acidogenic theory. Refer to the following table for description of theories.

S. No.	Name of the theory	Author	Description
1.	Chemicoparasitic or acidogenic	Miller	Dental caries is caused by acids resulting from the action of microorganisms on carbohydrates. It is characterized by decalcification of the inorganic portion and is accompanied or followed by disintegration of the organic substance of the tooth.
2.	Proteolysis theory	Gottlieb and Frisbie	Dental caries is caused by microorganisms which invade enamel lamellae and involve the dentin.
3.	Proteolysis-chelation theory	Schatz	Oral bacteria attack organic components of enamel and the breakdown products have chelating ability, which dissolve the tooth minerals.

2. **Oral bacteria attacks organic components of enamel and the breakdown products have the ability to dissolve the tooth minerals. This is**

   a. Proteolysis–chelation theory
   b. Proteolysis theory
   c. Acidogenic theory or chemicoparasitic theory
   d. Hypoplastic theory

Ans a.

Refer to the explanation and table of Q. No. 1.

3. **Proteolysis theory was proposed by**

   a. Miller
   b. Gottlieb and Frisbie
   c. Fitzerald
   d. Keyes

Ans b.

Refer to the explanation and table of Q. No. 1.

4. **Acids resulting from the action of micro-organisms on carbohydrates cause dental caries, which is characterized by decalcification of inorganic portion and followed by disintegration of organic substances. This theory is**

   a. Proteolysis–chelation theory
   b. Proteolysis theory
   c. Acidogenic theory or chemicoparasitic theory
   d. Hypoplastic theory

Ans c.

Refer to the explanation and table of Q. No. 1.

5. **Animals maintained in a germ-free environment did not develop caries even when fed on a high carbohydrate diet. This was proven by**

   a. Miller
   b. Gottlieb
   c. Orland and Fitzerald
   d. Loesche

Ans c.

Studies by Orland and by Fitzerald, Jordan and Achard demonstrated that dental caries will not occur in the absence of microorganisms. Animals maintained in a germ-free environment did not develop caries even when fed on a high carbohydrate diet. However, dental caries did develop in these animals when they were inoculated with microorganisms from caries-active animals and then fed cariogenic diets.

6. ***Streptococcus mutans* is present in the oral cavity of infants at birth. *Streptococcus mutans* is transmitted orally from mother to infant.**

   a. Both the statements are false
   b. Both the statements are true
   c. First statement is true and the second is false
   d. First statement is false and the second is true

Ans d.

Streptococcus mutans is not present in the oral cavity of infants at birth and can be detected only after the primary teeth begin to erupt. Transmission of *Streptococcus mutans* from mother to infant is confirmed by many investigators.

7. **The acids that initially decalcify the enamel have a pH of**

   a. 1–2
   b. 5.2–5.5
   c. 7–8
   d. 2.3–2.5

Ans b.

The answer is self-explanatory.

8. **Outer surface of enamel is far more resistant to demineralization by acids than deeper portion of enamel. Hence, the greatest amount of demineralization occurs 10–15 microns beneath the enamel surface.**

   a. Both the statements are false
   b. Both the statements are true
   c. First statement is true and the second is false
   d. First statement is false and the second is true

Ans b.

This demineralization that occurs 10–15 microns below the outer surface is called *subsurface demineralization.* The continuation of this process results in the subsurface enamel lesion that will first be observed as white spot lesion.

9. The time required for remineralization to replace the hydroxyapatite lost during demineralization is determined by

a. Age of the plaque
b. Nature of carbohydrate consumed
c. Presence or absence of fluoride
d. All of the above

Ans d.

In the presence of dental plaque that has developed for 12 hours or less, the enamel demineralization resulting from a single exposure to sucrose will be remineralized by saliva within about 10 minutes. A period of at least 4 hours is required by saliva to repair the damage to enamel resulting from a similar exposure to sucrose in the presence of dental plaque that is 48 or more hours old. Presence of fluoride greatly enhances the rate of remineralization and also helps in formation of fluor-hydroxyapatite.

10. In the presence of dental plaque that has developed for 12 hours or less, the enamel demineralization resulting from a single exposure to sucrose will be remineralized by saliva within about

a. 10 minutes
b. 60 minutes
c. 2 hours
d. 4 hours

Ans a.

Refer to the explanation of Q. No. 9.

11. The organic acids that are usually involved in demineralization are

a. Acetic acid
b. Pyruvic acid
c. Lactic acid
d. Both (a) and (b)
e. All of the above

Ans e.

Demineralization is produced by weak organic acids such as lactic acid, acetic acid and pyruvic acid.

12. The second primary molar has deeper and less completely coalesced pits and fissures. This results in a higher susceptibility of second primary molar to dental caries, even though the first primary molar erupts earlier.

a. Both the statements are false
b. Both the statements are true
c. First statement is true and the second is false
d. First statement is false and the second is true

Ans b.

The answer is self-explanatory.

13. Additional period required for enamel calcification after eruption is usually

a. 5 years
b. 1 year
c. 2 years
d. 8 years

Ans c.

Enamel calcification is incomplete at the time of eruption of the teeth and an additional period of about 2 years is required for the calcification process to be completed by exposure to saliva.

14. Which of the following secondary factors contribute to the etiology of dental caries?

a. Anatomic characteristics of teeth
b. Arrangement of teeth in the arch
c. Presence of dental appliances
d. Hereditary factors
e. All of the above

Ans e.

Permanent molars often have incompletely coalesced pits and fissures that allow dental plaque material to be retained at the base of the defect in contact with exposed dentin. Crowded and irregular teeth are not readily cleansed during the masticatory process. Dental appliances increase the risk for decay by retaining more microorganisms. Tooth morphology and enamel defects tend to follow a familial pattern. Hence, heredity may play an indirect role by genetically producing caries-susceptible surfaces.

15. Rampant caries is defined as suddenly appearing, widespread, rapidly burrowing type of caries, resulting in early involvement of the pulp, affecting those teeth usually regarded as immune to tooth decay. This definition is given by

a. Massler
b. Fitzerald
c. Keyes
d. Tinanoff

Ans a.

Question defines rampant caries.

16. Rampant caries can be caused by

a. High sucrose intake
b. Emotional disturbances
c. Patient under stress who takes tranquilizers and sedatives
d. Any of the above

Ans d.

Repressed emotions and fears, dissatisfaction with achievement, rebellion against a home situation, a feeling of inferiority, a traumatic school experience and continuous general tension have been observed in children and adults who have rampant dental caries. An emotional disturbance may initiate an unusual craving for sweets which in turn influence the incidence of dental caries. Patients who take tranquilizers have decreased salivary flow resulting in lowered caries resistance.

17. The physical state of carbohydrates and the frequency of ingestion contribute to the initiation and extension of dental caries. Fermentable carbohydrates taken in an adherent form are more cariogenic than those consumed in soluble form.

a. Both the statements are false
b. Both the statements are true
c. First statement is true and the second is false
d. First statement is false and the second is true

Ans b.

The answer is self-explanatory.

18. Acid production within dental plaque reaches demineralizing concentrations after ingestion of carbohydrates within

a. 4 minutes
b. 15 minutes
c. 30 minutes
d. 25 minutes

Ans a.

The answer is self-explanatory.

19. Acidogenic theory was proposed by

a. Miller
b. Schatz
c. Gotttlieb
d. Martin

Ans a.

W.D. Miller, probably the best known of the early investigators of dental caries, published extensively on the results of studies on dental caries since 1882. He proposed the acidogenic theory (refer table under Q. No. 1).

20. Model for demineralization and remineralization of white spot lesion was given by

a. Miller
b. Moreno
c. Martin
d. Massler

Ans b.

The physiochemical process of white spot lesions was difficult to understand until the *Moreno model* was described. In this model, acids formed by cariogenic bacteria dissolve the surface as well as subsurface enamel. The calcium and phosphate ions from the subsurface dissolution diffuse outward toward the surface and reprecipitate on the surface making the enamel surface appear unaltered.

21. Microorganisms primarily associated with smooth surface caries is

a. Lactobacilli
b. Mutans streptococci (*Streptococcus sobrinus*)
c. Actinomyces
d. *Streptococcus pyogenes*

Ans b.

Loesche conducted an extensive review of the literature regarding etiology of caries. He concluded that the evidence suggests that *Streptococcus mutans*, possibly *Streptococcus sobrinus*, and lactobacilli are human odontopathogens. He also observed that other aciduric species such as *Streptococcus sobrinus* may be more important in smooth-surface decay.

22. The microorganisms which are primarily involved in progression of caries in dentin are

a. Acidogenic microorganisms
b. Proteolytic microorganisms
c. Mucolytic microorganisms
d. Actinomyces

Ans b.

The high protein content of the dentin would favor the growth of those microorganisms which have the ability to utilize this protein for metabolism.

Thus proteolytic organisms would appear to predominate in deeper caries of the dentin, while acidogenic forms are prominent in early caries.

23. Lower anterior primary teeth are usually unaffected by caries in early childhood caries because of

a. Close proximity to submandibular ducts
b. Protection by tongue
c. Spacing present between the incisors
d. All of the above

Ans d.

Mandibular primary incisors seldom decay, probably because of the spacing that occurs in the area, protection of the tongue (while bottle-feeding) and their close proximity to the ducts of the submandibular salivary gland, which means that they benefit from the diluting and buffering properties of saliva.

24. According to Stephan, pH returns to normal following an exposure to fermentable carbohydrates in approximately

a. 15 minutes
b. 30–60 minutes
c. 60–120 minutes
d. 3 hours

Ans b.

Acidogenic bacteria in dental plaque can rapidly metabolize certain carbohydrates to acids. In the mouth, the resultant change in plaque pH over time is known as *Stephan curve.* Following exposure to fermentable refined carbohydrates, the pH reduces rapidly to reach a minimum in 5–20 minutes. However, this returns to its starting value within 30–60 minutes.

25. The pattern of caries progression appears to have a cone-shaped lesion with the base towards enamel surface and the apex towards dentinoenamel junction in

a. Dentinal caries
b. Enamel caries on smooth surface
c. Enamel caries on pits and fissures
d. White spot lesion

Ans b.

As the carious lesion progresses from smooth surface of enamel, towards the pulp, it tends to assume the shape of a triangle with the apex toward the pulp and the base toward the enamel.

26. An exchange of minerals between saliva and enamel is

a. Unimportant in tooth maintenance
b. Responsible for remineralization
c. Disrupted by fluoride
d. None of the above. This exchange does not occur

Ans b.

The presence of fluoride in the oral environment, even in very low concentration, can affect the equilibrium of demineralization in the opposite manner, leading to remineralization. This fluoride may come from the saliva, the plaque fluid or from the demineralized enamel itself. During remineralization, fluoride facilitates the diffusion of calcium and phosphorus back into the lesion (partially dissolved hydroxyapatite). This latter structure is now resistant to acid dissolution than were the original crystals. True "repair" of the original early lesion takes place.

27. Defensive reactions of the tooth to dental caries include

a. Remineralization of enamel
b. Formation of reparative and sclerotic dentin
c. Formation of reparative dentin and salivary ions
d. Formation of sclerotic dentin and salivary enzymes

Ans b.

The pulp–dentin complex responds to injury by formation of new hard tissue, mainly tertiary dentin, increasing the distance between the injury and the pulp and sometimes by decreasing the dentin permeability (sclerotic dentin). *Sclerotic dentin* is formed by the apposition of minerals into and between the tubules (intra and intertubular dentin).

28. When treating rampant dental caries, the first step is to

a. Restore all teeth with stainless steel crowns
b. Excavate softened tooth structure and temporize with zinc oxide-eugenol
c. Perform a diet analysis and apply topical fluoride solution to all teeth
d. Perform a prophylaxis, instruct in oral hygiene and watch for improved habits

Ans b.

When rampant caries occurs, the first step is to initiate treatment of all carious lesions, to stop or at least slow the progression of the disease and to identify the most important causes of the existing condition. If the restorative care is to be performed over several visits in the outpatient setting, gross caries excavation as an initial approach in the control of rampant dental caries has several advantages. The removal of the superficial caries and the filling of the cavity with a glass ionomer material or zinc oxide-eugenol cement (IRM) will at least temporarily arrest the caries process and prevent its rapid progression to the dental pulp.

29. Caries activity is directly proportional to each of the following except

a. Oral retention of fermentable carbohydrates
b. Frequency of eating fermentable carbohydrates
c. Total daily intake of fermentable carbohydrates
d. Physical form of food items containing fermentable carbohydrates

Ans c.

It was concluded from the studies that dental caries activity could be increased by the consumption of sugar if the sugar were in a form easily retained on the tooth. The more frequently this form of sugar was consumed between meals, the greater was the tendency for an increase in dental caries. Sweetened liquids provided to young children in nursing bottles can have enormous cariogenic potential. Frequent ingestion of carbonated soft drinks and other sweetened drinks are another form of snacking that can promote and accelerate caries progression. The least important determinant is the quantity of food intake.

Chapter 18

Early Childhood Caries

1. AAPD defines early childhood caries as the presence of one or more decayed, missing or filled tooth surfaces in any primary tooth in a child

a. 24 months of age or younger
b. 71 months of age or younger
c. 48 months of age or younger
d. 96 months of age or younger

Ans b.

AAPD defines *early childhood caries* as the presence of one or more decayed (noncavitated or cavitated), missing (due to caries), or filled tooth surfaces in any primary tooth in a child 71 months of age or younger. In children younger than 3 years of age, any sign of smooth surface caries is indicative of severe early childhood caries (S-ECC). From ages 3 through 5 years, one or more cavitated, missing (due to caries) or filled smooth surfaces in primary maxillary anterior teeth or a decayed, missing or filled score of (dmft) greater than 4 (age 3) greater than 5 (age 4) or greater than 6 (age 5) surfaces constitutes S-ECC.

2. The first window of infectivity for early childhood caries is between

a. 7 and 24 months
b. 24 and 48 months
c. 48 and 72 months
d. 72 and 96 months

Ans a.

Mutans Streptococci colonize the oral cavity of infants after the emergence of their first set of teeth. Typically, this happens during a period called window of infectivity, which is from 7 to 24 months, i.e. the period during the emergence of primary teeth.

3. Which of the following is a risk factor that predisposes an infant to early childhood caries?

a. Lack of oral hygiene measures
b. Sugars in drinks, milk and infant formulas during bedtime or naptime
c. Nursing bottles, pacifiers and prolonged "at will" feeding pattern
d. All of the above

Ans d.

All of the above factors can be a risk factor for development of early childhood caries in children.

4. The concept of window of infectivity was introduced by

a. Caufield
b. Harris
c. Garcia-Godoy
d. Tinnanoff

Ans a.

Caufield in 1993 monitored oral cavity levels of mutans streptococci in the oral cavity from birth up to 5 years. He noted the initial acquisition of Mutans streptococci and designated the time period as window of infectivity.

5. The stages of early childhood caries were described by

a. Harris and Garcia-Godoy
b. Tinnanoff and Sullivan
c. Caufield and Dasanayake
d. Caufield and Griffen

Ans a.

The stages of early childhood caries were described by Harris and Garcia-Godoy in 1999. The stages are very mild, mild, moderate and severe.

6. Which of the following primary teeth are most severely involved with nursing caries?

a. Canines
b. Second molars
c. Maxillary incisors
d. Mandibular incisors

Ans c.

Early childhood caries can develop as soon as the teeth erupt. Cavities may be visible as early as 10 months of age. It is typically present in children as white lines or spots on the maxillary incisors which are among the first teeth to erupt and least protected by saliva. Hence, maxillary incisors are the most severely affected set of teeth.

7. An 18-month-old child has dental caries on maxillary incisors and the first molars and canines. This child most probably has which of the following conditions?

a. Cretinism
b. Severe early childhood caries
c. Early childhood caries
d. Hereditary enamel hypocalcification

Ans b.

Any sign of smooth surface caries in children younger than 3 years is severe early childhood caries.

8. Recommended age for discontinuing bottle-feeding is

a. 12 months
b. 8 months
c. 20 months
d. 18 months

Ans a.

Prolongation of bottle-feeding beyond 12 months of age can result in early childhood caries.

9. Early childhood caries can occur because of

a. Prolonged bottle-feeding
b. At will breast feeding
c. Frequent use of sweetened syrupy medicines
d. Any of the above

Ans d.

All of the above-mentioned factors create a susceptible environment in the mouth by the presence of sucrose around the tooth, which results in early childhood caries.

10. Nursing caries affects primarily the lingual surfaces of primary maxillary incisors and occlusal surfaces of first primary molars. The mandibular incisors are characteristically unaffected.

a. Both the statements are true
b. Both the statements are false
c. First statement is true and the second is false
d. First statement is false and the second is true

Ans a.

The answer is self-explanatory.

Chapter 19

Role of Diet and Nutrition

1. Which of the following deficiency causes neural tube defects like anencephaly and spina bifida?

a. Iron
b. Folic acid
c. Zinc
d. Calcium

Ans b.

Folic acid deficiency causes neural tube defects like anencephaly and spina bifida.

2. The amount of folic acid required for prevention of neural tube defects is approximately

a. 100–200 µg/day
b. 200–250 µg/day
c. 200–400 µg/day
d. more than 600 µg/day

Ans c.

The amount of folic acid required to prevent neural tube defects is 200–400 µg/day.

3. Zinc deficiency can cause

a. Dwarfism
b. Hypogonadism
c. Delayed sexual maturation
d. Any of the above

Ans d.

Zinc plays an important role in growth and development. This trace element is also required for proper wound healing. Severe deficiencies result in dwarfism, hypogonadism and delayed sexual maturation.

4. **The daily dietary recommendation of calcium in children is**
   a. 600–800 mg
   b. 800–1200 mg
   c. 1200–1600 mg
   d. 1600–2000 mg

Ans b.

The daily dietary recommendation of calcium in children is 800–1200 mg.

5. **Anorexia nervosa is characterized by self-imposed weight loss, amenorrhea and distorted attitude toward eating and body weight. Binge eating and invariably self-induced vomiting characterize bulimia nervosa.**
   a. Both the statements are false
   b. Both the statements are true
   c. First statement is true and the second is false
   d. First statement is false and the second is true

Ans b.

During adolescence or before, some individuals (primarily girls) become preoccupied with their appearance and body weight and as a result, restrict their food intake. Anorexia nervosa results when this behavior is carried to the point of starvation. Bulimia nervosa is characterized by self-induced vomiting and it is more common than anorexia nervosa.

6. **Enamel erosion is common among bulimia nervosa patients. Fluoxetine hydrochloride appears to help control the obsessive–compulsive behavior involved in both anorexia nervosa and bulimia nervosa.**
   a. Both the statements are false
   b. Both the statements are true
   c. First statement is true and the second is false
   d. First statement is false and the second is true

Ans b.

Enamel erosion is common in patients with bulimia nervosa because of the exposure of the tooth surfaces to the highly acidic regurgitated gastric contents. Antidepressants may be helpful in some cases.

7. **The immature kidneys of a baby cannot concentrate waste efficiently. As a result, the infant must excrete relatively more water than an adult to eliminate a comparable amount of waste.**

a. Both the statements are false
b. Both the statements are true
c. First statement is true and the second is false
d. First statement is false and the second is true

Ans b.

The answer is self-explanatory. However, when dealing with infants, one must be careful about dehydration which has potentially serious consequences.

8. The most rapid growth occurs in humans during

a. Prenatal period
b. 6–12 months of age
c. Between 3 and 5 years of life
d. Beginning of teenage years

Ans a.

Prenatal period shows the most rapid growth in humans. The next rapid growth occurs during the first six months of life (also refer Q. No. 19 Chapter 5).

9. All the following statements are true except

a. Atherosclerosis begins early in life
b. Atherosclerosis of coronary arteries can produce myocardial infarction and coronary heart disease
c. Atherosclerosis is positively associated with elevated HDL (high density lipoprotein) levels
d. Hypercholesterolemia, hypertension and cigarette smoking are the three major risk factors for coronary heart disease

Ans c.

Atherosclerosis is negatively associated with elevated HDL concentrations and positively associated with elevated total serum cholesterol and elevated LDL (low density lipoprotein) levels. A prudent health goal will be to reduce the elevated levels of total and LDL cholesterol and increase the HDL levels.

10. Diagnostic criteria for anorexia nervosa include all the following except

a. Self-induced weight loss leading to maintenance of body weight less than 85% of that expected
b. Intense fear of weight gain
c. Recurrent episodes of binge eating
d. Endocrine changes manifesting as amenorrhea in females

Ans c.

Recurrent episodes of binge eating followed by self-induced vomiting or use of laxatives are diagnostic of bulimia nervosa.

11. One of the researchers pioneering in research related to vitamins and its role in enamel hypoplasia is

a. Mellanby
b. Sreebny
c. Nikiforuk
d. Pindborg

Ans a.

May Mellanby who did much work on the influence of vitamins on development of teeth was one of the pioneers in this field. She has observed that deficiency of vitamin D can lead to enamel hypoplasia.

12. One of the following nutrients when deficient is said to have deleterious effects on periodontium is

a. Vitamin E
b. Vitamin C
c. Vitamin A
d. Vitamin D

Ans b.

Vitamin C deficiency leads to scurvy. It results in early loss of teeth due to severe periodontal disease.

13. One of the following is a trace element

a. Fluorine
b. Vitamin C
c. Iron
d. Calcium

Ans a.

Elements known to have a role in metabolic processes of higher animals and whose daily requirement by humans is less than 100 mg are known as trace elements. Fluorine is a trace element.

14. Tooth mousse has a derivative of one of the following

a. Cod liver oil
b. Lactose
c. Casein
d. Maltose

Ans c.

Casein is a phosphoprotein present in milk and has been considered to be one of the ingredients responsible for caries protective effect. Tooth mousse has CPP-ACP (casein phosphopeptide and amorphous calcium phosphate) which is said to remineralize white spot lesions.

15. As per the recommendation of National Academy of Sciences, calories needed for a teenage boy is

a. 1000 calories/day

b. 1500 calories/day

c. 2800 calories/day

d. 3500 calories/day

Ans c.

According to the National Academy of Sciences, 2800 calories is right for teenage boys, many active men and some very active women.

Chapter 20

Recent Advances in Diagnosis of Dental Caries

1. Which device does not use the principle of fluorescence in diagnosis of caries?

a. DIAGNOdent
b. QLF
c. FOTI
d. Soprolife

Ans c.

FOTI : It uses fiberoptic transillumination. All the other three techniques use fluorescence.

2. What is the frequency of ultrasound?

a. >20 Hz
b. >200 Hz
c. >2000 Hz
d. >20,000 Hz

Ans d.

Ultrasound waves have a frequency of more than 20,000 Hz.

3. ICDAS criteria are for

a. Visual examination
b. Tactile examination
c. Radiographic examination
d. All of the above

Ans a.

International Caries Detection and Assessment System (ICDAS) uses visual examination.

4. For caries diagnosis, traditionally dentists have relied upon

a. Visual examination

b. Tactile examination
c. Radiographic examination
d. All the above

Ans d.

All the above-mentioned techniques have been traditionally used by the dentists.

5. The device that uses the principle of electric conductance for diagnosis of caries is

a. DIAGNOdent
b. QLF
c. CarieScan Pro
d. None of the above

Ans d.

Devices using electric conductance property are modified AC ohmmeter, Vanguard electronic caries detector, Caries meter, Modified electrochemical impedance spectroscopy, electrical impedance tomography.

Section VI

Restorative Dentistry and Endodontics

Chapter 21

Pit and Fissure Sealants and Preventive Resin Restorations

1. **The concentration of phosphoric acid used for acid etching usually is**
   a. 30–50% acid solution or gels
   b. 10–20% acid solution
   c. 70–80% acid solution or gels
   d. Less than 10%

Ans a.
The answer is self-explanatory.

2. **Generally, a 20 second etching time is recommended. Enamel that has been exposed to fluoride may be resistant to etching and may need to be exposed for longer periods.**
   a. Both the statements are false
   b. Both the statements are true
   c. First statement is true and the second is false
   d. First statement is false and the second is true

Ans b.
The answer is self-explanatory.

3. **Which of the following are advantages of light cured materials over chemical cure sealants?**
   a. Less chance of incorporation of air bubbles
   b. Working time is longer
   c. Better physical and mechanical properties
   d. All of the above

Ans d.
All of the above-mentioned factors are true regarding light cure materials.

4. **The sealed composite resin restoration (preventive resin restoration, PRR) is an alternative procedure for restoring young permanent**

teeth requiring only minimal tooth preparation for caries removal but also having adjacent susceptible fissures. This conservative cavity preparation with sealing for prevention is a successful approach for treating selected decayed teeth.

a. Both the statements are false
b. Both the statements are true
c. First statement is true and the second is false
d. First statement is false and the second is true

Ans b.
The answer is self-explanatory.

5. Acid etching was introduced by

a. Bowen (1965)
b. Buonocore (1955)
c. Wilson and Kent (1972)
d. Brown (1945)

Ans b.
Bowen introduced the Bis-GMA resin system. Buonocore introduced acid etching. Wilson and Kent introduced glass ionomer cement.

6. Bis-GMA resin was developed by

a. Bowen (1965)
b. Buonocore (1955)
c. Wilson and Kent (1972)
d. Brown (1945)

Ans a.
Refer to the explanation of Q. No. 5.

Bis-GMA resin is the chemical reaction product of bisphenol A and glycidyl methacrylate. It is the base resin to most of the current commercial sealants.

7. Match the following:

	Resin		Activator
A	Chemically curing resins	1	Benzoin methyl ether
B	UV curing resins	2	Diketones
C	Visible light curing resins	3	Tertiary amines

a. A-3, B-1, C-2
b. A-2, B-3, C-1
c. A-1, B-2, C-3

Ans a.

The answer is self-explanatory.

8. The condition that leads to the occurrence of dental caries is

a. A tooth with deep pit and fissure
b. Cariogenic bacteria
c. Suitable substrate for the bacteria to form acids
d. All of the above

Ans d.

A susceptible tooth, cariogenic bacteria and suitable substrate for the bacteria to form acids are all necessary for dental caries to occur.

9. The technique of prophylactic odontotomy was introduced by

a. Kline and Knutson
b. Bodecker
c. Hyatt
d. Buonocore

Ans c.

Prophylactic odontotomy, introduced by Hyatt in 1923, an invasive operative procedure, remains the treatment of choice for many clinicians well into the 1970s. This included filling the pits and fissures with silver or copper oxyphosphate cements as soon as the teeth erupts into oral cavity and small occlusal cavities are prepared when the teeth fully erupt into oral cavity and filled with silver amalgam.

10. Following types of fissures are not caries susceptible

a. I and K
b. K and V
c. U and I
d. U and V

Ans d.

U and V type fissures are usually shallow and wide, tend to be self-cleansable and are caries resistant.

11. Which type of PRR will require a local anesthesia and a liner?

a. Type A
b. Type B
c. Type C
d. All of the above

Ans c.

Type C PRR is characterized by the need for greater exploratory preparation in dentin. This would require local anesthesia and placement of a liner-like calcium hydroxide or GIC over the exposed dentin.

12. Diluted resin is used in

a. Type A PRR
b. Type B PRR
c. Type C PRR
d. All of the above

Ans b.

Diluted composite resin (combination of unfilled and filled bonding agent and filler resins) is used for Type B PRR.

13. The disadvantages of clear resin when used as a sealant is

a. Esthetically unpleasant
b. Low strength
c. Poor retention
d. Difficult to detect on recall examinations

Ans d.

Patients are asked to report for regular recalls after sealant placement. If the sealant is lost completely or partially, it should be replaced. Clear and tooth colored sealants are esthetic but are difficult to detect on recall examinations.

14. The success of a sealant retention depends mainly on

a. Proper isolation
b. Proper washing of occlusal surface
c. Etching
d. Washing after etching

Ans a.

Typically, resin adhesion to etched enamel requires a clean, dry enamel surface. Resins used as sealants are typically not moisture tolerant.

15. Caries on the occlusal and buccal or palatal surfaces of teeth account for what % of the caries experienced by children and adolescents?

a. 20%
b. 40%
c. 60%
d. 90%

Ans d.

In general, caries on occlusal and buccal/palatal surfaces account for almost 90% of caries experienced in children and adolescents. The reason for this high rate of caries relates specifically to the pit and fissure morphology of occlusal and buccal/palatal surfaces that are not affected by the caries preventive effects of systemic and topical fluorides.

16. Sealant retention to buccal and palatal pits and fissures of molars compared to occlusal pits and fissures

a. Is considerably lower
b. Is the same
c. Is considerably higher
d. Has never been evaluated

Ans a.

Sealant retention to buccal and palatal pits and fissures of molars is lower than the occlusal surfaces.

17. Difficult-to-seal teeth include all the following except

a. The fully erupted premolar
b. The partially erupted permanent first molar
c. The partially erupted permanent second molar
d. The partially erupted premolar

Ans a.

Isolation of field and access to the pits and fissures contribute to sealant success. Teeth should therefore be fully erupted into the oral cavity before attempting the placement of a resin sealant.

18. A caries diagnosis for pits and fissures using a sharp explorer has been discarded in recent years in favor of

a. Radiographic evidence
b. Visual changes in the appearance of enamel
c. New diagnostic devices
d. All of the above

Ans d.

The concept of using a sharp explorer for the detection of pit and fissure caries has been discarded in favor of the visual appearance of enamel, radiographic diagnosis and new types of diagnostic devices.

19. Three different variations in the appearance of pits and fissures in cross-section include all of the following except

a. V type
b. U type
c. S type
d. I type

Ans c.

Nango described three variations in pits and fissures according to their appearance in cross-section, namely V type, U type and I type pits and fissures.

20. Based on a review of published sealant data, one can expect what percent of sealant loss per year?

a. 5–10%
b. 20–25%
c. 40–45%
d. 60–65%

Ans a.

A basic concept of 5–10% of sealant loss per year has been seen when one reviews published sealant data. This data reveals the importance of re-evaluating teeth with sealants on a periodic basis and to reapply if necessary.

21. Clinical success with sealants is based upon

a. Technique
b. Fissure morphology
c. Characteristics of the sealant
d. All of the above

Ans d.

The answer is self-explanatory.

22. DIAGNOdent is a diagnostic device for assessing the presence or absence of pit and fissure caries. DIAGNOdent is a

a. Fiberoptic transilluminator
b. Portable digital X-ray device
c. Laser fluorescence device
d. Electronic explorer

Ans c.

The DIAGNOdent laser fluorescence unit takes advantage of the fact that the light reflecting and fluorescing properties of normal, healthy enamel differs from the characteristics of enamel surfaces in pits and fissures affected by dental caries.

23. All the following are types of sealants except

a. Colored sealants

b. Self-cure sealants
c. Light-cure sealants
d. Heat-cured sealants

Ans d.

There are no heat-cured sealants. Broadly, sealants can be categorized as either resin based or glass ionomer based.

24. When placing a sealant, the adhesion to the enamel surface can be enhanced by cleaning the occlusal surface with

a. A nonfluoride, pumice prophylaxis paste
b. An air abrasion device
c. Alcohol on a cotton roll
d. Both (a) and (b)

Ans a.

Following isolation of the tooth, the tooth surface must be cleaned. For this, a water–pumice paste with a prophylaxis cup in a slow speed handpiece is used. The adhesion of sealant to enamel surfaces can be enhanced by cleaning the occlusal surfaces with a nonfluoride, pumice prophylaxis paste or by using an air abrasion device.

25. In cases where the dentition is fully erupted and sealants are indicated, it may be necessary to perform a fissurotomy in the pits and fissures to create room for a thickness of sealant to be successful.

a. True
b. False

Ans a.

The answer is self-explanatory.

26. The sealant should be placed to cover all pits and fissures and extend onto the cusp ridges. The sealant should be applied to a minimum thickness of

a. 0.1 mm
b. 0.3 mm
c. 1.0 mm
d. 2.0 mm

Ans b.

Sealant is applied to the occlusal surface using the canula tip supplied by the manufacturer. After dispensing, the sealant was placed to extend onto the cusp ridges using a brush type applicator. The final sealant thickness upon application should be at least 0.3 mm.

27. Some sealant manufacturers recommend the use of an additional step with a separate intermediate adhesive resin. A disadvantage of doing this when compared to any potential benefit is

a. It is more costly because it requires an additional bottle of bonding agent
b. It is more costly because it requires more time for application of the sealant
c. It increases the number of steps which can lead to the potential for contamination during the procedure
d. All of the above

Ans d.

The answer is self-explanatory.

28. Sealants constitute a highly effective preventive measure for reducing pit and fissure caries.

a. True
b. False

Ans a.

The answer is self-explanatory.

Chapter 22

Atraumatic Restorative Treatment

1. **Atraumatic restorative treatment (ART) is a procedure based on removing carious tooth tissues using hand instruments alone and restoring the cavity with an adhesive restorative material. At present the restorative material is glass ionomer cements.**
   a. Both the statements are true
   b. Both the statements are false
   c. The first statement is true and the second is false
   d. The first statement is false and the second is true

Ans a.
The statements describe the ART technique.

2. **The type of GIC used for ART is**
   a. Type I GIC
   b. Type II GIC
   c. Type III GIC
   d. Type IX GIC

Ans d.
Type IX GIC is the material of choice for ART restorations. It is a high strength restorative with high fluoride release.

3. **The initial trials of ART was carried out in all of the following countries except**
   a. Thailand
   b. Zimbabwe
   c. Tanzania
   d. India

Ans d.
This technique was pioneered in the mid-1980s in Tanzania. Then in 1991, field trial was carried out and later in Zimbabwe in 1993.

Chapter 23

Pediatric Operative Dentistry

1. Use of rubber dam offers the following advantages

a. Saves time
b. Provides protection
c. Controls saliva
d. All of the above

Ans d.

The time required for application of rubber dam ranges from 15 seconds to 6 minutes. This time required for the placement will be invariably made up and additional time is also saved through the elimination of rinsing and spitting by the pediatric patient. It prevents foreign objects from coming into contact with oral structures. It also prevents swallowing or aspiration of foreign objects and materials. Rubber dam effectively controls the saliva, helping the operator to identify small pulp exposures easily and place restorative materials on the tooth without contamination.

2. The latex sheets used for rubber dam is usually of ________ size.

a. 5 × 5 inch
b. 2 × 2 inch
c. 1 × 1 inch
d. 6 × 6 inch

Ans d.

The armamentarium of rubber dam consists usually 6 × 6 inch latex sheets. Smaller sheets are available for pediatric patients (5 × 5 inches).

3. The framework used for rubber dam application is otherwise called

a. Clark's frame
b. Young's frame
c. Barnum's frame
d. Nicholos frame

Ans b.

The answer is self-explanatory.

4. The smallest punch hole created by rubber dam punch is used to isolate

a. Mandibular premolars
b. Primary incisors
c. Mandibular permanent incisors
d. Both (b) and (c)

Ans d.

The large punch hole is used for the clamp-bearing tooth and for the most permanent molars. The medium-sized punch holes are generally used for the premolars and primary molars. The second smallest hole is used for maxillary permanent incisors, whereas the smallest hole is adequate for the primary incisors and the lower permanent incisors.

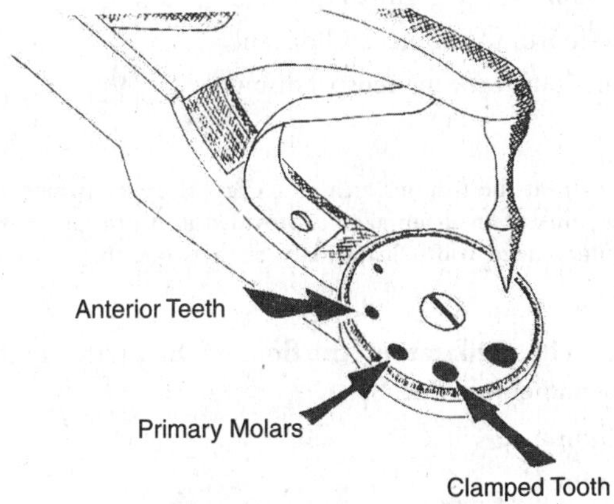

Fig. 23.1 Rubber dam punch.

5. Rounded angles throughout the cavity preparation (Class II) will result in

a. Less concentration of stresses
b. Complete condensation of amalgam (more bulk)
c. Both (a) and (b)
d. Prevention of thermal stimulus injuring the pulp

Ans c.

Rounded angle throughout the cavity preparation will result in less concentration of stresses and will permit better adaptation of the materials into the extremities of the preparation.

6. **All of the following are true regarding Class II cavity preparation in primary molars except**
   a. Buccal and lingual extension carried to self-cleansing areas
   b. Flat pulpal floor
   c. Greater buccal and lingual extension at the cervical area
   d. Lesser buccal and lingual extension at the cervical area

Ans d.

In traditional Class II cavity preparation, the buccal and lingual extensions should be carried to self-cleansing areas. The cavity design should have greater buccal and lingual extension in the cervical area of primary teeth because of the broad, flat contact areas and the distinct buccal bulge in the gingival third.

7. **Ideally, the width of the isthmus should be**
   a. Half the intercuspal distance
   b. One-third the intercuspal distance
   c. One-fourth the intercuspal distance
   d. Three-fourth the intercuspal distance

Ans b.

The strength at the isthmus area of a Class II cavity is three times greater when the bulk of amalgam alloy is provided in depth rather than in width. The recommended width in primary teeth is one-third of the intercuspal distance.

8. **During cavity preparation, the floor of the cavity is extended into dentinoenamel junction by**
   a. 0.05 mm
   b. 0.5 mm
   c. 5 mm
   d. 0.2 mm

Ans b.

Limiting the cavity to 0.5 mm pulpal to dentinoenamel junction reduces the chance of inadvertent pulp exposure.

9. **All of the following are true regarding Class I cavity preparation except that the**
   a. Preparation includes all susceptible grooves and fissures
   b. Depth of the cavity is carried to 0.5 mm below DE junction
   c. Undermining marginal ridges strengthen the tooth
   d. All unsupported enamel rods are removed

Ans c.

If the marginal ridges are undermined, the enamel is more susceptible to fracture.

10. A Class II cavity preparation comprises of

a. Occlusal preparation
b. Proximal box
c. Isthmus
d. All of the above

Ans d.

The answer is self-explanatory.

11. The buccal and lingual walls of the proximal box in a Class II preparation should

a. Diverge towards the cervical region
b. Converge towards the cervical region
c. Diverge towards the occlusal region
d. None of the above

Ans a.

Refer to the explanation of Q. No. 6.

12. The most common cause for failure of an amalgam restoration is

a. Proximal ditch
b. Delayed expansion
c. Failure at occlusal preparation
d. Due to poor handling of amalgam alloy

Ans a.

Breakdown of the material in the proximal wall region results in a defect known as *proximal ditch*. This leads to marginal leakage and secondary caries resulting in failure of the restoration..

13. An MOD amalgam has a better survival rate in

a. Mandibular second primary molar than first primary molar
b. Mandibular first primary molar than second primary molar
c. All primary molars
d. None of the above

Ans a.

An MOD has a better survival rate in mandibular second primary molars. However, multisurface decay is better managed by the placement of a stainless steel crown.

14. One of the following is incorrectly defined

a. Class I—preparation involving pits and fissures in posterior teeth
b. Class II—preparation involving occlusal and proximal surfaces
c. Class III—preparation in proximal surfaces of anteriors involving the incisal edge
d. Class V—preparation in the cervical region of teeth

Ans c.

Class III is preparation which involves the proximal surfaces of the anterior teeth without involving the incisal edge. Preparation involving the incisal edge is classified as Class IV cavity preparation.

15. The modified Class III preparation uses a dovetail on the lingual side in

a. Maxillary canine
b. Mandibular canine
c. Mandibular premolar
d. Maxillary premolar

Ans a.

The modified Class III preparation uses a dovetail on the lingual or occasionally on the labial surfaces of the tooth. A lingual lock is normally considered for the maxillary canine, whereas the labial lock may be more conveniently cut on the mandibular teeth where the esthetic requirement is not so important.

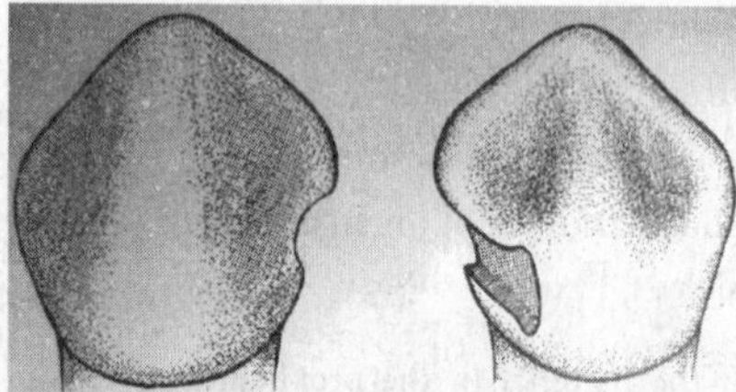

Fig. 23.2 Class III in mandibular canine—Labial dovetail (lingual and labial views).

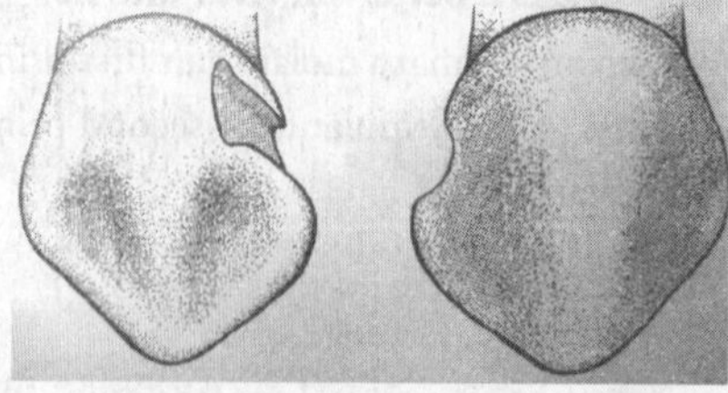

Fig. 23.3 Class III in maxillary canine—Lingual dovetail (lingual and labial views).

16. In a Class II preparation in permanent first molar, retention of the proximal box

a. Depends on retention of the occlusal preparation
b. Is independent of the occlusal preparation
c. Is not necessary
d. Is because of the occlusal divergence of the box

Ans b.

Retention of the restoration results from the mechanical undercut obtained by the extension into the fissures of the occlusal part and the converging walls of the proximal box. It is important that retention of the interproximal box and the occlusal part are independent of each other, as they may be subjected to different displacement forces.

17. Outline of the cavity for amalgam restoration is determined by

a. Size of the carious lesion
b. The need for extension for prevention
c. Occlusal anatomy of the tooth
d. All of the above

Ans d.

All the above-mentioned factors have to be considered while determining the outline form for cavity preparation.

18. The most commonly used base in deep cavities after removal of deep caries is

a. Calcium hydroxide powder
b. Hard setting calcium hydroxide
c. Zinc oxide eugenol
d. Polycarboxylate cement

Ans b.

With deep carious lesions and near pulp exposures, the depth of the cavity should be covered with a biocompatible base material to provide adequate thermal protection to the pulp. A hard setting calcium hydroxide is generally used for this purpose.

19. The primary purpose of applying cavity varnish is to prevent

a. Thermal damage to the pulp
b. Marginal leakage
c. Discoloration of tooth
d. Pulp exposure

Ans b.

Cavity varnishes are used to prevent marginal leakage and bases are used to provide thermal protection to the pulp.

20. Preservation of primary dentition will always prevent a malocclusion. Early loss of primary molars causes more severe effects than early loss of primary incisors.

a. First statement is false and the second is true
b. First statement is true and the second is false
c. Both the statements are true
d. Both the statements are false

Ans a.

Preservation of primary dentition prevents malocclusion but not always. Early loss of primary incisors does not usually cause space loss.

21. Enamel rods in the gingival one-third of primary teeth incline

a. Horizontally
b. Occlusally
c. Apically
d. Gingivally

Ans b.

Enamel rods incline occlusally in primary teeth in the cervical region; hence, bevelling of gingival seat is not required in Class II cavity preparations. However, in permanent teeth they incline gingivally. When a gingival seat is prepared in this region, it results in unsupported enamel, which requires bevelling.

22. All of the following are true regarding contact areas in primary teeth except

a. Broad contact area
b. Flatter contact area
c. Situated more occlusally
d. Need to be broken in Class II cavity preparation

Ans c.

The contact areas between the primary molars are broader, flatter and situated farther gingivally than those between the permanent molars.

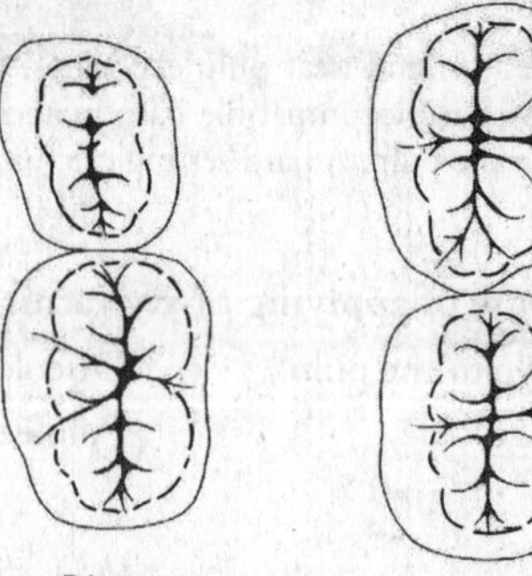

Fig. 23.4 Picture depicting broad contact areas in primary teeth.

23. The pulp horns of primary teeth are less prominent and relatively far from the surface. The distobuccal pulp horn of mandibular first primary molar is exposed often during restorative procedures.

a. Both the statements are true
b. Both the statements are false
c. First statement is true and the second is false
d. First statement is false and the second is true

Ans b.

The reverse is true. The pulp horns of primary teeth are more prominent than those of permanent teeth and are relatively closer to the surface when the thinner primary enamel is considered. The mesiobuccal pulp horn of mandibular first primary molar is exposed often during restorative procedures.

24. All of the following are true regarding primary teeth except

a. Crowns of primary molars are wider mesiodistally
b. Primary molars have a very narrow occlusal table
c. Less marked cervical prominence
d. Enamel is thinner in primary teeth than the permanent teeth

Ans c.

The primary teeth show a marked cervical prominence.

25. There is a marked increase in the incidence of interproximal caries during the age of

a. 2–3 years
b. 3–5 years
c. 7–9 years
d. 6–8 years

Ans b.

Occlusal lesions are more common than interproximal lesions in preschool children. In these young children, posterior contact may not close until 3 years of age, which may explain this observation. Once the proximal contacts are established, the incidence of interproximal caries may increase.

26. Whenever possible, facial and lingual walls of the proximal box of a Class II cavity in the primary molar should be

a. Flared as much as possible
b. Rounded as much as possible
c. Kept as parallel as possible
d. Parallel to the respective external surfaces of tooth

Ans d.

The facial and lingual walls of the proximal box of a Class II cavity in the primary molar should be parallel to the respective external surfaces of the tooth (refer explanation of Q. No. 6).

27. In which of the primary molars does the anatomy of the pulp contraindicate an MOD preparation for the placement of an amalgam restoration?

a. Maxillary first molar
b. Maxillary second molar
c. Mandibular first molar
d. Mandibular second molar

Ans c.

Mandibular first primary molar has a prominent cervical bulge, which makes it a poor candidate for MOD preparation (refer explanation of Q. No. 13).

28. Rubber dam was introduced by

a. S.C. Barnum
b. Sturdevant
c. Broadbent
d. Marzouk

Ans a.

The answer is self-explanatory.

29. The length of the floss taken to tie to the rubber dam clamp is approximately

a. 15 cm
b. 45 cm
c. 1 m
d. 10 cm

Ans b.

A 45 cm length of dental floss is taken and tied to the bow of the clamp as a safety measure. The floss will enable us to retrieve the clamp if it is dislodged.

30. Routine use of slow speed (micromotor) is recommended for cavity preparation in the age group of

a. 2.5 to 3.5 years
b. 4 to 6 years
c. 5 to 7 years
d. 3 to 5 years

Ans a.

The noise of an airotor and the water spray can be extremely disturbing to a young child (less than 3 years of age). The author routinely uses slow speed contra-angle handpiece on young children (2.5 to 3.5 years of age) who sit on the dental chair with or without their parents. The slow speed handpiece can first be tried on their nails so that they can feel the vibration associated with it. Use of slow speed is highly recommended for providing restorative care for anterior teeth in young children as use of high speed airotor may spray water into their nostrils. This makes them restless and the dentist may have to discontinue the procedure.

31. Class IV cavities are best restored with

a. Amalgam
b. Composite resin restoration
c. Composite resins with strip crowns
d. Glass ionomer cement

Ans c.

The most common sites for caries in the maxillary central incisors are the mesial and buccal surfaces in frequency. Sometimes the caries was so extensive that Class IV restorations are required. The long term survival of these restorations was poor and dentists are reluctant to undertake them. Furthermore, small restorations in small teeth are difficult. The advent of strip crowns for primary incisors has now meant that these teeth can be easily restored with good prognosis. Hence, when caries involves the incisal edge/angle, use of strip crowns, anterior stainless steel crowns and open faced stainless steel crowns are recommended.

32. The pulpal floor is kept flat in amalgam cavity preparation because

a. It distributes the occlusal stress evenly
b. Filling can be condensed easily
c. Pulpal outline is flat towards the occlusal surface
d. Lining can be given easily

Ans a.

Uneven distribution of forces into the pulp can cause pulpal damage. Hence the pulpal floor is kept flat for uniform distribution of stresses (refer explanation of Q. No. 8).

33. A diagnosis of small occlusal cavities is most readily made by the use of

a. Bite-wing radiographs
b. Periapical radiographs
c. Panoramic radiographs

d. Transillumination
e. An explorer and compressed air

Ans e.

Traditionally, dentists have relied upon a visual-tactile-radiographic procedure (Radike technique) for the detection of dental caries. This procedure involves the visual identification of demineralized areas (typically white spots) or suspicious pits or fissures and the use of the dental explorer and compressed air to determine the presence of a loss of continuity or breaks in the enamel and assess the softness or resilience of the enamel.

34. The rubber dam is particularly adaptable to the primary second molar because the

a. Occlusocervical height favors its retention
b. Cervical constriction of the crown favors its retention
c. Mesiobuccal bulge favors its retention
d. Smaller diameter of the crown (as compared with permanent teeth) favors its retention

Ans b.

The answer is self-explanatory.

35. Incipient proximal decalcification in primary molars can first be seen in the radiograph

a. At the point of contact of approximating teeth
b. Just gingival to the point of contact
c. Just occlusal to the point of contact
d. None of the above. There is no most frequent location

Ans b.

The Class II lesions occur after primary molar contacts have been established. Incipient Class II lesions in primary molars can be diagnosed only with bite-wing radiographs. The flat, broad, elliptical contact areas of these teeth defy clinical exploration. The lesion will appear as a radiolucent triangle in enamel towards the amelodentinal junction with the base at or just below the contact area.

36. The approximate ideal depth for the amalgam preparation in a primary molar is

a. Just into the dentin
b. 1 mm into the dentin
c. To the dentinoenamel junction
d. Never into the dentin

Ans a.

A cavity depth of 1.5 mm will usually provide sufficient bulk of restorative material for strength. As primary enamel is 1.0 mm thick, the use of the no. 330 bur to the full length of the cutting head (1.5 mm) will prepare a cavity of approximately 0.5 mm into dentin (refer to the explanation of Q. No. 8 and 32).

37. An advantage of the rubber dam is that it

a. Muffles any screams the child may emit
b. Aids in the management of child behavior
c. Enables the operator to salvage silver scraps
d. Reduces the necessity for a carefully carved cervical margin

Ans b.

The upset child often settles down once the rubber dam is in place. It may be that the child mentally dissociates the tooth from the rest of the body, which could explain an improvement in the child's behavior. More likely, the child realizes that he or she is in no danger of choking from the water of the high-speed air turbine; also, they are not embarrassed by the taste of particles and the like and thus respond favorably to the increased comfort afforded by the rubber dam (refer to the explanation of Q. No. 1).

38. A 4-year-old child has severe, acute, dental pain. So many teeth are carious that the determination of the offending tooth is difficult. The best diagnostic tool to use is

a. Percussion
b. Radiographs
c. Electric pulp testing
d. Have the mother identify the offending tooth

Ans a.

Pain from pressure on a tooth indicates that supporting periodontal structures are inflamed. Percussion can be done by applying finger pressure on the tooth and observe the child's response by watching the eyes. Constricted pupils are indicative of pain. Radiographs, despite their immense diagnostic value, can deceive the clinician into thinking that periapical or interradicular pathosis is absent when in fact it may be histologically present. This is because the microscopic lesion must be of certain dimensions before it is manifested radiographically. Furthermore, superimpositions of permanent successors mask the true appearance, particularly in maxillary primary teeth. Vitality tests, either thermal or electrical, are of little value in primary teeth.

39. Bitewing radiographs of a 5-year-old child show interproximal caries just short of the dentinoenamel junction. The dentist should recommend

a. Restoration of the teeth as soon as possible
b. Prophylaxis and topical fluoride application
c. Disking of the affected areas
d. Three-month recall for re-evaluation
e. Both (b) and (d)

Ans a.

Early diagnosis and treatment of Class II lesions enables the clinicians to prepare a cavity of conservative extensions and dimensions. In such cases, the resulting well-supported margins will give the best chance for the restoration to endure for the life of the tooth.

40. When the gingival wall of a Class II cavity preparation in a primary molar extends too far gingivally, a satisfactory gingival wall is difficult to obtain because the

a. Proximal contact is broad and flat
b. Cervical enamel rods incline occlusally
c. Facial and lingual surfaces are tapered
d. Primary molar always has a marked cervical constriction

Ans d.

There is a marked cervical prominence of enamel in primary molars gingival to which is an equally marked cervical constriction. The placement of the floor of the interproximal box in a Class II cavity is dictated by these anatomical features. When the gingival floor of the interproximal box is placed too far cervically, it becomes too narrow. The operator may then be tempted to re-establish the gingival floor by moving the axial wall farther pulpally, unfortunately at the risk of exposing the pulp.

41. Properly contoured restorations for primary teeth serve to

a. Maintain interarch relationships
b. Maintain proximal contacts and length of the dental arch
c. Maintain vertical dimension by preventing
d. All of the above

Ans b.

Space maintenance begins with good restorative dentistry. The dentist should strive for ideal restoration of all interproximal contours. Early restoration of interproximal caries ensures that no space loss occurs.

42. A radiopaque area is observed in the dentin underlying a 3-month-old Class II restoration. Which of the following bases was used in this restoration?

a. Calcium hydroxide
b. Zinc oxyphosphate cement
c. Zinc oxide and eugenol
d. Zinc oxide and eugenol and formocresol

Ans a.

In certain cases, such as a Class II preparation that involves the restoration of an angle or of a deep depression, it may be necessary to cover a calcium hydroxide base with a layer of stronger zinc phosphate or glass ionomer cement. Dentinal bridge will be formed at the base of the cavity after 6–8 weeks and this gives the radiopaque appearance.

43. The most common cause of failure of a Class II amalgam restoration in a primary molar is

a. Pulp exposure
b. Recurrent caries
c. Fractured isthmus
d. Margin failure in the proximal box

Ans c.

Fracture of the isthmus of a Class II amalgam restoration is a common problem that may result from the restoration being left high in occlusion or from insufficient bulk of amalgam in the isthmus, because the preparation is too shallow or because the amalgam has been over-carved. A narrow isthmus gives greater fracture resistance to the tooth and better marginal integrity to the restoration (refer explanation of Q. No. 12).

44. The area in a Class II restoration in a primary molar most likely to fracture is the

a. Isthmus
b. Gingival margin
c. Lingual margin of the occlusal aspect
d. Facial margin of the interproximal aspect

Ans a.

Refer to the explanation of Q. Nos. 12 and 43.

45. The modified Class III preparation for an amalgam restoration in a primary canine is typified by its

a. Lack of esthetics
b. Facial or lingual dovetail
c. Elimination of the need for a matrix
d. Elimination of the need for anesthesia

Ans b.

Refer to the explanation of Q. No. 15.

46. The dental pulp first becomes influenced by dental caries when the carious lesion reaches

a. The dental pulp
b. The dentinoenamel junction
c. Halfway through the dentin
d. A point 1–2 mm away from the pulp

Ans b.

Brannstron and his associates demonstrated the alarming rapidity with which bacteria penetrate the enamel. From incipient carious lesions, without cavitation on the enamel surface, microorganisms can reach the dentinoenamel junction. It is quite conceivable that a degree of pulp inflammation could develop well before a visual or radiographic break in the enamel becomes apparent. Seltzer et al have described these pulp changes, from early irritation dentin formation under initial caries, to frank chronic inflammatory exudate under deep carious lesion.

Chapter 24

Pulp Therapy of Primary and Young Permanent Teeth

1. **A tooth that has been treated successfully with a pulpotomy technique should have after 1 year**
   a. A normal periodontal ligament and lamina dura
   b. Radiographic evidence of a calcified bridge if calcium hydroxide had been used as a capping material
   c. No radiographic evidence of internal resorption
   d. All of the above

Ans d.

All of the above-mentioned factors are true regarding success of a pulpotomized tooth.

2. **A patient aged 7 years complains of severe toothache at night in relation to 75. The mode of treatment probably will be**
   a. Pulpotomy
   b. Pulpectomy
   c. Direct pulp capping
   d. Indirect pulp capping

Ans b.

Nocturnal pain indicates irreversible pulpitis. Hence the treatment options can be pulpectomy or extraction. The nocturnal pain associated with the tooth increases at night because of the patient's posture which increases the blood flow to the head and neck. This in turn increases the intrapulpal pressure, which results in severe toothache (refer explanation of Q. No. 48).

3. **A severe toothache at night usually means extensive degeneration of the pulp. This calls for more than a conservative type of pulp therapy.**
   a. Both the statements are false
   b. Both the statements are true
   c. First statement is true and the second is false
   d. First statement is false and the second is true

Ans b.

The answer is self-explanatory (refer to the explanation of Q. No. 2).

4. **All of the following statements are true regarding gingival abscess except**
   a. A gingival abscess or draining fistula associated with deep carious lesion is an obvious clinical sign of irreversibly diseased pulp
   b. Such infections can be resolved only by successful endodontic therapy or extraction of the tooth
   c. Gingival abscess is also known as parulis
   d. A gingival abscess or a draining fistula associated with a tooth with a deep carious lesion is an obvious clinical sign of reversibly diseased pulp

Ans d.

The answer is self-explanatory.

5. **A gingival abscess or a draining fistula associated with a tooth with a deep carious lesion is an obvious clinical sign of**
   a. Reversibly diseased pulp
   b. Irreversibly diseased pulp
   c. Beginning of pulpal degeneration
   d. Healthy radicular pulp and infected coronal pulp

Ans b.

Gingival abscess or parulis (gum boil) is because of the degenerated pulp or necrosed pulp.

6. **The proximity of carious lesions to the pulp cannot always be determined accurately in the X-ray film. What often appears to be an intact barrier of secondary dentin protecting the pulp may actually be a perforated mass of irregularly calcified and carious material.**
   a. Both the statements are false
   b. Both the statements are true
   c. First statement is true and the second is false
   d. First statement is false and the second is true

Ans b.

The answer is self-explanatory.

7. **Which of the following conditions are relative contraindications for endodontic therapy in children?**

a. Susceptibility to subacute bacterial endocarditis
b. Nephritis
c. Leukemia
d. All of the above

Ans d.

In case of children with conditions which render them susceptible to subacute bacterial endocarditis or those with nephritis, leukemia, solid tumors or idiopathic cyclic neutropenia, extraction of the involved tooth after proper premedication with antibiotics should be the treatment of choice rather than pulp therapy.

8. The teeth selected for indirect pulp treatment should fulfill which of the following criteria?

a. No history of spontaneous unprovoked toothache
b. No tenderness to percussion
c. No abnormal mobility
d. No radiographic evidence of radicular disease
e. No evidence of internal or external resorption
f. All of the above

Ans f.

Spontaneous pain indicates irreversible pulpitis. Tenderness to percussion indicates inflammation of the periapical tissues. Abnormal mobility indicates periodontal breakdown. Hence in the above situations, endodontic treatment becomes necessary. Also, radiographic evidence of radicular disease, internal or external resorption indicates the need for more invasive procedures.

9. The size of the exposure, the appearance of the pulp and the amount of bleeding are valuable observations in diagnosing the condition of primary pulp. The most favorable condition for vital pulp therapy is the small pinpoint exposure surrounded by sound dentin.

a. Both the statements are false
b. Both the statements are true
c. First statement is true and the second is false
d. First statement is false and the second is true

Ans b.

The answer is self-explanatory.

10. Vital pulp therapy can be carried out if which of the following criteria are fulfilled?

a. Small exposures that have been accidentally produced by trauma or during cavity preparation

b. Absence of pain with the possible exception of discomfort caused by the intake of food
c. Lack of bleeding at the exposure site as is often the case in a mechanical exposure or an amount of bleeding that would be considered normal in the absence of hyperemic or an inflamed pulp
d. Any of the above

Ans d.

All of the above-mentioned situations can be treated by vital pulp therapy.

11. The material of choice for direct pulp capping in permanent molars is

a. Calcium hydroxide
b. Zinc oxide eugenol
c. Glass ionomer cement
d. Reinforced zinc oxide eugenol (IRM)

Ans a.

Calcium hydroxide stimulates formation of reparative dentin. Hence, this is the material of choice for pulp capping.

12. The material of choice for pulpotomy in primary molars is

a. Calcium hydroxide
b. Zinc oxide eugenol
c. Formocresol or glutaraldehyde
d. Reinforced zinc oxide eugenol (IRM)

Ans c.

Formocresol or glutaraldehyde is the material of choice for pulpotomy. Calcium hydroxide should not be used for pulpotomy as it causes internal resorption in primary teeth.

13. The material of choice for pulpotomy in permanent molars is

a. Calcium hydroxide
b. Zinc oxide eugenol
c. Formocresol or glutaraldehyde
d. Reinforced zinc oxide eugenol (IRM)

Ans a.

The material of choice for pulpotomy in permanent teeth is calcium hydroxide because of its ability to induce secondary dentin formation.

14. **Who introduced calcium hydroxide?**

   a. Herman
   b. Jordan
   c. Robert Bunon
   d. Wilson and Kent

Ans a.

Herman introduced calcium hydroxide. Wilson and Kent introduced glass ionomer cement in 1972.

15. **The pH of calcium hydroxide is**

   a. 12
   b. 7
   c. 3
   d. 10

Ans a.

Because of its alkalinity, it is so caustic that when placed in contact with vital pulp tissue, the reaction produces a superficial necrosis of the pulp.

16. **The immediate reaction of the pulp tissue beneath the calcium hydroxide in direct pulp capping is**

   a. Inflammation
   b. Necrosis
   c. Fatty degeneration
   d. Gangrene formation

Ans b.

Refer to the explanation of Q. No. 15.

17. **After the pulp capping procedure, a calcified bridge is evident radiographically in**

   a. 2 weeks
   b. 4 weeks
   c. 12 weeks
   d. 2 months

Ans b.

One month after the pulp capping procedure, a calcified bridge is evident radiographically. This bridge continues to increase in thickness during the next 12-month period. The pulp tissue beneath the calcified bridge remains vital and is essentially free of inflammatory cells.

18. Which of the following is not an advantage of glutaraldehyde over formocresol as a pulpotomy agent?

a. Formaldehyde reactions are reversible but glutaraldehyde reactions are not
b. Formaldehyde is a small molecule that penetrates the apical foramen, whereas glutaraldehyde is a larger molecule that does not
c. Formaldehyde requires a long reaction time and an excess of solution to fix tissue, whereas glutaraldehyde fixes the tissue instantly and excess solution is not required
d. The amount of glutaraldehyde absorbed systemically is more

Ans d.

The systemic absorption of glutaraldehyde is less when compared to formocresol. Hence the fourth choice is not correct regarding glutaraldehyde.

19. The concentration of glutaraldehyde used for pulpotomy is

a. 4%
b. 8%
c. 2%
d. 6%

Ans c.

The answer is self-explanatory.

20. Which of the following is an indication of failure after vital pulp therapy?

a. Internal resorption
b. Alveolar abscess
c. Early exfoliation after pulp treatment
d. Any of the above

Ans d.

Radiographic evidence of internal resorption occurring within the pulp canal several months after pulpotomy procedure is the most frequently seen evidence of an abnormal response in primary teeth. An alveolar abscess occasionally develops some months after the pulp therapy has been completed. The child may present with a fistulous opening indicating the chronicity of the infection. Occasionally, a pulpally treated tooth previously believed to be successfully managed will loosen and exfoliate prematurely for no reason. It is believed that such a condition results from low grade, chronic, asymptomatic and localized infection.

21. Internal resorption appears first in the radiograph as

a. Interproximal bony loss
b. Small granules in the pulp chamber
c. A small area around the apex of the root
d. An encroaching radiolucency on the medial surfaces of the roots
e. Small radiolucent enlargement of the pulp cavity in a localized area

Ans e.

Internal resorption is a destructive process generally believed to be caused by osteoclastic activity. If the inflammation is extended to the entrance of the pulp canal, osteoclasts may have been attracted to the area; if it were possible to examine the tooth histologically, a small bays of resorption will be evident. This bays of resorption appears as a small radiolucent enlargement of the pulp cavity in a localized area.

22. Indirect pulp capping procedure on primary molars are indicated when

a. Removal of decay has exposed the pulp
b. A tooth has a large, long standing lesion with a history of continuous pain
c. The carious lesion has just penetrated the dentinoenamel junction
d. The carious lesion is suspected of having produced an exposure of the pulp

Ans d.

The technique is to remove all decay, except that which, in the clinicians' experience, would expose the pulp if it were removed. A pulp protecting base, such as zinc oxide or calcium hydroxide, is placed over the deep aspects of the cavity, whose margins are well supported and finished. For this treatment to be successful, the pulp must be vital and free of inflammation; at least if any inflammation is present, it must be reversible so that the secondary dentin can act as a barrier to further insult.

23. The cotton pellet applied to the pulpal stumps in the formocresol pulpotomy technique should be

a. Slightly dampened with formocresol
b. Saturated with formocresol
c. Left in place for 15 minutes
d. Left in place after the second visit

Ans a.

The cotton pellets are first saturated with formocresol and later compressed between gauze to remove excess formocresol so that they are just moistened with the liquid. Excess formocresol is undesirable since it serves no purpose other than to increase the likelihood of a soft tissue burn.

24. The treatment of choice for a nonvital permanent incisor with immature root development is

a. Pulpotomy
b. Silver point placement
c. Lateral condensation with gutta-percha
d. Retrograde root canal therapy with amalgam
e. Filling the canal with calcium hydroxide and CMCP

Ans e.

The principle of treatment is to debride and sterilize the canal before filling it with calcium hydroxide paste and CMCP; saturating the periapical tissues with calcium ions, together with elimination of bacteria, stimulate physiologic calcific repair of the apex. When the repair is complete, conventional root canal treatment can be performed using lateral and apical condensation against the repaired, calcified apical tissues. This technique is called *apexification.*

25. A nonvital primary incisor (abscess due to trauma) in a 4-year-old patient can be effectively treated by

a. Pulpectomy
b. Extraction
c. 5-minute formocresol puplotomy
d. 7-day formocresol pulpotomy

Ans a.

The degree of repair that is possible with abscessed primary teeth as long as there has not been too much root resorption is remarkable. Teeth that are mobile, tender to percussion and with considerable cellulitis present can be restored to full function with the use of antibiotics and pulpectomy.

26. If a successful puplectomy cannot be accomplished in a 5-year-old child with a chronically infected primary molar, which of the following is the most acceptable treatment?

a. Treat with an antibiotic and allow the tooth to remain in place
b. Allow the tooth to remain in the mouth for a space maintainer
c. Allow the tooth to remain in the mouth unless it is creating pain for the patient
d. Extract the tooth to prevent damage to the surrounding bone and the developing permanent tooth

Ans d.

It is unwise to maintain untreated infected primary teeth in the mouth. They may be open for drainage and often remain asymptomatic for an indefinite period. However, they are a source of infection and should be treated or removed. The morphology of root canals in primary teeth makes endodontic treatment difficult and often impractical. If the canal cannot be properly cleansed of necrotic material, sterilized and adequately filled, endodontic therapy is more likely to fail. Failure of treating the infection can also lead to Turner's hypoplasia.

27. Following removal of a relatively large area of decay in recently erupted permanent molar, an exposure of the pulpal tissue is noted. The dentist decides to perform a pulpotomy using calcium hydroxide to treat the tissue remaining in the root canals. The dentist would expect a dentin bridge to form at

a. A level somewhat below the amputation

b. A level halfway between the apex and the amputation

c. The exact level of the amputation

d. The apical site

Ans a.

Calcific bridge forms over the vital pulp tissue below the level at which amputation of pulp was done.

28. Pulpal infection in primary mandibular posterior teeth is first manifested on a radiograph in the area

a. Of bifurcation

b. At the apex of the root

c. Around the permanent tooth bud

d. Near the crest of the alveolar bone

Ans a.

Radiolucency in primary molars is usually seen in the furcation and not at the periapex. The high incidence of furcation radiolucency in primary molars has been attributed to the presence of accessory canals in the bifurcation region of primary molars. Also, the pulpal floor in infected primary molars may be more porous and permeable. The accessory canals and porous pulpal floor, which is thinner in primary than in permanent teeth, may permit the diffusion of inflammatory exudate more readily; this would explain the high incidence of interradicular rather than periapical pathology in necrotic primary teeth.

29. The most successful treatment for a vital primary second molar with a large carious pulpal exposure is

a. Indirect pulp treatment

b. Pulpotomy with formocresol

c. Pulpotomy with calcium hydroxide
d. Pulp capping with calcium hydroxide

Ans b.

The size of the exposure, appearance of the pulp and the amount of bleeding are valuable observations in diagnosing the conditions of the primary pulp. The most favorable condition for vital pulp therapy is a small pinpoint pulp exposure (direct pulp capping) surrounded by sound dentin. However, a true caries exposure even of pinpoint size or large exposure will be accompanied by inflammation of the pulp, the degree of which is usually directly related to the size of the exposure. Under these circumstances, pulpotomy (using formocresol, ferric sulphate or glutaraldehyde) has to be performed. Pulpotomy with calcium hydroxide is contraindicated in primary teeth as it can cause internal resorption.

30. In performing the pulp amputation for a pulpotomy, it is wise to use a spoon excavator to avoid

a. Perforation of the pulpal floor
b. Pulling out the radicular portion of the pulp
c. Macerating the pulp at the amputation site
d. All of the above

Ans d.

Care must be excised not to perforate either the thin pulpal or interproximal wall, or the floor of the pulp chamber, by using excessive force with a round bur. A large, round bur run at a slow speed with a light touch is recommended or a large, sharp spoon excavator; there is less danger of inadvertently forcing these down the canals as their dimensions would exceed those of the canal entrance in most instances.

31. Radiographic examination of a permanent molar with an early acute pulpal abscess would reveal

a. Involvement of the bifurcation
b. Little change from normal structure
c. A large area of periapical bone rarefaction
d. A disturbance in the integrity of the periodontal ligament

Ans b.

The clinician must remember that the initial acute periapical abscess often presents no radiographic change because a significant amount of bone must first be resorbed before a change can be demonstrated on the radiograph.

32. Internal resorption is most frequently seen

a. With replanted teeth
b. In nonfluoridated areas

c. As a part of the devitalizing process
d. With $Ca(OH)_2$ pulpotomies on primary teeth

Ans d.

Refer to the explanation of Q. No. 21.

33. Uncontrollable hemorrhage after amputation of the coronal portion of the pulp may indicate that

a. The blood level of vitamin K is deficient
b. There is incomplete amputation of pulp tissue
c. Endodontic treatment or removal of the tooth is needed
d. Advanced degeneration of the pulp extends into the canals

Ans d.

Extraction or pulpectomy is to be carried out if uncontrollable hemorrhage after amputation of the coronal pulp is observed. This indicates advanced degeneration of the pulp extending into the radicular pulp.

34. Pulp extirpation in primary teeth is mechanically difficult because of

a. Sensitivity of primary pulps
b. Lack of cooperation of children
c. Tortuous anatomy and branching of canals
d. All of the above

Ans c.

Subsequent deposition of secondary dentin throughout the life of the primary teeth cause a change in the morphologic pattern of the root canal, producing variations and eventual alterations in the number and size of the canals. The variations included lateral branching, connecting fibrils, apical ramifications and partial fusion of the canals. These findings explain the complications often encountered in root canal therapy of primary teeth.

35. Direct pulp capping is indicated for a primary molar with an exposure when there is

a. Pain from the tooth when eating
b. A history of unprovoked or spontaneous toothache
c. Radiographic evidence of internal resorption
d. Little or no hemorrhage from the exposure site

Ans d.

Refer to explanation of Q. No. 29.

36. Which of the following cell types is most prominent in an area of repair following drainage of a perapical abscess?

a. Fibroblast
b. Osteoblast
c. Lymphocyte
d. Erythrocyte
e. Karyocyte

Ans a.

Fibroblasts are the crucial reconstructive cells in the progression of wound healing because they produce the most of the structural proteins, e.g. collagen. Collagen is first detected in the wound about the third day after injury. The fibroblasts produce Type III collagen initially and then, as the wound matures, Type I collagen.

37. The most common cause of sinus tracts in gingival tissues of children is

a. Pericementitis
b. Periapical cyst
c. Acute periapical abscess
d. Chronic periapical abscess

Ans d.

It is important to perform a thorough clinical examination in a pediatric patient. Pulpal pathology in primary teeth is often painless and symptomless. Only clinical finding may be the presence of a gumboil or a fistulous tract on the attached gingiva adjacent to the corresponding tooth. A gingival abscess or a draining fistula associated with a deep carious lesion is an obvious clinical sign of an irreversibly diseased pulp.

38. A healthy 5-year-old child has a necrotic pulp in a primary second molar that has a permanent successor. The primary second molar should be

a. Treated endodontically
b. Allowed to remain in the mouth, unless it is creating pain for the patient
c. Allowed to remain in the mouth, but treated with an antibiotic to eliminate infection
d. Drained through an opening through the crown into the pulp chamber, but allowed to remain in the mouth to serve as a space maintainer
e. None of the above

Ans a.

Necrotic pulp in a primary second molar should be treated endodontically (pulpectomy) and the tooth should be preserved.

39. Formalin-containing drugs are often advocated for pulp therapy in cariously exposed vital primary pulps. Which of the following pulpal reactions to the drug can be expected?

a. A calcified bridge will develop
b. There will be a massive infiltration of inflammatory cells
c. There will be a surface fixation of the pulpal tissue accompanied by degeneration of the odontoblasts
d. The pulp will remain vital throughout and relatively unchanged; however, all microorganisms will be destroyed

Ans c.

The clinical success experienced in the treatment of primary pulps with these materials is possibly related to the drug's germicidal action and fixation qualities rather than to its ability to promote healing.

40. Which of the following is the best indicator of success of a pulpotomy in an immature permanent tooth?

a. Patient comfort
b. Stable vitality readings
c. Continuation of root formation
d. Formation of a dentinal bridge covering the pulp stumps in the root canal

Ans c.

Formation of calcific bridge, continued apical development, absence of internal resorption and periapical radiolucency are radiographic evidences of success of pulpotomy procedure in permanent teeth.

41. A healthy 8-year-old child has a fractured permanent central incisor. The pulp is widely exposed and vital. From radiographs, root ends appear incompletely calcified. The recommended procedure is to

a. Cap the pulp
b. Extract the tooth
c. Perform a pulpotomy
d. Remove the entire pulp

Ans c.

A large vital exposure in permanent teeth with incompletely formed apices warrant treatment by calcium hydroxide pulpotomy. The aim is to remove the infected coronal pulp and place calcium hydroxide over the healthy radicular stumps after the inflamed coronal pulp has been amputated. This procedure will facilitate physiological root closure.

42. Successful management of deep caries and pulpally involved teeth in children is mainly contingent on

a. Radiographic findings
b. Extent of inflammation in the pulp
c. Proximity of caries to the pulp
d. Responses of the child to various clinical tests

Ans b.

The most important and also the most difficult aspect of pulp therapy is determining the health of the pulp or its stage of inflammation so that an appropriate decision can be made regarding the best form of treatment.

43. Which of the following diagnostic criteria is least reliable in assessing pulp status in the primary dentition?

a. Swelling
b. Pulp testing
c. Spontaneous pain
d. Internal resorption

Ans b.

The reliability of the pulp test for the young child can be questioned sometimes because of the child's apprehension, associated with the test itself. The value of electric pulp test in determining the condition of the pulp of primary teeth is questionable, although it will give an indication of whether the pulp is vital or not. The test does not provide reliable evidence of the degree of inflammation of the pulp. A complicating factor is the occasional positive response to the test in a tooth with a necrotic pulp if the content of the canals is liquid.

44. Compared to permanent tooth abscess, a primary tooth abscess is a more diffuse infection because

a. Surrounding alveolar bone is less dense
b. Roots of the primary tooth are farther apart
c. Pain is less and, therefore, the abscess is not detected early
d. Young patients are less resistant to infection

Ans a.

Alveolar bone is less dense in children leading to faster and diffuse spread of infection.

45. Apexification is obtaining physiologic root closure with a medicament. Apexogenesis is inducing a barrier formation in a nonvital tooth.

a. Both the statements are true
b. Both the statements are false
c. First statement is true and the second statement is false
d. First statement is false and the second statement is true

Ans b.

Apexogenesis is facilitating physiological root closure in a tooth with vital pulp and apexification is inducing a barrier formation in a nonvital tooth.

46. Which of the following methods can assess any temperature changes in the pulp?

a. Pulp oximeter
b. Doppler flowmeter
c. Hughes probe eye camera
d. Electric pulp testing

Ans c.

Hughes probe eye camera is capable of detecting very small temperature changes and has been used to measure pulp vitality experimentally. This equipment is capable of detecting temperature changes as small as 0.1°C.

47. The normal intrapulpal pressure is said to be

a. 2–4 mm Hg
b. 5–14 mm Hg
c. 20–30 mm Hg
d. 40–60 mm Hg

Ans b.

Tissue pressure in the pulp is a result of vascular pressure and it is normally about 15 cm H_2O. This was previously reported by Van Hassel as 5–14 mm Hg.

48. Pulp is said to undergo irreversible damage when the intrapulpal pressure increases up to

a. 10 mm Hg
b. 5 mm Hg
c. 12 mm Hg
d. 35 mm Hg

Ans d.

During irreversible pulpitis, the pulpal pressure goes up to 35 mm Hg.

49. MTA can be used for

a. Pulp capping
b. Pulpotomy
c. Apexification
d. All of the above

Ans d.

Mineral trioxide aggregate can be used for all the above-mentioned procedures.

50. Buckley's formocresol contains all except

a. Formaldehyde
b. CMCP
c. Tricresol
d. Glycerine

Ans b.

Formocresol was introduced by Buckley in 1904. Buckley's formocresol is a solution of 19% formaldehyde and 35% tricresol in a vehicle of 15% glycerine and water.

51. Ledermix is a combination of

a. Prednisolone and calcium hydroxide
b. Calcium hydroxide and iodoform
c. Formocresol and calcium hydroxide
d. Formocresol and prednisolone

Ans a.

Ledermix is a combination of prednisolone and calcium hydroxide. Though many such combinations have been tried, they have been shown to preserve chronic inflammation and reduce reparative dentin formation.

Chapter 25

Crowns in Pediatric Dentistry

1. Stainless steel crowns were popularized by

a. Croll (1981)
b. Kennedy (1983)
c. Humphrey (1950)
d. Mink and Hill (1971)

Ans c.

Preformed metal crowns, also referred to as stainless steel crowns, were introduced to Pediatric Dentistry by Humphrey in 1950.

2. The most commonly used crowns are

a. Stainless steel crowns
b. Nickel-chromium crowns
c. Tin base crowns
d. Aluminium base crowns

Ans a.

Stainless steel crowns have become an invaluable restorative material in the treatment of badly broken down primary teeth. They are generally considered superior to large multi-surface amalgam restorations and have a longer clinical life span than 2 or 3 surface amalgam restorations. The crowns are manufactured in different sizes as a metal shell with some preformed anatomy and are trimmed and contoured as necessary to fit individual teeth.

3. The required amount of occlusal reduction for stainless steel crown is

a. 1 mm
b. 1.5 mm
c. 1.5 to 2.0 mm
d. 4 mm

Ans c.

According to Nash (1981), 69L or 169L bur is used to reduce the occlusal surface by 1.5 to 2.0 mm following the cuspal outline and maintaining the original contour of the cusp. However, the amount of occlusal reduction varies with authors as follows:

1. Humphrey (1950)—occlusal reduction if necessary, preserving as much tooth structure as possible
2. Rapp (1966)—occlusal surface is reduced such that 4 mm of tooth structure is available from gingival margin
3. Mink and Bennet (1968)—1 to 1.5 mm
4. Troutman (1976)—1 mm
5. Kennedy (1976)—1.5 to 2 mm

4. The crown margin on the buccal surface of first primary molar is like

a. Smile shape
b. Flat shape
c. Stretched out "S"
d. Frown

Ans c.

The buccal gingiva of the first primary molar has a different outline. Because of the mesiobuccal cervical bulge, the gingival margin dips down as it is traced from distal to mesial which resembles a stretched "S".

5. The most ideal full coronal restoration for anterior teeth is

a. Stainless steel crowns
b. Resin-veneered stainless steel crowns
c. Strip crowns (celluloid crowns)
d. Polycarbonate crowns

Ans c.

Celluloid crowns are a popular method of restoring primary anterior teeth. These crowns provide superior esthetics than other forms of anterior coronal coverage restorations. If these crowns are chipped or fractured, repair is possible.

6. Nickel–chromium crowns belong to

a. Untrimmed/uncontoured crowns
b. Pretrimmed crowns
c. Precontoured crowns
d. None of the above

Ans c.

They are similar to pretrimmed crowns in height of the crowns but they are more rounded in the gingival margin and they simulate the normal appearance of the tooth.

7. **All are bonded type of anterior full coronal restorations except**
   a. Strip crowns
   b. Art glass crowns
   c. Pedo jackets
   d. Polycarbonate crowns

Ans d.

S.No.	Bonded type	Preformed and held by luting cement
1.	Strip crowns	Stainless steel crowns
2.	Pedo jackets	Facial cut-out stainless steel crowns
3.	New millennium crowns	Resin-veneered stainless steel crowns
4.	Art glass crowns	Polycarbonate crowns

8. **Resin-veneered crown with crimped labial gingival margin is**
   a. Nusmile crown
   b. Cheng crown
   c. Dura crown
   d. Kinder crown

Ans c.

Recently a new resin-veneered *Dura crown* was introduced which has labial gingival margin crimped and resin adapted to the gingival edge of the anterior aspect of the crown.

9. **The only disadvantage of anterior stainless steel crown is**
   a. Less wear resistance
   b. Unsightly silver appearance
   c. Bonding failure
   d. More prone to fracture

Ans b.

Preformed anterior stainless steel crowns are the most durable and reliable for restoring severely fractured primary incisors. Croll described that stainless steel crowns are easy to place, fracture proof, wear resistant and attached firmly to the tooth until exfoliation. The main disadvantage is the unsightly silver metallic appearance.

10. **The plier used to produce contact point is**
   a. Johnson plier no. 114

b. Abell ball and socket plier no. 112
c. Gordon plier no. 137
d. Crimper no. 800-417

Ans b.

The answer is self-explanatory. Refer the following table:

S. No.	Plier	Use
1.	Abell ball and socket plier no. 112	To produce contact points
2.	Gordon plier no. 137	To contour the cervical margin
3.	Crimper no. 800-417	To crimp the last 1–2 mm of the gingival margin
4.	Johnson plier no. 114 (wide) 115 (medium)	For general contouring of the stainless steel crowns

11. In festooning and trimming a stainless steel crown, special attention must be paid to the greater length necessary in the region of the mesiobuccal bulge in the

a. Primary first molar
b. Primary second molar
c. Maxillary primary canine
d. Maxillary lateral primary incisor

Ans a.

Two prominent features of the mandibular first primary molar are the deep central pit and the marked buccogingival ridge. This ridge reaches its greatest curvature at the mesiobuccal angle where it is also most prominent.

12. In the tooth preparation for a steel crown, the surface requiring the least amount of reduction is the

a. Distal
b. Buccal
c. Mesial
d. Lingual
e. Occlusal

Ans d.

Buccolingual reduction for the stainless steel crown preparation is often limited to the bevelling of the bucco-occlusal and occlusogingival line angles and is confined to the occlusal one-third of the crown. The prominence (unprepared) on the lingual surface helps in retention of the stainless steel crown.

13. A stainless steel crown should normally extend below the gingival crest approximately

a. 1.0 mm

b. 1.5 mm

c. 2.0 mm

d. 2.5 mm

Ans a.

Crowns are manufactured longer than necessary for the average tooth and hence many may require some trimming. A properly trimmed crown will extend approximately 1 mm into the gingival sulcus.

14. Which of the following permanent restorations is indicated for use after a pulpotomy has been completed on a primary molar?

a. A stainless steel crown placed at the same appointment, or as soon as possible

b. A stainless steel crown placed in 6 weeks when a radiograph indicates no internal resorption

c. An amalgam placed at the same appointment

d. An amalgam placed in 6 weeks when a radiograph indicates no bone destruction between roots

Ans a.

Primary molar is small, and the buccal and lingual retaining walls become thin and weak with little remaining supporting dentin after the access opening for pulp therapy. The tooth is susceptible for fracture because of this. Hence, it is advisable to place a stainless steel crown at the same appointment.

Section VII

Injuries to the Teeth—Prevention and its Management

Chapter

26 Traumatic Injuries of Teeth and its Supporting Structures

1. **A dental disturbance that has a greater psychological impact on both the parents and child is**
   a. Multiple decayed teeth
   b. Discolored front tooth
   c. Fracture or loss of an anterior tooth
   d. Mucocele

Ans c.

Fracture or loss of an anterior tooth due to trauma is a tragic experience for the young patient as well as the parents.

2. **Facial fractures in children have a very low incidence because**
   a. Of the elastic nature of the child's facial bones
   b. Of lack of exposure to alcohol-associated motor vehicle accidents
   c. Of anatomic protection offered by prominent calvaria
   d. Any of the above

Ans d.

All of the above factors contribute to the decreased incidence of facial fractures in children. Because of the resilient bones surrounding the primary teeth, injuries usually comprise of tooth luxations.

3. **A fracture can be defined as a sudden violent breach of continuity of bone, which may be complete or incomplete in character. Contusion is produced by blunt trauma that results in edema and hematoma formation in the subcutaneous tissues.**
   a. Both the statements are true
   b. Both the statements are false
   c. The first statement is true and the second is false
   d. The first statement is false and the second is true

Ans a.

The question defines the terms fracture and contusion.

4. **An abrasion results from friction along a surface, removing or peeling of the superficial layers of the skin that results in a raw exposed or bleeding surface. On the other hand, laceration is one which causes a discontinuity in the skin or mucosal surface, which can be simple, stellate, jagged, beveled or flap-like.**
   a. Both the statements are true
   b. Both the statements are false
   c. The first statement is true and the second is false
   d. The first statement is false and the second is true

Ans a.
The statements mentioned above differentiate abrasion from laceration.

5. **Which of the following is the commonest type of injury in the orofacial region?**
   a. Laceration
   b. Contusion
   c. Abrasion
   d. Avulsion

Ans a.
Laceration is the commonest type of injury after trauma in the oro-facial region.

6. **Trauma to primary dentition occurs most commonly in __________ age group.**
   a. Less than 1 year
   b. 1 to 2.5 years
   c. 2.5 to 3.5 years
   d. 4 to 6 years

Ans b.
Trauma to primary dentition occurs most commonly in 1 to 2.5 years age group because the child starts walking between 10 and 20 months during which the child falls frequently.

7. **Children with accident-prone facial profiles belong to __________ category of malocclusion.**
   a. Class I
   b. Class II, div. 1
   c. Class II, div. 2
   d. Class III

Ans b.

Injuries to the teeth are common in children with protruding anterior teeth. In Class II, div. 1 malocclusion, the protrusion of maxillary incisors makes these teeth more susceptible to injury.

8. Children with cerebral palsy are a special group with more predilections to dental trauma. This is because many children with cerebral palsy have protruding anterior teeth and they are subject to frequent falls.

a. Both the statements are true
b. Both the statements are false
c. The first statement is true and the second is false
d. The first statement is false and the second is true

Ans a.

The answer is self-explanatory.

9. All of the following are true of direct trauma except

a. When the tooth itself is struck against a surface or when an object strikes a tooth or teeth
b. Example for direct trauma is hitting against table chair or playground
c. This usually involves anterior dentition
d. This type of trauma favors crown or crown root fractures in the premolar or molar region; also possibility of jaw fractures

Ans d.

Indirect trauma such as injuries to chin transmits the forces to the posterior teeth resulting in crown or crown root fractures in the premolar or molar region.

10. High velocity blows cause the greatest damage to the supporting structures of the dentition but tooth fractures are less frequent. Low velocity impacts result in crown fractures and are usually not associated with damage to the supporting structures.

a. Both the statements are true
b. Both the statements are false
c. The first statement is true and the second is false
d. The first statement is false and the second is true

Ans b.

The reverse is true. Low velocity blows cause the greatest damage to the supporting structures of the dentition but tooth fractures are less frequent.

High velocity impacts result in crown fractures and are usually not associated with damage to the supporting structures.

11. All of the following factors involved in traumatic injury to the teeth are described correctly except

a. Sharp impact favors clean crown fractures with minimum tooth displacement because the energy spreads rapidly over a limited area
b. Enamel is fractured easily when the direction of impacting force is parallel to the enamel rods and with dentin, it fractures easily when the force is perpendicular to the dentinal tubules
c. Low velocity impact causes more tooth fractures than damage to the supporting tissues
d. If a tooth is struck with a resilient or a cushioned object, the risk of luxation and alveolar fracture is increased

Ans c.

Refer to the explanation of Q. No. 10.

12. In the primary dentition, teeth are more frequently displaced or luxated than they are fractured. This is because the alveolar bone in the young child has large marrow spaces and is relatively pliable.

a. Both the statements are true
b. Both the statements are false
c. The first statement is true and the second is false
d. The first statement is false and the second is true

Ans a.

The alveolar bone in the young child is more elastic and resilient. Hence, it can absorb forces and allow displacement or luxation more frequently.

13. Whose classification of traumatic injuries is based on the system adopted by WHO in its application of international classification of diseases to Dentistry and Stomatology?

a. Rabinowitch (1956)
b. Ellis and Davey (1960)
c. Andreasen (1981)
d. Ulfohn (1985)

Ans c.

Andreasen's classification of traumatic injuries is based on WHO classification of injuries to teeth. Classification of traumatic injuries to teeth:

Rabinowitch

- Fractures of enamel/slightly into dentin
- Fractures into the dentin
- Fractures into the pulp
- Fractures of the root
- Comminuted fractures
- Displaced teeth

Ulfohn

- Fracture of enamel
- Fracture of the crown with indirect pulp exposure through the dentin
- Fracture of the crown with direct pulp exposure

Ellis and Davey

- Class 1—Simple fracture of the crown involving enamel and little or no dentin
- Class II—Extensive fracture of the crown, involving considerable dentin but not the dental pulp
- Class III—Extensive fracture of the crown, involving considerable dentin and exposing the dental pulp
- Class IV—Traumatized teeth that becomes nonvital with or without loss of crown structure
- Class V—Teeth lost as a result of trauma
- Class VI—Fracture of the root with or without loss of crown structure
- Class VII—Displacement of a tooth without fracture of crown or root
- Class VIII—Fracture of crown enmasse and its replacement
- Class IX—Traumatic injuries to deciduous teeth

14. Teeth lost as a result of trauma is classified by Ellis and Davey as

a. Class I
b. Class VII
c. Class VI
d. Class V

Ans d.

Refer to the explanation of Q. No. 13.

15. Nonvital teeth belongs to ___________ of Ellis and Davey's classification.

a. Class I
b. Class VI
c. Class IV
d. Class VIII

Ans c.

Refer to the explanation of Q. No. 13.

16. Accident in which a child has fallen with an object in mouth results in

a. Crown-root fracture
b. Dislocation of the teeth in a labial direction
c. Fracture of root without crown fracture
d. Fracture of crown enmasse

Ans b.

The object in the mouth tends to displace the anterior teeth in a labial direction.

17. Subconjunctival hemorrhage with periorbital ecchymosis and edema suggests a fracture of zygoma, nasal bone or frontal bone. Sublingual hematoma is diagnostic of mandibular fracture.

a. Both the statements are true
b. Both the statements are false
c. The first statement is true and the second is false
d. The first statement is false and the second is true

Ans a.

The answer is self-explanatory.

18. When deviation of the mandible is seen during opening and closing movements, zygomatic arch fracture should be suspected. Trismus or inability to close the mouth may be an indication of a condylar injury.

a. Both the statements are true
b. Both the statements are false
c. The first statement is true and the second is false
d. The first statement is false and the second is true

Ans b.

Deviation of the mandible is seen during opening and closing movements in condylar injuries. Trismus or inability to close the mouth may be indicative of a depressed zygomatic arch fracture.

19. Following a trauma, if the tooth reacts to hot, cold, sweet or sour food, it indicates exposure of dentin or pulp. If there is sensitivity to pressure on eating or touch, it suggests an occlusal disturbance.

a. Both the statements are true
b. Both the statements are false
c. The first statement is true and the second is false
d. The first statement is false and the second is true

Ans a.

The answer is self-explanatory.

20. Match the following:

	View		Fracture location
A	Water's view	1	Frontal sinus, Frontal bone, Ethmoidal cells, Zygomatic frontal suture
B	Caldwell view	2	Body of the mandible, Angle
C	Towne's view	3	Condyle, Alveolar segment
D	Panoramic view	4	Orbital, Nasal fracture
E	Orbital and nasal films	5	Midface, Zygoma, Maxilla, Maxillary orbital floors and Nasal pyramid

a. A-5, B-1, C-2, D-3, E-4
b. A-1, B-2, C-3, D-4, E-5
c. A-3, B-4, C-5, D-2, E-1
d. A-4, B-3, C-5, D-2, E-1

Ans a.

The answer is self-explanatory.

21. Which of the following recent methods are used to assess pulp circulation (vitality)?

a. CT scan
b. MRI
c. Laser Doppler flowmeter
d. Pulseoximeter
e. Both (c) and (d)

Ans e.

Laser Doppler flowmeter and pulseoximeter are the recent equipments used to assess pulp circulation.

22. The maxilla is the final facial bone to complete normal growth and development. The condylar head is an important growth center of the mandible.

a. Both the statements are true
b. Both the statements are false
c. The first statement is true and the second is false
d. The first statement is false and the second is true

Ans d.

The mandible is the final facial bone to complete normal growth and development.

23. Condylar injury before the age of 3 years is likely to result in a significant mandibular growth distortion. After 12 years of age, condylar injury has little effect on mandibular growth.

a. Both the statements are true
b. Both the statements are false
c. The first statement is true and the second is false
d. The first statement is false and the second is true

Ans a.

The answer is self-explanatory.

24. It is not advisable to consider permanent crowning until the child is 17 years. This is because the development of the dentofacial structures would not be complete by then.

a. Both the statements are true
b. Both the statements are false
c. The first statement is true and the second is false
d. The first statement is false and the second is true

Ans a.

Use of metal ceramic crowns or ceramic crowns are avoided in children less than 17 years because the final occlusion and gingival margins are not established by that time.

25. In direct pulp capping, the prime requisite of pulp healing is an adequate seal against oral fluids. Therefore a restoration should be placed immediately, which will protect the pulp capping material until the healing process is well advanced.

a. Both the statements are true
b. Both the statements are false
c. The first statement is true and the second is false
d. The first statement is false and the second is true

Ans a.

In other words, after pulp capping a permanent restoration is done in the same visit with cements like GIC, which does not allow marginal leakage. This ensures the success of capping procedure.

26. According to Frank, which of the following is a successful result of apexification?

a. Continued closure of the canal and apex to a normal appearance
b. A dome-shaped apical closure with the canal retaining a blunderbuss appearance
c. No apparent radiographic change but a positive stop in the apical area
d. A positive stop and radiographic evidence of a barrier coronal to the anatomic apex of the tooth
e. Any of the above

Ans e.

Calcium hydroxide and mineral trioxide aggregates are some of the materials used to induce apexification. These procedures are carried out in a nonvital tooth. Apexogenesis occurs in a vital tooth where the root end closes physiologically.

27. A tooth receiving an injury that causes coronal fracture may have a better pulpal prognosis than a tooth that sustains a severe blow without fracturing the crown. This is because a part of the energy of the blow dissipates as the crown fractures rather than all the energy being absorbed by the tooth's supporting tissues.

a. Both the statements are true
b. Both the statements are false
c. The first statement is true and the second is false
d. The first statement is false and the second is true

Ans a.

The answer is self-explanatory.

28. A 9-year-old child reports to the office with a maxillary permanent central incisor having a small hypoplastic spot on the labial surface as the chief complaint. The child gives a history of fall when he was 4 years old, which resulted in a fracture of his maxillary primary incisor. The most probable diagnosis is

a. Hypoplasia due to systemic disease
b. Fluorosis
c. Turner's tooth
d. Amelogenesis imperfecta

Ans c.

Any trauma or infection to primary tooth can result in damage to the succedaneous permanent tooth. This results in hypoplasia of the permanent tooth (Turner's hypoplasia).

29. Primary anterior teeth intruded as the result of a blow may often re-erupt within

a. 3–4 weeks
b. 6–8 weeks
c. 8–12 weeks
d. 7–10 days

Ans a.

Treatment of intrusion of a primary teeth is to wait and watch when there is no impingement on the permanent tooth germ. In such instances, the primary tooth usually re-erupts within 3–4 weeks.

30. Primary teeth that are displaced but not intruded should be repositioned as soon as possible after the accident to prevent interference with occlusion. Frequently, the severely loosened primary tooth remains mobile and undergoes rapid root resorption.

a. Both the statements are true
b. Both the statements are false
c. The first statement is true and the second is false
d. The first statement is false and the second is true

Ans a.

When a primary tooth crown is displaced lingually, the apex and cortical bone moves labially (i.e. away from the developing tooth germ). This tooth is left untreated if there is no interference with occlusion. Over a period of 1 to 2 months, tongue pressure will reposition the tooth. If interference exists, repositioning needs to be done.

31. When a permanent tooth is intruded, the tendency for the injury to be followed by rapid root resorption, pulp necrosis or ankylosis is greater. To prevent this, pulp tissue is extirpated and calcium hydroxide is placed inside the root canal as an interim dressing. This is usually done

a. Within 2 weeks after the injury
b. Within 6 weeks after the injury
c. Immediately after the trauma (in the first visit itself)
d. Within 8 weeks after the injury

Ans a.

Intracanal calcium hydroxide has the ability to arrest or delay the onset of external resorption or ankylosis. Hence it is used whenever there is a possibility of ankylosis or external resorption.

32. The success of the replantation procedure is undoubtedly related to the length of time that elapses between the loss of the tooth and its replacement in the socket. The condition of the tooth and particularly the condition of the periodontal ligament tissue remaining on the root surface are also important factors that influence the success of replantation.

a. Both the statements are true
b. Both the statements are false
c. The first statement is true and the second is false
d. The first statement is false and the second is true

Ans a.

The answer is self-explanatory.

33. Avulsion injuries are more common in children of 7 to 9 years of age when the incisors are erupting. This is because of the loosely structured periodontal ligament around the erupting teeth which favors complete avulsion.

a. Both the statements are true
b. Both the statements are false
c. The first statement is true and the second is false
d. The first statement is false and the second is true

Ans a.

The answer is self-explanatory.

34. The best medium to preserve an avulsed tooth is

a. Milk
b. Isotonic saline
c. Patients oral cavity
d. HBSS (Hank's balanced salt solution)

Ans d.

The answer is self-explanatory.

35. Primary teeth replantation is contraindicated even in the most ideal conditions. This is because of the poorer prognosis and the additional risk of further injury to the succedaneous tooth.

a. Both the statements are true
b. Both the statements are false
c. The first statement is true and the second is false
d. The first statement is false and the second is true

Ans a.

In management of traumatic injuries to the primary dentition, the foremost objective is to prevent the damage to the underlying permanent tooth. Any procedure which is likely to cause damage to the permanent tooth should be avoided.

36. Stabilization by splinting is usually done for 7 to 14 days after avulsion. Rigid stabilization can induce replacement resorption of the root.

a. Both the statements are true
b. Both the statements are false
c. The first statement is true and the second is false
d. The first statement is false and the second is true

Ans a.

The different type of injuries and the recommended duration of splinting:

S. No.	Type of injury	Splinting duration
1.	Subluxation	1–2 weeks
2.	Lateral luxation	4–6 weeks
3.	Root fracture	8–12 weeks

37. All replanted permanent teeth with complete root development should have a pulpectomy soon after replantation regardless of the length of time the tooth was out of the mouth. The pulp is extirpated before the splint is removed preferably within one week after the injury.

a. Both the statements are true
b. Both the statements are false
c. The first statement is true and the second is false
d. The first statement is false and the second is true

Ans a.

Performance of pulpectomy of an avulsed tooth should be carried out in the mouth within the first week. Pulpectomy should not be carried out in the first visit before replantation as this process prolongs the extraoral period time of the tooth. Also, performing a pulpectomy in a splinted tooth is easier than doing it holding the tooth in hand.

38. In root fractures, the best prognosis is with

a. Coronal third fracture
b. Middle third fracture
c. Apical third fracture
d. Fracture between middle and coronal third

Ans c.

Generally, apical third fracture of the root does not need any treatment. Middle third fracture may need splinting for 4 to 6 weeks. Coronal third fracture has the poorest prognosis, as this fracture line tends to communicate with the oral cavity and complicate the healing process.

39. Following a root fracture, healing takes place by which of the following means?

a. Healing with calcified tissue
b. Healing with interposition of connective tissue
c. Healing with interposition of bone and connective tissue
d. Healing with interposition of granulation tissue
e. Any of the above

Ans e.

Healing of root fracture can take place by any of the above-mentioned means.

40. Which of the following is the least favorable form of repair after root fracture?

a. Healing with calcified tissue
b. Healing with interposition of connective tissue
c. Healing with interposition of bone and connective tissue
d. Healing with interposition of granulation tissue

Ans d.

Healing with granulation tissue is the least favorable form of healing of a root fracture.

41. A relatively long stabilization period is required for teeth with fractured roots. This seems to encourage the more favorable type of healing with calcified tissue.

a. Both the statements are true
b. Both the statements are false

c. The first statement is true and the second is false
d. The first statement is false and the second is true

Ans a.

The answer is self-explanatory. Refer to the explanation of Q. No. 40.

42. Splints for root fractures should be more rigid than the splints used for stabilization after other types of displacement injuries. The usual duration for splinting of root fractures is for

a. 3 months
b. 3 weeks
c. 2–3 weeks
d. 1 month

Ans a.

Refer to the explanation of Q. No. 41.

43. Which type of tissue necrosis is predominant in oral electrical burns?

a. Fat necrosis
b. Liquefaction necrosis
c. Coagulation necrosis
d. Caseation necrosis

Ans c.

A common cause of oral burns is electrical trauma. The most frequently encountered electrical injury to children is a burn around the mouth. These burns occur often in children between 6 months and 3 years of age and are equally common among boys and girls.

44. Eschar is

a. The necrotic tissue after an electrical burn
b. Scar tissue which forms after minor oral surgeries like frenectomies
c. Scar tissue in the palate
d. An organized clot

Ans a.

Within a few hours after the burn injury there may be a great increase in edema. In 7–10 days the edema begins to subside. The necrotic tissue known as eschar becomes charred or crusty in appearance and begins to separate from the surrounding viable tissue.

45. After electrical burns, a burn appliance is given to prevent contracture of healing tissue and to serve as a framework on which a normal appearing commissure may be created and preserved. This is usually delivered between

a. 2–3 days after the injury
b. 10–14 days after injury
c. 6–8 weeks after injury
d. 1–2 days after injury

Ans b.

This burn appliance is given 10–14 days after injury to prevent a contracture and preserve a normal appearing commissure.

46. Which of the following is true about the burn appliance?

a. It has to be worn 24 hours a day for 9–12 months except for eating and cleaning
b. The appliance is a static base with wings extending laterally to provide contact with both commissures
c. The shape and location of the wings are important not only in preventing contracture or cohesion of the lips during healing but also in shaping the affected commissure to duplicate the unaffected side
d. All of the above

Ans d.

The answer is self-explanatory.

47. If during extraction of a primary molar, the permanent tooth bud is accidentally totally withdrawn from the mouth, the treatment of choice is to

a. Discard the tooth bud
b Curette this area thoroughly
c. Perform pulpotomy and replant the tooth bud
d. Perform pulpectomy and replant the tooth bud
e. Replace the tooth bud deep into the alveolus from which it came

Ans e.

The answer is self-explanatory.

48. A severe blow to the anterior permanent tooth, not causing fracture, frequently leads to

a. Permanent looseness

b. Immediate pulpal death
c. Pulpal death, but only if treatment is delayed too long
d. Pulpal death regardless of treatment
e. None of the above. In the absence of fracture no permanent damage could result

Ans d.

A severe blow to a permanent anterior tooth not causing fracture can interrupt the blood supply to the pulp through the apex leading to ischemia and pulpal death.

49. The radiograph of a traumatized tooth is necessary to

a. Assess the stage of the root development
b. Determine the presence or absence of root fractures
c. Have a base from which comparisons can be made with future radiographs
d. All of the above

Ans d.

Radiographs of a traumatized tooth is necessary to detect root fractures, extent of root development, size of the pulp chamber, periapical radiolucencies, resorption, degree of tooth displacement, position of unerupted teeth, jaw fractures and presence of tooth fragments and other foreign bodies in the soft tissues. Generally, follow-up radiographs are taken to detect inflammatory root resorption (3 weeks) and replacement resorption (6–7 weeks).

50. An 8-year-old girl has lost both maxillary incisors in an accident. The best treatment would be

a. Do nothing except observe
b. Move lateral incisor into central incisor position
c. Construct and place a space maintainer with bands cemented on the lateral incisors
d. Place a temporary prosthesis supplying artificial crowns for the lost central incisors
e. Construct and install a permanent bridge using lateral incisors as abutments

Ans d.

When incisors are lost to trauma, usually the space is maintained using temporary prosthesis with artificial crowns and ultimately restorative or implant solutions are used when the growth is completed.

51. Which of the following is most diagnostic of ankylosis of a primary molar?

a. Change in color
b. Cessation of eruption
c. Cushioned sound on percussion
d. Radiographic density of lamina dura
e. Loss of vitality on electric pulp testing

Ans b.

Ankylosis, the fusion of tooth to bone is common in primary dentition. The ankylosed tooth cannot erupt further but the unaffected adjacent teeth will continue to erupt. This creates an illusion that the ankylosed tooth is submerged in bone. Prevalence of ankylosed teeth in primary dentition is between 7 and 14%. The sequence of commonly ankylosed teeth is:

1. Mandibular primary first molar
2. Mandibular primary second molar
3. Maxillary primary first molar
4. Maxillary primary second molar

52. An ankylosed primary molar may result in all the following except

a. Loss of arch length
b. A serious problem of extraction
c. Delayed eruption of succeeding premolar
d. Failure of calcification of the permanent successor

Ans d.

Ankylosis of a primary tooth at an early age may result in large marginal ridge discrepancies, tipping of adjacent teeth and vertical bone loss and all these problems except space loss resolves when the succedaneous tooth erupts.

53. Ankylosis occurs most frequently in which of the following tooth?

a. Permanent maxillary lateral incisor
b. Primary mandibular canines
c. Primary mandibular first molars
d. Primary maxillary second molars

Ans c.

Refer to the explanation of Q. No. 51.

54. The chief cause of failure of replantation of permanent tooth is

a. Ankylosis
b. Infection
c. Pulpal necrosis resorption
d. External resorption
e. Internal resorption

Ans d.

The chief cause of failure of replantation of permanent teeth is external resorption. The primary therapeutic concern in avulsed teeth is to maintain the vitality of periodontal ligament fibers and the longer they are out of the mouth, the worse the prognosis for their survival. PDL cells on avulsed teeth that have been stored dry for more than one hour are necrotic and they will eventually resorb. As soon as this external resorption is detected radiographically, pulp tissue is extirpated followed by copious irrigation with sodium hypochlorite which helps in the dissolution of organic debris in the canal followed by placement of interim intracanal medicament with calcium hydroxide.

55. A primary incisor that is traumatized often discolors subsequent to the injury as a result of

a. Degeneration of the pulp
b. Pressure of the developing permanent tooth
c. Extravasation of blood elements in to the dentinal tubule
d. Loss of union between the periodontal ligament and the tooth

Ans c.

As a result of trauma, when pulpal hemorrhage occurs red blood cells undergo lysis and release hemoglobin. Hemoglobin and hemoglobin derivatives such as hematin molecules that contain iron ions invade the dentin tubules and stain the tooth dark. The colors are traditionally divided into pink, red, yellow and dark.

S. No.	Color	Significance
1.	Pink discoloration	Is observed shortly after the injury and may represent intrapulpal hemorrhage
2.	Red discoloration	A reddish hue noticed long after the injury is and usually due to internal resorption in the pulp chamber
3.	Yellow discoloration	Can be seen when the dentin is thick and the pulp chamber narrows than usual (Pulp canal obliteration)
4.	Dark discoloration	Is the most controversial posttraumatic complication in terms of the significance of the change in tooth color. Term "dark" refers to a variety of shades including black, grey, brown and intermediate hues.

56. The most frequent cause of fracture of root tips in the extraction of primary molar is

a. Improper use of cowhorn forceps
b. Ankylosis of the primary molar
c. Presence of a supernumerary premolar
d. Resorption of the root between apex and bifurcation
e. Asymmetrical resorption of the molar roots in which only one root is completely resorbed

Ans d.

The answer is self-explanatory.

57. Fractured maxillary anterior teeth generally occur most often in children with

a. Maxillary retrusion
b. Class I malocclusion
c. Class II, div. 1 malocclusion
d. Class II, div. 2 malocclusion
e. Class III malocclusion

Ans c.

Presence of a Class II, div. 1 malocclusion is indicative of an accident-prone dental profile and a causal factor for sports-related dental injuries. Clinical presence of narrow maxillary arch and inadequate lip seal and excessive overjet, overbite, protruding maxillary incisors, labial inclination and spacing between maxillary incisors increases the potential for fracture. Also refer to the explanation of Q. No. 7.

58. In a root fracture of the apical one-third of a permanent anterior tooth, the tooth usually

a. Requires endodontic treatment
b. Remains in function and is vital
c. Undergoes pulpal necrosis and becomes ankylosed
d. Is indicated for extraction and prosthetic replacement

Ans b.

The prognosis for root fracture is best when the fracture occurs in the apical one-third of the root. The prognosis worsens progressively with fractures that occur cervically on the root. Bender and Freedland reported that more than 75% of the teeth with intra-alveolar (apical third) root fractures maintain their vitality. Also refer to the explanation of Q. No. 38.

59. Primary teeth discolored by trauma with no clinical signs of infection should be

a. Bleached
b. Pulp tested
c. Receive root canal therapy
d. Examined by periodic radiograph

Ans d.

Traumatically injured teeth with avascular necrosis may remain asymptomatic both clinically and radiographically and exfoliate uneventfully. Hence the discoloration alone in the absence of clinical signs of infection should be observed periodically with radiographs. Tooth should be treated only if there are any clinical signs (gum boil, periapical radiolucency, pain, nocturnal pain, swelling) of infection.

60. A 9-year-old boy has a traumatized permanent central incisor with a pulp exposure of 2 mm in diameter. The injury occurred 4 weeks ago; the tooth now has a necrotic pulp. Radiographs show that the root has developed to two-thirds of its length and has a wide open apex. No other significant signs and symptoms exist. Treatment of choice is to

a. Extract the tooth and place a prosthesis
b. Induce apexification and fill the root canal
c. Fill the root canal and place a retrograde amalgam
d. Perform complete orthodontic treatment and fill the root canal with cement

Ans b.

Apexification is a method of treatment for immature permanent teeth in which root growth and development ceased due to pulp necrosis. Its purpose is to allow the formation of an apical barrier. Apexification is traditionally performed using a calcium hydroxide dressing that disinfects the root canal and induces apical closure. Nowadays, MTA is widely used for this purpose.

61. A 4-year-old child has a traumatized central incisor with a Class IX (Ellis) fracture. The injury occurred about a month ago, and examination indicates that the pulp is necrotic. There are no other pathological findings. Treatment of choice is

a. Watchful observation
b. Extraction and use of space maintainer
c. Pulpectomy and root canal filling using gutta- percha points and cement
d. Endodontic treatment and root canal filling with a resorbable paste

Ans d.

Several treatment options are available for crown fracture with pulp exposure in primary teeth, including pulpotomy, pulpectomy and extraction. The vitality of the tissue and the time elapsed since the injury dictate the treatment of choice.

62. Examination reveals a large pulp exposure in a fractured permanent incisor that has a fully formed apex. Indicated treatment is

a. Pulpotomy
b. Direct pulp capping
c. Indirect pulp capping
d. Full root canal treatment
e. No treatment until pulp dies

Ans d.

Size of the exposure is a determinant on the treatment planning. A large exposure usually needs a full root canal treatment.

63. A primary maxillary anterior tooth in a 4-year-old child was traumatically intruded into the tissues so that only half the tooth is visible. The most appropriate treatment is to

a. Extract the tooth
b. Perform a pulpotomy
c. Administer no treatment
d. Place orthodontic bands on adjacent teeth and draw the tooth down with elastics

Ans c.

Intruded primary incisors that do not cause permanent tooth damage can be left to spontaneously re-erupt. Re-eruption begins within 2–3 weeks but occasionally can be delayed for more than 6 months. In many cases, the teeth do not erupt back to their original position but into a rotated alignment. Also refer to the explanation of Q. No. 29.

64. Treatment of root fracture in the apical third of a permanent central incisor includes

a. Extraction
b. Calcium hydroxide pulpotomy
c. Immobilization for 2–4 weeks
d. Immobilization for 2–4 months

Ans c.

Optimal results are obtained if the coronal fragment is repositioned and splinted as soon as possible. Former recommendations called for firm immobilization with a splint for several months. Recent evidence indicates that root fractured teeth may heal better if splinted for only 3–4 weeks with a functional splint that allows for some mobility of the teeth (refer Q. No. 58).

65. A 9½-year-old child has a white spot on the facial surface of a permanent maxillary central incisor. This condition is most probably due to

a. Hypocalcification secondary to trauma to the primary dentition in the area
b. Hypoplastic defect secondary to a systemic infection at 6–12 months of age.
c. Disturbance during the morphodifferentiation stage of tooth development
d. Hypocalcified enamel secondary to increased calcium uptake in the tooth at 6–12 months age

Ans a.

Intrusive luxation of a primary incisor is potentially one of the most serious traumatic injuries to the underlying developing permanent tooth bud. If the traumatic insult occurs during the apposition stage, when the deposition of dentin and enamel matrix takes place, a localized enamel hypoplasia of the crown of the permanent tooth may result. It is also known as Turner's hypoplasia. It can be caused by long standing infection associated with a primary tooth too. Also refer to Q. No. 28.

66. A 11-year-old patient fractured a permanent incisor 2 hours ago. An Ellis Class III mesioangular fracture is now evident. The treatment of choice is to

a. Perform a pulpotomy
b. Perform a partial pulpectomy
c. Institute a gutta-percha endodontic procedures
d. Place calcium hydroxide and perform a composite restoration

Ans d.

Direct pulp capping using calcium hydroxide is indicated in small pulpal exposures that can be treated within few hours of the injury. The objective of the treatment is to preserve vital pulp tissue that is free of inflammation and physiologically walled off by calcific barrier.

67. A traumatized primary tooth turns pink over a period of time. The pathologic change that has occurred is

a. Ankylosis
b. Enamel hypoplasia

c. Complete necrosis
d. Internal resorption

Ans d.

Internal resorption is a destructive process generally believed to be caused by odontoclastic action. It may be observed radiographically in the pulp chamber or canal within a few weeks or months after an injury. The destructive process may progress slowly or rapidly. If progression is rapid, it may cause a perforation of the crown or root within a few weeks. Mummery described this condition as "pink spot" because when the crown is affected, the vascular tissues of the pulp shine through the remaining thin shell of enamel (refer explanation of Q. No. 55).

68. Which of the following statements is correct regarding the "submerged" primary molar?

a. The tooth is non-vital
b. The tooth is ankylosed
c. There is no permanent successor
d. Resorption of roots is not evident
e. The periodontal ligament is thickened

Ans b.

Refer to the explanation of Q. Nos. 52, 53 and 54.

69. A 7-year-old girl has a Class II fracture (2 × 4 mm of dentin exposed) of a maxillary central incisor. The tooth is vital, and there are no other pathologic signs or symptoms. The immediate treatment of choice is to

a. Perform a pulpotomy using calcium hydroxide
b. Restore the tooth with a permanent restoration
c. Smooth the margins of the tooth and observe
d. Apply calcium hydroxide to the exposed dentin and restore the tooth with a permanent restoration

Ans d.

The primary issue in managing fractures that expose the dentin is to prevent bacterial irritants from reaching the pulp. Thus, the exposed dentin is covered with calcium hydroxide or GIC to seal out oral flora, followed by permanent restoration.

70. A child with a dental age of 11 years traumatized a central incisor 6 months prior to a visit to the dental office. The chief complaint is intermittent swelling and pain. Examination discloses periapical pathosis. Suggested treatment is

a. Pulpotomy
b. Observation
c. Root canal therapy
d. Extraction of the tooth

Ans c.

A pulpectomy is indicated when root maturation is complete. Occasionally a patient has a periapical abscess associated with a traumatized tooth. If an abscess is present, it must be treated first. If there is acute pain and swelling of soft tissues, drainage through pulp canal will give the child almost immediate relief.

71. How reliable are electric pulp tests of traumatized, young permanent anterior teeth taken immediately after injury?

a. Never reliable
b. Seldom reliable
c. Usually reliable
d. Highly reliable if multiple readings are made
e. Highly reliable if an adjustment is made for the degree of recuperation

Ans b.

Following traumatic injuries, the tooth may be in a state of shock and can give false response. Hence, the reading after the injury should not be taken as the only reading; further testing should be performed on subsequent visits.

72. A 9-year-old patient has a noncarious primary maxillary right first molar in infraocclusion. The radiograph shows lack of periodontal ligament and a radiolucent area that may be normal resorption. The first premolar is present. The first molar is best treated by

a. Observation
b. Extraction only
c. Routine extraction and space maintenance
d. Surgical removal and space maintenance

Ans a.

An ankylosed tooth discovered during the developmental stage should not be removed routinely unless a large marginal ridge discrepancy develops between the tooth and the unaffected adjacent teeth. If a marginal ridge discrepancy exists, the adjacent teeth may tip into the space occupied by the ankylosed tooth and cause space loss. Under such circumstances, the ankylosed tooth may be considered for extraction.

73. A 11-year-old child comes to the dental office one hour after injury to a maxillary central incisor. The tooth is vital and slightly mobile. Radiographic examination reveals a fracture at the apical third of the root. The indicated treatment at this time is to

a. Render palliative therapy
b. Extract the tooth
c. Relieve the occlusion and splint the tooth
d. Perform immediate root canal treatment and splint

Ans c.

A tooth with fractured root is usually mobile and its coronal fragment is often displaced. Hence splinting with relieving the occlusion will help in good prognosis. Also refer to the explanation of Q. No. 64.

74. A maxillary central incisor of an 8-year-old boy was completely displaced. The avulsed tooth was found, and the patient was seen by his dentist 20 minutes after the injury. Immediate treatment of choice is to

a. Clean the tooth with saline, then replant the tooth in its socket
b. Plant the root to remove necrotic tissue, then replant the tooth in its socket
c. Sterilize the tooth in a strong cold sterilizing solution, then replant the tooth in its socket
d. Perform endodontic treatment and root canal filling, then replant the tooth in its socket

Ans a.

The tooth should be rinsed carefully with a stream of saline from a syringe. Special care should be taken to rinse the apical part of the pulp as well. Due to very patent apical foramen, revascularization of the pulp is considered possible. Basic requirement for optimal healing are that the tooth is out of the socket for as short a period as possible, that the extra-alveolar storage is in physiologic medium and the contamination of the tooth is eliminated, reduced and controlled by antibiotics.

75. Which one of the following is a numerical classification?

a. Andreasen's classification
b. Ellis and Davey classification
c. WHO classification
d. SHY Wei classification

Ans c.

The World Health Organization has adopted a system of classification in its application of international classification of disease to Dentistry and Stomatology in 1978. Every injury has a code number.

76. Trauma to the teeth resulting in loosening but no displacement is

a. Concussion
b. Subluxation
c. Luxation
d. Avulsion

Ans b.

Subluxation is defined as evidence of abnormal movement in horizontal and/or vertical direction with sensitivity to percussion and occlusal forces. There is usually clinical evidence of hemorrhage around the gingival margin indicating damage to the periodontal ligament .

77. A 4-year-old boy had a fracture in the upper central incisors involving the enamel and dentin with pulpal involvement. It is

a. Ellis Class III
b. Ellis Class II
c. Ellis Class I
d. Ellis Class IX

Ans d.

Refer to the explanation of Q. No. 13.

78. An incomplete fracture of enamel without loss of tooth structure is

a. Crown infraction
b. Crown infarction
c. Enamel fracture
d. Ellis Class I fracture

Ans a.

Enamel infraction is defined as an incomplete fracture of the enamel without loss of tooth substances. The fracture lines can be detected by the use of trans-illumination or staining of teeth with disclosing solution. The infraction appears as a vertical or horizontal crack or craze on the tooth. The injury does not require any initial therapy but the injured tooth should be periodically evaluated for the possible sequelae of trauma as explained earlier.

79. Hemorrhage around the gingival margin indicates damage to the

a. Gingiva
b. Tooth
c. Periodontal ligament
d. Pulp

Ans c.

Greater impact to the teeth will result in subluxation, whereby some periodontal ligament fibers will be ruptured and the tooth loosened, but not displaced. There is often slight bleeding from the gingival sulcus.

80. Avulsion/exarticulation is classified in Ellis and Davey's classification as

a. Ellis Class IV
b. Ellis Class V
c. Ellis Class VI
d. Ellis Class VII

Ans b.

Refer to the explanation of Q. No. 13.

81. A 9-year-old girl has Ellis Class III fracture in 11 with a sinus opening. The treatment of choice is

a. Apexogenesis
b. Apexification
c. Direct pulp capping
d. Cvek's pulpotomy

Ans b.

Refer to the explanation of Q. No. 60.

82. A 12-year-old boy has a fracture line in 21 involving the enamel, dentin, pulp and cementum. It is described as

a. Complicated crown fracture
b. Uncomplicated crown fracture
c. Complicated crown root fracture
d. Uncomplicated crown root fracture

Ans c.

Fracture involving enamel, dentin, cementum with pulp involvement is called complicated crown root fracture. Whenever there is pulpal involvement, it is called "complicated".

Chapter 27

Sports Dentistry for Children and Adolescents

1. Which of the following is the primary reason for dental injuries being under-reported?

a. They contribute to only 10% of the orofacial injuries
b. The lack of standardized national and international reporting norms
c. Because sports dentistry is not a field of sports medicine
d. They are less important as a health entity

Ans b.

The answer is self-explanatory.

2. According to Fusilier, the presence of impacted third molars can place the individuals at a higher risk of fracture of

a. body of the mandible
b. angle of the mandible
c. ramus of the mandible
d. symphysis of the mandible

Ans b.

The presence of impacted third molars can put the individual at a higher risk of fracture at the angle of the mandible. Hence, the younger athletes can go for an assessment of third molars around the athletic activity.

3. The predictive index for sports-related injuries is based on the

a. Intensity and velocity of the sport
b. Intensity and frequency of the sport
c. Velocity and frequency of the sport
d. Intensity, velocity and frequency of the sport

Ans a.

Peter J. Fos has given a detailed description of development of a "predictive index" for sports-related traumatic injuries. Sport activities can be characterized according to two dimensions, the velocity and intensity of the sport. Each dimension can be divided further into three levels: high, moderate and low. Using these dimensions, a sports classification matrix was constructed.

4. **In the predictive index, hockey is placed as a**
   a. High intensity and high velocity sports
   b. Low intensity and low velocity sports
   c. High intensity and low velocity sports
   d. Low intensity and high velocity sports

Ans a.

Hockey is a high intensity contact sport with high velocity. Hence, this sport can be categorized as high risk category in the predictive index.

5. **One of the following parts of the body is not protected by a helmet without a face mask:**
   a. Occipital bone
   b. Zygoma
   c. Ears
   d. Skull

Ans b.

Face mask is designed to protect the eyes, nose and zygoma from any traumatic injuries. Most of the organized sports like boxing, ice hockey and football mandate the use of helmets, face masks and mouth guards during practice and competition. Helmet without a face mask will not protect the zygoma.

6. **The Academy for Sports Dentistry states that the "properly fitted mouth guard" should fulfill the following criteria:**
   a. A fit that is retentive and not dislodged on impact
   b. Adequate thickness in all areas to provide for the reduction of impact force
   c. Speech considerations equal to the demands of the playing status of the athlete
   d. All of the above

Ans d.

The answer is self-explanatory.

7. **One of the following is not a disadvantage of stock mouth guards**
   a. Least retentive
   b. Bulky
   c. Interfere with the athlete's ability to speak
   d. Have an unpleasant odour and taste

Ans d.

The answer is self-explanatory.

8. **One of the following is not a disadvantage of mouth-formed mouth guards**

a. Least retentive
b. Too bulky
c. Uncomfortable to wear
d. Have an unpleasant odour and taste

Ans a.

The mouth-formed mouth guards are fabricated with impression taken from the subject. Hence, these mouth guards have the best retention.

9. Which of the following are the advantages of boil and bite mouth guards?

a. Easy to use
b. Its fit can be modified
c. Comes in a wide variety of styles and colors
d. All of the above

Ans d.

The answer is self-explanatory.

10. Which of the following is a disadvantage of custom-fabricated mouth guards?

a. Its fit can be modified
b. Multiple dental visits are needed for fabrication
c. Least retentive
d. Have an unpleasant odor and taste

Ans b.

The answer is self-explanatory.

11. One of the following is not true regarding maintenance of mouth guards

a. Mouth guards should be washed with hot water
b. Mouth guards should be cleansed with a toothbrush and toothpaste
c. Mouth guards should be stored in a plastic container
d. Mouth guards should be periodically inspected for perforations and distortions

Ans a.

Mouth guards should be washed after each use in cold or lukewarm water to minimize accumulation of debris. Washing with hot water should be avoided as it may cause deformation of the mouth guard.

Section VIII
Pediatric Orthodontics

Chapter 28

Preventive and Interceptive Orthodontics

1. Cephalometer was introduced by

a. Simon
b. Racini and Carerra
c. Broadbent
d. Tweed

Ans c.

Broadbent introduced the cephalometer in 1931. In 1922, Simon introduced gnathostatics, a photographic technique that related the teeth and their respective bony bases to each other as well as to specific craniofacial structures. Racini and Carerra obtained the first X-ray films of the skull by the standard lateral view in 1926. Tweed, Steiner and Ricketts developed the clinical application of cephalometrics and developed the techniques that permit the observation of discrepancies observed in the mandible, maxilla, dental units and soft-tissue profile.

2. While taking a cephalometric radiograph, the distance between the subject (midsagittal plane) and the X-ray tube is

a. 60 inches
b. 120 inches
c. 180 inches
d. 30 inches

Ans a.

While taking a cephalometric radiograph, the head of the subject is stabilized by a cephalostat (head holder) and the X-ray tube is positioned at a distance of 60 inches from the midsagittal plane of the subject.

3. Frankfort horizontal plane is

a. Imaginary line from lower border of nose to lower border of ear
b. Imaginary plane from lower border of the orbit to tragus of ear
c. Imaginary plane from lower border of nose to tragus of ear
d. Imaginary line from upper border of orbit to tragus of ear

Ans b.

Refer the following table describing the cephalometric points and planes.

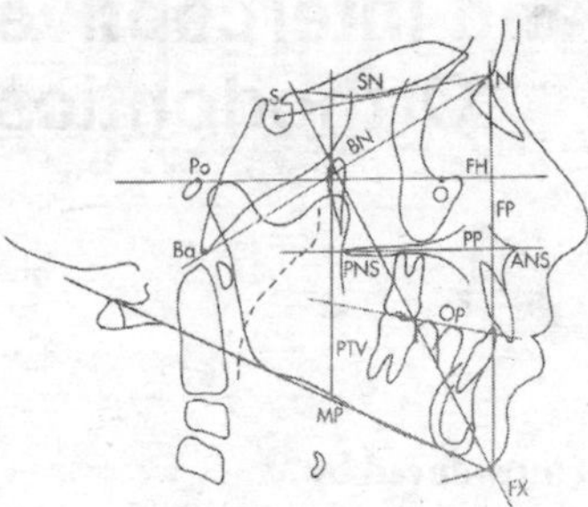

Fig. 28.1 Cephalometric points and planes.

Cephalometric points	Description
Sella turcica (S or Sella)	The midpoint of hypophyseal fossa.
Nasion (N)	The external junction of nasofrontal suture in the median plane. If the suture is not visible, this point is located at the deepest concavity of the two bones.
Orbitale (O)	The most inferior point on the external border of the orbit.
Condylion (Cd)	The most superior point on the articular head of the condyle.
Anterior nasal spine (ANS)	The most anterior projection of the anterior nasal spine of the maxilla in the median plane.
A point (subspinale or A)	The deepest point of the curvature of the anterior maxilla between ANS and the alveolar crest. Although A point may change with treatment, it represents the most forward point of the maxilla.
B point (supramentale or B)	The most posterior point on the outer curve of the mandibular alveolar process between the alveolar crest and the bony chin. B point delineates the most anterior point of the mandible in the median plane.
Pogonion (Pg)	The most anterior point on the midsagittal mandibular symphysis.
Menton (M)	The most inferior point of the mandibular symphysis.
Gnathion (Gn)	A constructed point that is formed by the intersection of the facial and mandibular planes.

Gonion (Go)	A constructed point that is represented by the intersection of the lines tangent to the posterior margin of the ascending ramus and the mandibular plane.
Articulare (Ar)	The point of intersection of the posterior margin of the ascending ramus and the outer margin of the cranial base.
Porion (Po)	A point located at the most superior point of the external auditory meatus or the superior aspect of metal ring that is a component of the left ear rod of the cephalostat.
Basion (Ba)	The most inferior posterior point on the occipital bone that corresponds to the anterior margin of the foramen magnum.
Pterygomaxillary fissure (Ptm)	A teardrop shaped fissure of which the anterior borders of the pterygoid plates of the sphenoid bone create the posterior wall and the anterior wall represents the posterior border of the maxilla (maxillary tuberosity). The tip of the fissure denotes the posterior extent of the maxilla.
Posterior nasal spine (PNS)	The tip of the posterior spine of palatine bone. This landmark is usually not visible on well-exposed lateral head films; therefore it is a constructed point that is represented by the intersection of a continuation of the anterior wall of the pterygopalatine fossa and the floor of the nose. It also denotes the posterior limit of the maxilla.
Pt point (Pt)	The intersection of the inferior border of the foramen rotundum with the posterior wall of Ptm.
CF point (center of face)	The cephalometric landmark formed by the intersection of the Frankfort horizontal plane and a perpendicular line through Pt.
Frankfort horizontal plane (FH)	This plane is constructed from porion to orbitale and represents the basic horizontal plane of the head.
Pterygoid vertical plane (PTV)	A line perpendicular to the Frankfort horizontal plane through the Pt point represents this plane. Studies have shown that the intersection of FH and PTV is very stable, since growth has little effect on this point.

Basion Nasion plane (BN)	This plane passes through basion and nasion. This plane represents cranial base and is the dividing plane between the cranium and the face.
Sella Nasion plane (SN)	A line connecting the sella and the nasion represents this plane. It denotes the anteroposterior extent of the anterior cranial base. This reference plane is of questionable diagnostic value in true mandibular prognathism.
Occlusal plane (OP)	This plane separates the mandibular and maxillary permanent molars (or in younger patients the primary second molars) and passes through the contact between the most anterior maxillary and mandibular incisors. If the incisors do not contact, the line passes midway between the incisal edges. OP is nearly parallel to both the palatal plane and the Frankfort horizontal plane.
Facial plane (FP)	A line constructed through the nasion perpendicular to the Frankfort horizontal plane represents this plane.
Mandibular plane(MP)	The mandibular plane is constructed as a tangent to the inferior border of the mandible.
Facial axis (FX)	This line is constructed from Pt point through gnathion. FX ideally crosses the basion nasion plane at a right angle.
Palatal plane (PP)	This plane extends through the anterior nasal spine and posterior nasal spine. The relationship of this plane to FH is useful in evaluating the treatment changes occurring in the maxilla.

4. The normal SNA is

a. 90–92 degrees
b. 80–82 degrees
c. 60–62 degrees
d. 70–72 degrees

Ans b.

SNA is the angle between SN plane and A point. The clinical norm for SNA is 82 degrees. This establishes the horizontal location of the maxilla.

5. The normal ANB is

a. 8–10 degrees
b. 2–4 degrees
c. 12 degrees
d. 0 degree

Ans b.

ANB is the difference between SNA and SNB angles. The clinical norm for ANB is 2 degrees. This indicates the horizontal relationship between maxilla and mandible. Positive values indicate that the maxilla is forward of the mandible, whereas negative values indicate a Class III skeletal relationship.

6. The normal incisor mandibular plane angle (IMPA) is

a. 60–64 degrees
b. 90–94 degrees
c. 120–124 degrees
d. 34 degrees

Ans b.

IMPA is the inner angle between the long axis of the mandibular incisor and mandibular plane. The clinical norm is 90 degrees. This is an evaluation of the angular position of the incisor to the mandibular basal bone.

7. The normal mandibular plane angle (FMA) is

a. 26 degrees (1 degree decreases every 4 years during normal growth)
b. 26 degrees (1 degree increases every 4 years during normal growth)
c. 46 degrees (4 degrees decrease every 2 years during normal growth)
d. 56 degrees (4 degrees decrease every 2 years during normal growth)

Ans a.

FMA is the angle formed by the intersection of Frankfurt horizontal plane and mandibular plane. The clinical norm is 26 degrees. This will decrease 1 degree every 4 years during normal growth. Values in excess of 31 degrees may indicate clockwise growth with dolichofacial growth trends, whereas values less than 21 degrees imply vertical deficiency often seen in brachyfacial growth patterns.

8. Convex facial profile is characteristic of which malocclusion?

a. Class I malocclusion
b. Class II malocclusion (div. 1)
c. Class III malocclusion
d. Class I with crowding

Ans b.

Class I malocclusion generally has a straight profile. Concave profile is characteristic of Class III malocclusion. Convex profile is usually seen in Class II, div. 1 malocclusion.

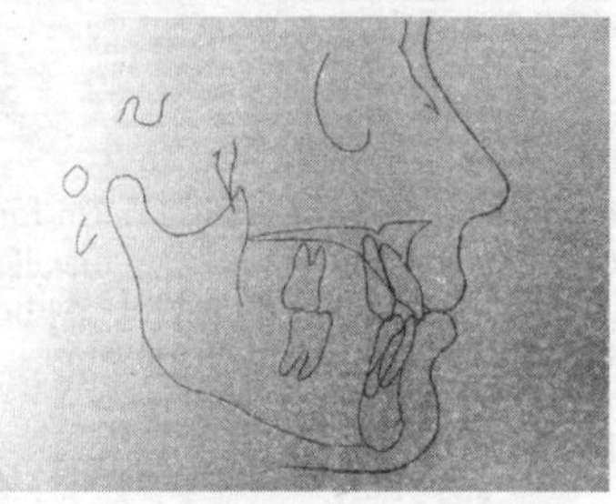

Fig. 28.2 Straight profile.

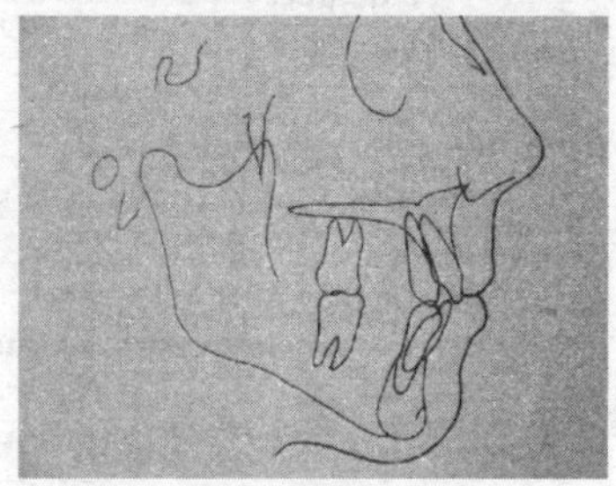

Fig. 28.3 Convex profile.

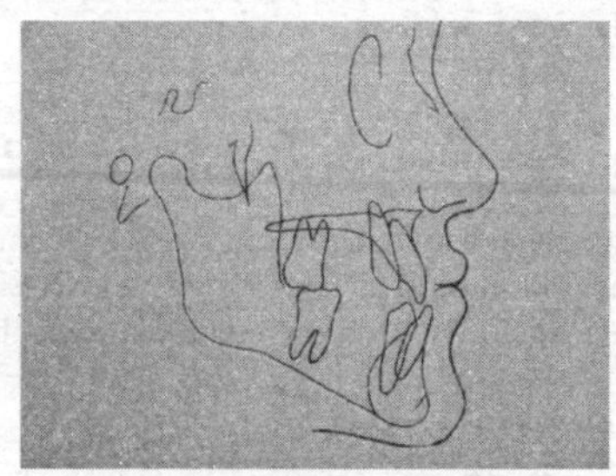

Fig. 28.4 Concave profile.

9. Dolichofacial facial pattern is more common in patients with

a. Class I malocclusion
b. Class II malocclusion (div. 1)
c. Class III malocclusion
d. Class I with crowding

Ans b.

The faces of these patients are usually long and of weak musculature because of the tendency for vertical growth. The molar occlusion is often of the Class II, div. 1 variety.

10. Brachyfacial pattern of face is more common in patients with

a. Class I malocclusion
b. Class II malocclusion (div. 1)
c. Class III malocclusion
d. Class II malocclusion (div. 2)

Ans d.

The short faces and wide square mandibles of these patients are most often associated with Class II, div. 2 malocclusions. These patients typically exhibit excessive anterior overbites and strong chins.

11. Open bites can be caused by

a. Abnormal habits
b. Deviant growth patterns
c. Forward tongue position
d. Any of the above

Ans d.

Abnormal habits like thumb sucking, digit sucking and tongue thrusting can result in anterior open bite. Forward tongue position can cause anterior open bite, which is more commonly seen in children with Down syndrome.

12. Anterior crossbite involving one of the permanent incisors should be corrected

a. As soon as it is detected
b. At the age of 7 years
c. Before the eruption of permanent canines
d. After the eruption of permanent canines

Ans a.

Anterior crossbite of one or more of the permanent incisors should be treated as soon as it is detected. Delayed treatment can lead to serious complications such as loss of arch length, gingival stripping, etc.

13. Delayed treatment of anterior crossbite can lead to

a. Loss of arch length
b. Gingival stripping because of traumatic occlusion
c. Wear facets on the labial and incisal surfaces of involved incisors
d. Any of the above

Ans d.

Delayed treatment of anterior crossbite can lead to any of the above-mentioned complications.

14. Anterior crossbite is caused by

a. Presence of a supernumerary tooth
b. Trauma to primary teeth resulting in displacement of permanent teeth
c. An arch length deficiency
d. All of the above

Ans d.

All of the above-mentioned causes can lead to anterior crossbite. A labially positioned supernumerary tooth may cause lingual deflection of an incisor, which may erupt in a crossbite relationship. Trauma to primary tooth or delayed exfoliation of primary tooth can lead to displacement of permanent tooth and eruption in crossbite. An arch length deficiency in the maxillary arch can cause the maxillary lateral incisor to erupt palatally resulting in anterior crossbite.

15. Which of the following factors should be present to correct anterior crossbite by simple appliances?

a. Sufficient room should be present mesiodistally to move the tooth into its correct position
b. Sufficient overbite should be present to hold the tooth in its new position
c. The apical portion of the in locked tooth should be relatively in the same position as that of the normal tooth
d. The patient should have normal occlusion in the molar and canine areas
e. All of the above

Ans e.

If all of the above-mentioned factors are present, then the case may be considered uncomplicated and anterior crossbite can be corrected with simple appliances.

16. Teeth in the initial stage of eruption with a minimal degree of interlocking (crossbite) can be repositioned within 24 hours by using

a. Lower cemented bite plane
b. Tongue blade therapy
c. Appliance with double cantilever spring
d. Fixed appliance.

Ans b.

In children who are cooperative and have proper encouragement and guidance at home, an anterior crossbite (developing crossbite) can be corrected with a narrow wooden tongue blade. The child is instructed to place the tongue blade behind the inlocked tooth and use the chin as fulcrum to exert pressure on the tooth toward the labial side. This procedure should be practiced at least 5 minutes each hour as often as possible during the day. But the results of this therapy are often disappointing because of lack of cooperation. Lower cemented bite plane (inclined plane) is indicated when the posterior teeth are not present for retention for removable Hawley's appliance with double cantilever spring. A removable Hawley's appliance with double cantilever spring is the widely used treatment option to correct anterior crossbite. Fixed appliance is used to correct anterior crossbite when adequate space is not available for the tooth to move in a labial position (severe arch length deficiency).

17. Which of the following is true about tongue blade therapy?

a. The tongue blade is used, using the chin as fulcrum and exerting pressure on the tooth towards the labial side
b. The procedure should be practiced at least 5 minutes every hour during the day
c. It is used to correct the teeth in the initial stage of eruption with minimal degree of interlocking
d. All of the above

Ans d.

All the above-mentioned factors are true regarding tongue blade therapy.

18. Which of the following is true regarding the inclined plane?

a. The inclination of the inclined plane is 45 degrees to the long axis of the lower incisors
b. After placing the inclined plane, the posterior teeth should be out of contact by 2–3 mm
c. Patient should be seen every 2–3 days
d. All of the above

Ans d.

All the above-mentioned factors are true regarding inclined plane. Also the child should be encouraged to follow a normal diet and the physical activities should be restricted.

19. W-arch (Porter appliance) and quadhelix appliances are used for crossbite correction. A fixed acrylic jackscrew appliance causes palatal expansion and less dental tipping.

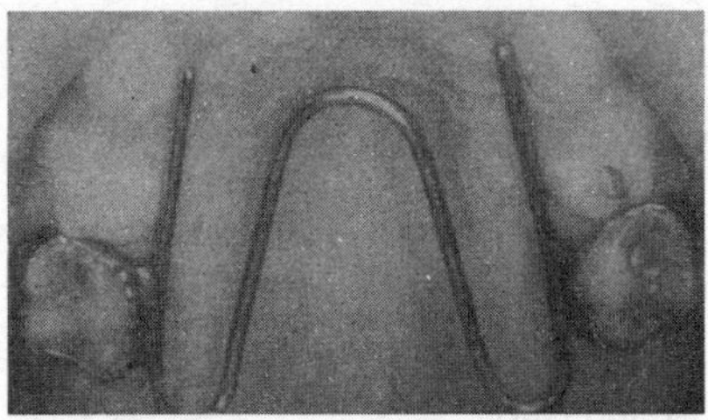

Fig. 28.5 Soldered W-arch for maxillary expansion.

a. Both the statements are false
b. Both the statements are true
c. First statement is true and the second is false
d. First statement is false and the second is true

Ans b.

The soldered W-arch or Porter appliance is an efficient appliance for correction of posterior crossbite. This may sometimes function as a reminder appliance in some cases of posterior crossbite associated with thumb sucking.

20. A low tongue position can result in the application of unequal forces to the maxillary posterior teeth and can allow these teeth to assume crossbite relationship with mandibular teeth. In patients who breathe through their mouths, the tongue can assume a low position in the mouth resulting in muscle imbalance and subsequently a buccal crossbite.

a. Both the statements are false
b. Both the statements are true
c. First statement is true and the second is false
d. First statement is false and the second is true

Ans b.

The answer is self-explanatory.

21. A functional crossbite results from the mandible shifting into an abnormal but often more comfortable position. If there is no evidence of a discrepancy in the upper and lower midline when the mandible is at rest but there is a deviation of the mandible toward the side of the crossbite when the teeth are brought into occlusion, the malocclusion is considered functional.

a. Both the statements are false
b. Both the statements are true
c. First statement is true and the second is false
d. First statement is false and the second is true

Ans b.

The answer is self-explanatory.

22. If the first permanent molar (only) is in crossbite in one of the sides, the method of choice for correction of posterior crossbite is

a. W-soldered arch
b. Quadhelix appliance

c. Cross elastic technique
d. Expansion appliance with jackscrew

Ans c.

When the posterior crossbite is involving a single tooth, the treatment of choice is cross elastics. Normally, the correction can be achieved in 4–8 weeks with this technique.

23. Ectopic eruption of first permanent molars is more common in the mandible. It is more frequently observed in girls than in boys.

a. Both the statements are false
b. Both the statements are true
c. First statement is true and the second is false
d. First statement is false and the second is true

Ans a.

The reverse is true. Ectopic eruption of first permanent molars is more common in the maxilla. It is more frequently observed in boys than in girls.

24. Ectopic eruption of first permanent molars can be corrected by

a. Helical spring
b. Open coil spring
c. Brass ligature wire
d. Any of the above

Ans d.

Ectopic eruption can be corrected by any of the above-mentioned treatment options.

25. At what age is the child expected to have 12 primary teeth and 12 erupted permanent teeth?

a. 5 years
b. 7 years
c. 9 years
d. 12 years

Ans c.

At 9 years, the primary canines, first and second primary molars are usually present. This in each quadrant represents the 12 primary teeth. In permanent teeth, the first molars, central and lateral incisors are present at 9 years, which is totally 12 permanent teeth.

26. Serial extraction is referred (Dewel) to as orderly removal of selected primary and permanent teeth in a predetermined sequence. Serial

extraction is indicated primarily in severe Class I malocclusion in the mixed dentition that has insufficient arch length for the amount of tooth material.

a. Both the statements are false
b. Both the statements are true
c. First statement is true and the second is false
d. First statement is false and the second is true

Ans b.

The answer is self-explanatory.

27. Which of the following is not true of "mature swallow"?

a. Relaxation of lips
b. Placement of tongue behind maxillary incisors
c. Elevation of mandible
d. This usually occurs before 3 years of age

Ans d.

Relaxation of lips, placement of tongue behind maxillary incisors and elevation of mandible is characteristics of mature swallow. However, this pattern of swallowing is not established before 3 years of age.

28. Dental arch circumference reduces during

a. Primary dentition period
b. Late transition period
c. Permanent dentition period
d. Both (b) and (c)

Ans d.

In late transition period due to the early and late mesial shift, reduction of the arch length occurs. In permanent dentition, continuous proximal wear results in reduction in arch length.

29. Which of the following factors contribute to accommodation of larger permanent incisors?

a. Presence of interdental spaces in the primary anterior teeth
b. The more labial placement of the crowns increasing the arch circumference
c. Increase in intercanine diameter
d. All of the above

Ans d.

All the above-mentioned factors contribute to the larger permanent incisors. This is known as *incisal liability*.

30. Maximum intercanine width in mandible is completed by

a. 4–5 years
b. 7–8 years
c. 9–10 years
d. 10–12 years

Ans c.

The answer is self-explanatory.

31. Crossbites are often seen in the developing dentition in the molar region. Treatment should always be as follows:

a. Both molars should be moved equal amounts for correction
b. One molar should be moved the entire distance for correction
c. The possibility of functional interference and shift of the mandible should be considered
d. One molar should be extracted

Ans c.

The most common transverse problem in the preadolescent is maxillary constriction with a posterior crossbite. A posterior crossbite with an associated mandibular shift should be managed as soon as possible to prevent soft tissue and dental compensation. In a few cases, the mandibular shift is due to interference caused by the primary canines. These can be diagnosed by repositioning the mandible and noting the interference. Selective removal of enamel with a diamond bur eliminates the interference and the lateral shift into crossbite.

32. The major etiologic factor responsible for Class II malocclusion is

a. Sleeping habits
b. Growth discrepancy
c. Thumb and tongue habits
d. Tooth-to-jaw size discrepancy

Ans b.

In Class II malocclusion, more than irregular teeth, lack of space is involved. In most instances, there is an actual anteroposterior discrepancy in the jaw relationship.

33. A 10-year-old patient has mandibular canines trying to erupt into a space insufficient by 2 mm. Primary second molars are large

and firmly in place. First premolars are erupting. An acceptable preventive orthodontic procedure for this would be

a. Disking the mesial proximals of the mandibular primary second molars
b. Extracting the mandibular primary second molars
c. Placing a removable bite opener
d. Extracting the first premolars

Ans a.

There is an occasional need for disking of oversized first or second deciduous molars to allow eruption of contiguous permanent teeth. If it appears, then a maxillary canine will not have enough space in the dental arch and it will thus erupt to the labial side and if the second premolars are not ready to erupt, the needed arch length may be attained by slicing the proximal end of the second molar.

34. Most Class II malocclusions can be prevented by

a. Maintaining the integrity of the primary dentition
b. Preventing the deleterious habits (such as thumb sucking, lip biting, etc.)
c. Breast feeding
d. No known techniques
e. (a), (b) and (c) above

Ans d.

The role of hereditary is strong in Class II malocclusion. Hence the possibility for prevention is less.

35. For an 8-year-old patient with good posterior occlusion, no arch length deficiency, one central incisor severely rotated and a large midline diastema present, the procedure of choice is to

a. Have the labial frenum excised
b. Rotate the tooth with an appliance
c. Examine for a supernumerary tooth
d. Inject thyroid hormone to stimulate eruption of the lateral incisors
e. None of the above

Ans c.

Of major concern to the dentist is the frequency of deflection or noneruption of the maxillary permanent central incisors as a result of supernumerary teeth. In many cases, supernumerary teeth do not have to be in contact with the permanent incisors to prevent it from erupting normally. The careful removal of a supernumerary tooth usually allows the permanent tooth to erupt, though it may be malposed.

36. An 8-year-old patient has an end-on molar relation and normal vertical and horizontal overlap. The mandibular lateral incisors are erupting slightly lingually. The dentist should

a. Insert a lingual arch
b. Refer him to an orthodontist
c. Continue routine dental care and developmental supervision
d. Institute orthodontic therapy to reposition the lateral incisors and to correct the Class II molar relation

Ans c.

Children can have various amounts of irregularity without any real arch length shortage when the leeway space is included. Mild irregularity is even considered normal in patients who have no arch length discrepancy. Longitudinal studies of persons with ideal occlusions show that there is a period when up to 2 mm of transitional irregularity occurs early in the mixed dentition and eventually resolves. Observation is usually the best course.

37. In correcting an anterior crossbite, the appliance to be used is determined by the

a. Amount of overbite
b. Age of the patient
c. Cooperation of the patient
d. All of the above

Ans d.

As with all removable appliances, the child must cooperate by wearing the device full time (except during eating) to allow the appliance accomplish the desired tooth movement. Fixed appliances do not require much cooperation from the child. A decision must be made as to whether the teeth should be tipped into position or bodily moved into place.

38. The optimal time to employ an orthodontic appliance that takes advantage of growth is during

a. Late primary dentition
b. Early mixed dentition
c. Late mixed dentition
d. Early permanent dentition

Ans c.

All growth modification treatments are usually carried out in the late mixed dentition. However, the data are not totally clear that one must treat children when they are at a certain rate of facial growth to be successful, and experience has shown that most skeletal and dental problems can be managed a bit later in one phase during the transition from the mixed dentitions. For these reasons, a single stage of orthodontic treatment is most popular and adequately effective.

39. A child has an extreme open bite. Only the most posterior teeth contact those in the opposite arch. The best procedure for the dentist would be to

a. Refer the child to an orthodontist for treatment
b. Remove the posterior tooth in each quadrant
c. Make an overlay denture to create occlusion
d. Place the bands on the teeth and place elastics to close the bite

Ans a.

Extreme open bite may be due to skeletal problems. Skeletal open bite patients should be referred to a specialist.

40. A 7-year-old child has normal occlusion except for a marked lingual eruption of a maxillary central incisor. Which of the following is the best orthodontic therapy?

a. Crossbite elastics
b. Home therapy with a tongue blade
c. Maxillary acrylic inclined plane
d. Myofunctional therapy
e. A maxillary appliance to apply labial force

Ans e.

Maxillary Hawley's appliance with posterior bite plane and double cantilever spring is the appliance of choice to correct anterior crossbite. For single tooth posterior crossbite, a simple crossbite elastic is used to correct the crossbite. If there is a simple local problem with adequate space for the tooth in crossbite to be moved into its correct position, several approaches are possible. The use of a tongue blade may be sufficient to intercept the developing crossbite.

41. A 13-year-old child has a 3 mm maxillary midline diastema and a heavy fibrous midline frenum. The child exhibits an otherwise normal occlusion. Which of the following is the best approach to manage this problem?

a. Band the central incisors and use a space-closing device
b. Band the central incisors and close the space with extra oral force
c. Excise the tissue between the central incisors and close the diastema orthodontically
d. Excise the tissue between the central incisors and permit the space to close on its own

Ans c.

Simple orthodontic procedures may close the space with a reasonable chance of success, provided that the occlusion is normal otherwise. If the frenal attachment is thought to be the cause of the diastema, frenectomy can be completed at the end of the active appliance phase or during the retention phase. Before stepping in with surgery, however, one should be sure that the diastema is not in a transient "ugly duckling" stage of development as the canines and lateral incisors maneuver for erupting space in the alveolar process. If there is any doubt, one must wait until the permanent canines have fully erupted before incising the frenum.

42. A malocclusion is characterized by contraction of the maxillary denture, labioversion of the maxillary incisors, deep overbite and overjet. These are typical characteristics of a malocclusion of which of the following categories of Angle's classifications?

a. Classs I
b. Class II, div. 1
c. Class II, div. 2
d. Class III

Ans b.

The answer is self-explanatory.

43. A child of age 7½ years has a 2.5 mm space between the permanent maxillary central incisors. The lateral incisors are half erupted. Advice to the parents should be that

a. The condition should be corrected because it is hindering the eruption of the lateral incisors
b. Research has not at this time found a reason for the condition, but it will be self-correcting
c. At this stage the condition is not regarded as abnormal
d. The lingual frenum should be resected immediately

Ans c.

It may be a self-correcting malocclusion (ugly duckling stage). Hence wait and watch is the best approach.

44. A major disadvantage of treatment using a cervical head gear is

a. Psychological trauma due to the appearance
b. Potential deformity of the neck
c. Extrusion of the maxillary molars
d. Extrusion of maxillary incisors
e. Impaction of maxillary canines

Ans c.

Cervical headgear provides predominantly distal and occlusal forces. Traditionally, one avoids using a head gear that tends to extrude the posterior teeth in a long faced person or person with limited over bite. On the other hand, a headgear that extrudes the molars is often useful in a patient with a short face and a deep bite.

45. In patient with severe Class II skeletal malocclusion, the cephalometric ANB angle would most likely approximate

a. –3 degrees
b. 0 degree
c. 2 degrees
d. 8 degrees

Ans d.

Normal ANB angle is 2 degrees. If the angle is 2–4 it is skeletal Class I, if it is less than 2, it is Class II and if it is greater than 4, it is Class III.

46. A single force applied perpendicularly to the facial surface of an anterior tooth will cause it to

a. Translate
b. Tip about its apex
c. Move bodily away from the force
d. Tip about a point one-third the length of the root from the apex

Ans d.

If a force is applied against the crown of a tooth, and if this force has a "one-point contact", then a tipping effect is produced. Tipping, the most simple form of tooth movement, will have a center of rotation approximately at a point one-half the root length from the apex.

47. Serial extraction is indicated primarily in

a. Class I malocclusion
b. Class II malocclusion
c. Class III malocclusion
d. None of the above

Ans a.

If teeth are removed, in severe Class I malocclusions, much of the irregularities may actually be reduced automatically by the spontaneous drift of the remaining teeth into the empty space. Serial extraction offers a great opportunity for the orthodontist who recognizes Class I malocclusions early and thus provides the space needed for self-adjustment.

48. It is important to delay the treatment of unilateral crossbite until the permanent dentition because the crossbite cannot be corrected with any degree of permanence until all permanent teeth have erupted.

a. Both the statement and reason are correct and related
b. Both the statement and reason are correct but not related
c. The statement is correct but the reason is not
d. The statement is not correct but the reason is an accurate statement
e. Neither the statement nor the reason is correct

Ans e.

Management of maxillary constriction can begin as soon as the problem is discovered, if the child is mature enough to accept the treatment. Treatment has the potential to eliminate crossbites of the succedaneous teeth, increased arch length and simplify future diagnostic decisions that can be complicated by functional shifts.

49. A family dentist, after completing restorative procedures on an 11-year-old patient who has moderate crowding of anterior teeth, observes that the primary molars are in various states of exfoliation. His advice to the patient should be to return

a. In 3 months for observation
b. In 6 months for regular examination
c. In 1 year
d. After all permanent teeth have completely erupted

Ans a.

Arch length discrepancy of less than 5 mm indicates moderate crowding (already there is space loss and to avoid further space loss with exfoliation of primary teeth and to check any delay in eruption of permanent tooth, it is necessary to observe and periodically to correct the situation at the earliest).

50. When a permanent first molar erupts ectopically toward the mesial in an intact arch without excessive resorption of the primary molar roots, the treatment of choice is to

a. Extract the involved primary molar
b. Wait for exfoliation of the primary molar
c. Disk the distal surface of the primary molar
d. Place brass separating wire to move the permanent molar distally

Ans d.

The goal of the treatment is to move the ectopically erupting tooth away from the tooth it is resorbing, allow it to erupt and retain the primary second molar. If a small amount of movement is needed and little or none of the permanent molars are clinically visible, a 20-mm brass wire can be passed around the contact between the permanent molar and the primary second molar. The brass wire is tightened every 2 weeks until the permanent molar can slip past the primary molar and erupt.

51. The major criterion to differentiate between a true Class III and pseudo-Class III malocclusion is the

a. Existence of a forward shift of the mandible during closure
b. Occlusal relationship between maxillary and mandibular first molars
c. Presence of a bilateral crossbite
d. Degree of anterior crossbite

Ans a.

In pseudo-Class III malocclusion, there is a functional protrusion as the incisors meet in an end-to-end relationship at point of initial contact and the mandible is then guided forward into an anterior crossbite relationship by tooth guidance. The dramatic change in 2 to 3 months from Class III to normal occlusion is accomplished merely by tipping the maxillary incisors labially a little and retracting the mandibular incisors, eliminating the premature tooth contact and guidance. True Class III malocclusions with normal path of closure cannot be expected to respond in this manner.

52. When an uncontrolled tipping force is applied to the crown of a single-rooted tooth, the fulcrum is usually located

a. At the apex
b. At the cervical line
c. 5 mm beyond the apex
d. One-third of the root length from the apex

Ans d.

Refer the explanation of Q. No. 46.

53. Cephalometrics is useful in assessing which of the following relationships?

a. Tooth-to-tooth
b. Bone-to-bone
c. Tooth-to-bone
d. All of the above

Ans d.

Analysis of lateral cephalometrics head film is a diagnostic aid used to determine the relationship between the skeletal and dental structures (i.e. tooth–tooth, tooth–bone, bone–bone).

54. Orthodontic correction of which of the following is most easily retained?

a. Diastema
b. Rotation
c. Expansion
d. Anterior crossbite
e. Generalized spacing

Ans d.

If the patient exhibits a positive over bite and overjet after treatment, retention is probably not necessary because the occlusion generally holds the tipped incisors in its new position.

55. Gonion, menton and pogonion are cephalometric landmarks located on the

a. Midline
b. Mandible
c. Bony chin
d. Skeletal profile

Ans b.

Gonion—the point on the jaw angle which is most inferiorly, posteriorly and outwardly directed.

Menton—the lowest point on the symphysial shadow as seen in norma lateralis.

Pogonion—most anterior point in the contour of the chin.

Also refer the table in this chapter.

56. Which of the following procedures is used to prevent relapse after correction of a rotated permanent maxillary canine?

a. Recontour of the crown
b. Supracrestal fiberotomy
c. Establishment of cuspid-protected occlusion
d. Removal of all functional contacts with canine in lateral and protrusive excursions

Ans b.

Gingival fibers (supracrestal fibers) reorganize very slowly following rotational movement of teeth and in some cases irregularity returns even if retention is well conceived. Some clinicians have suggested that if the periodontium is healthy, a circumferential supracrestal fiberotomy may be performed to reduce relapse. When treatment is complete or nearly complete, the supracrestal fibers are cut with a scalpel and a no. 12B blade under LA. Theoretically, the stretched gingival fibers will not need to reorganize but will reattach in a new position after being cut.

Chapter 29

Space Maintainers and Regainers

1. Which of the following considerations is important to a dentist when space maintenance is considered?

a. Time elapsed since loss of tooth
b. Amount of bone covering the unerupted tooth
c. Dental age of the patient
d. All of the above

Ans d.

All the above-mentioned factors have to be evaluated while considering space maintainers. Premature loss of primary teeth can lead to space loss in the arches. If space loss occurs, it usually takes place during the first 6 months after the extraction. It is wise to insert a space maintainer as soon as the tooth is lost. Erupting premolars usually require 4 to 5 months to move through 1 mm of the bone. Hence, the bone covering the unerupted permanent tooth has to be assessed before placing a space maintainer. Studies by Gron have indicated that the loss of primary molar before the age of 7 years (chronologic) will lead to delayed eruption of succedaneous tooth, whereas the loss after 7 years of age leads to an early emergence.

2. Primate spaces are present

a. Mesial to maxillary canines and distal to mandibular canines
b. Mesial to mandibular canines and distal to maxillary canines
c. Mesial to maxillary and mandibular canines
d. Distal to maxillary and mandibular canines

Ans a.

Primate spaces are present mesial to maxillary canines and distal to mandibular canines. They are known as simian spaces or anthropoid spaces.

3. Primate spaces are otherwise called

a. Simian spaces
b. Primate spaces by Baume
c. Anthropoid spaces
d. All of the above

Ans d.

All the above-mentioned names are used alternatively to denote primate spaces. Baume first reported this in 1950.

4. Flush terminal plane refers to the relationship of the distal surfaces of the

a. Primary cuspids
b. First permanent molars
c. Permanent second molars
d. Second primary molars

Ans d.

When the distal surfaces of second primary molars are in a straight line, it is referred to as flush terminal plane. When the distal surface of the lower second primary molar is mesial to the same surface of the maxillary molar, it is known as mesial step. In distal step, the distal surface of the lower second primary molar is distal to the same surface of the maxillary molar.

5. Spaces between anterior primary teeth are

a. Uncommon and undesirable
b. Common and undesirable
c. Common and desirable
d. Uncommon and desirable

Ans c.

Spacing between primary anterior teeth is commonly seen and desirable. This is known as physiological spacing. These spaces help the larger sized permanent teeth to erupt in normal alignment. Whenever these spaces are not present in primary dentition, it results in crowding of the permanent dentition.

6. Which of the following is not an example of unilateral fixed space maintainer?

a. Distal shoe
b. Band and loop
c. Nance arch
d. Crown and loop

Ans c.

Nance arch is a bilateral fixed space maintainer indicated when there is bilateral tooth loss in the maxilla. Distal shoe, Band and loop and Crown and loop are all examples of unilateral fixed space maintainers. Distal shoe is a unilateral fixed space maintainer used when the primary second molar is lost prematurely before the eruption of first permanent molar. Band and loop is a unilateral fixed space maintainer used when there is premature loss of primary molar on one side of the arch. Crown and loop is a unilateral fixed space maintainer indicated when there is unilateral tooth loss. Usually, crown and loop is preferred over band and loop when the abutment tooth had pulp treatment (pulpotomy or pulpectomy) before.

Classification of space maintainers and few examples

Fixed	Band and loop
Removable	Acrylic partial denture
Unilateral	Crown and loop
Bilateral	Nance arch, lingual arch
Active	Wilson arch
Passive	Band and loop
Functional	Acrylic partial denture
Non-functional	Band and loop

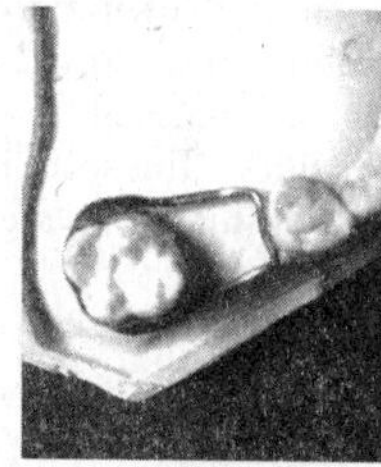

Fig. 29.1 Band and loop space maintainer.

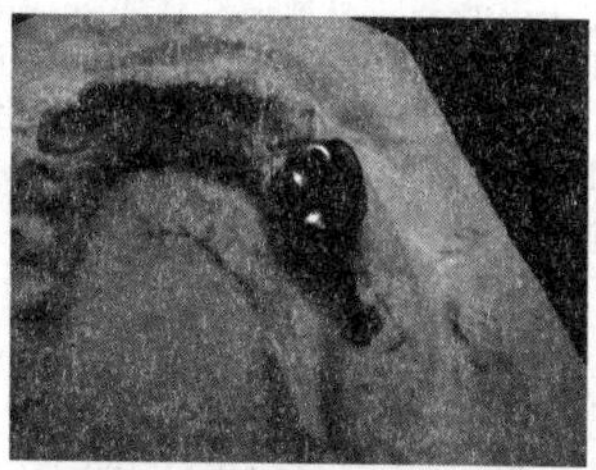

Fig. 29.2 Distal shoe space maintainer.

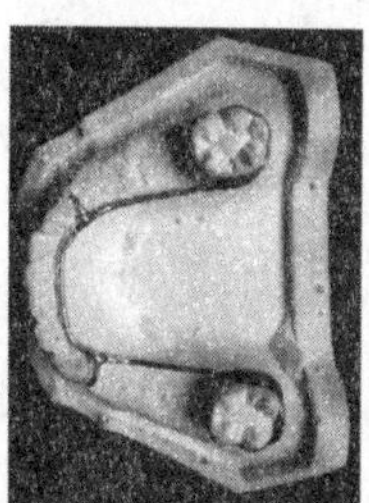

Fig. 29.3 Lingual arch space maintainer.

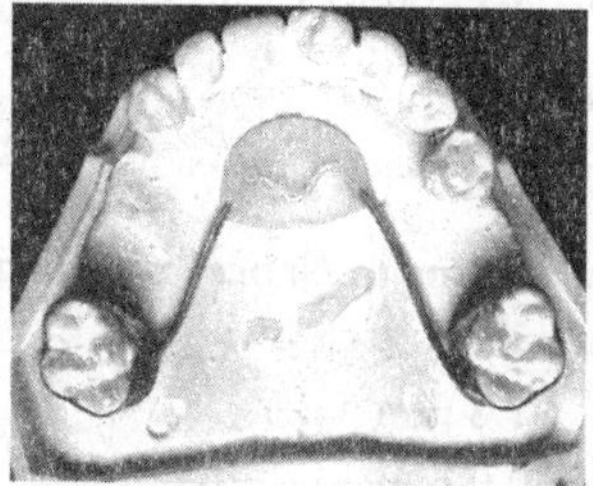

Fig. 29.4 Nance palatal arch space maintainer.

7. **Most common cause of malocclusion is**

   a. Hypothyroidism
   b. Presence of supernumerary tooth
   c. Early loss of primary teeth
   d. Congenital absence of third molars

Ans c.

The most common cause of malocclusion is premature loss of primary teeth. This amounts to 60–70% of the malalignments encountered.

8. Early mesial shift utilizes

a. Leeway space of Nance
b. Primate spaces
c. Meyers space
d. Von Ebner's space

Ans b.

Primate spaces are spaces present mesial to the maxillary canines and distal to the mandibular canines. They are used for early mesial shift. There is no space called Meyer's or von Ebner's space.

Leeway space of Nance—The combined mesiodistal width of primary canines, first and second molars is greater than the combined mesiodistal width of unerupted permanent canines and premolars. The difference in the maxilla is 1.8 mm and in the mandible is 3.4 mm (both the sides). This space is utilized by late mesial shift to achieve Class I molar relationship when the primary teeth do not have primate spaces.

9. Late mesial shift utilizes

a. Leeway space of Nance
b. Primate spaces
c. Meyer's space
d. Von Ebner's space

Ans a.

Refer to the explanation of Q. No. 8.

10. According to Nance, average amount of leeway space present in the maxillary arch is

a. 1.8 mm
b. 0.9 mm
c. 1.7 mm
d. 3.4 mm

Ans a.

The amount of leeway space present in the maxilla is 0.9 mm on either side. Hence the total leeway space present in the maxilla is 1.8 mm.

11. A distal step relationship of the second primary molars is indicative of

a. Class I malocclusion

b. Class II malocclusion
c. Class III malocclusion
d. Class II, div. I

Ans b.

In distal step relationship, the distal surface of the mandibular second primary molar is distal to the maxillary second molar. This results in the eruption of maxillary first permanent molar mesial to the mandibular first permanent molar resulting in a Class II molar relationship.

Mesial step. First permanent molar erupts in class I molar relationship (mandibular second molar mesial to maxillary second molar).

Distal step. First permanent molar erupts in Class II molar relationship.

Flush terminal plane (with primate spaces). First permanent molar erupts in end on relationship. Class I molar relationship is achieved by early mesial shift.

Flush terminal plane (without primate spaces). First permanent molar erupts in end on relationship. Class I molar relationship is achieved by late mesial shift.

12. Advantage of Moyer's mixed dentition analysis over Nance is

a. It can be performed only in the maxillary arch
b. It does not require a radiograph
c. It can be done before the eruption of permanent incisors
d. It can be performed in the primary dentition itself

Ans b.

Moyer's mixed dentition analysis uses a probability chart and does not need a radiograph. This can be performed both in the maxilla and the mandible. To perform a mixed dentition analysis, mandibular permanent incisors must be present. Moyers, Nance, and Tanaka and Johnson analysis uses the mesiodistal width of mandibular permanent incisors as standards. All the mixed dentition analyzes use mesiodistal width of mandibular permanent incisors as standards because of its early eruption and less susceptibility for morphological variations. It cannot be performed in primary dentition because of the absence of mandibular permanent incisors.

13. While using Moyer's probability chart, the percentage level of probability used for space prediction is

a. 25%
b. 50%
c. 75%
d. 100%

Ans c.

The percentage level used for space prediction using Moyer's probability chart is 75%.

14. In Tanaka and Johnson analysis, the value that is added for prediction of required space in maxillary arch is

a. 11
b. 10.5
c. 12
d. 9.5

Ans a.

The formula used for space prediction in Tanaka and Johnson analysis is as follows:

In maxilla

$$\frac{\text{Combined mesiodistal width of mandibular central and lateral incisors}}{2} + 11$$

In mandible

$$\frac{\text{Combined mesiodistal width of mandibular central and lateral incisors}}{2} + 10.5$$

15. A 4-year-old child who has to undergo removal of severely decayed second primary molar would require a

a. Band and loop space maintainer
b. Crown and loop space maintainer
c. Distal shoe space maintainer
d. Reverse band and loop space maintainer

Ans c.

As the first permanent molars would not have erupted by then, the space maintainer indicated in this situation is distal shoe space maintainer. It will guide the eruption of first permanent molar. Refer to the explanation of Q. No. 6.

16. An 8-year-old patient who has lost all the four maxillary primary molars would require

a. Nance arch space maintainer
b. Lingual arch space maintainer
c. Passive lingual arch space maintainer
d. Band and loop

Ans a.

Nance arch space maintainer is indicated when there is premature bilateral loss of primary molars in the maxilla. In a similar situation in the mandible, the choice of space maintainer will be passive lingual arch. On the other hand, band and loop space maintainer is indicated when there is unilateral loss of primary tooth either in the mandible or in the maxilla.

17. A 6-year-old child who has lost all the four mandibular primary molars (lower permanent incisors have not erupted) and the permanent first molars are partially erupted, would require a

a. Nance arch space maintainer
b. Lingual arch space maintainer
c. Removable acrylic partial denture
d. Band and loop

Ans c.

Presence of mandibular permanent incisors is a prerequisite for a lingual arch space maintainer as the lingual arch rests on the cingulum of permanent incisors. As the lower permanent molars are partially erupted, banding of these teeth for a lingual arch is not possible. Nance arch space maintainer is used in the maxilla and band and loop space maintainer in unilateral tooth loss situations. Therefore, removable partial denture (as a functional type) is the treatment of choice.

18. In a 6-year-old child who has lost mandibular right first primary molar and has an endodontically treated second primary molar, the space maintainer of choice will be

a. Band and loop
b. Crown and loop
c. Lingual arch
d. Reverse crown and loop

Ans b.

As the endodontically treated mandibular second molar can serve as an abutment, crown and loop space maintainer will be the treatment of choice. Reverse crown and loop space maintainer is indicated when the second primary molar is lost after the eruption of first permanent molar (partially erupted) in which the first primary molar is endodontically treated.

19. All of the following are examples of nonfunctional space maintainer except

a. Band and loop
b. Crown and loop
c. Acrylic partial denture
d. Lingual arch

Ans c.

Space maintainers that have components participating in mastication are called *functional space maintainers.* In other words, the space maintainer should replace the function of the tooth, which is lost prematurely. Of the space maintainers mentioned above, only the acrylic partial denture can have teeth on it, which can help the patient chew.

20. One of the following space maintainer is otherwise called eruption-guiding appliance.

a. Band and loop
b. Crown and loop
c. Distal shoe
d. Reverse crown and loop

Ans c.

Distal shoe space maintainer is otherwise called eruption guiding appliance and intra-alveolar appliance because the intra-alveolar extension of the distal shoe space maintainer guides the eruption of unerupted first permanent molar.

21. Major disadvantage of removable space maintainer is that it

a. Is difficult to keep it clean
b. Cannot be made esthetic
c. Will not maintain the vertical dimension
d. May not be worn

Ans d.

The major drawback of a removable space maintainer is that the patient may not wear it consistently.

22. An 8-year-old patient has an end on molar relation and normal vertical and horizontal overlap. The mandibular lateral incisors are erupting slightly lingually. The dentist should

a. Insert a lingual arch
b. Refer him to an orthodontist
c. Continue routine dental care and developmental supervision
d. Institute orthodontic therapy to reposition the lateral incisors to correct the Class II molar relationship

Ans c.

As the mandibular incisors are erupting lingually the patient should be under developmental supervision, as he may need serial extraction or proximal stripping in due course of time.

23. In a mixed dentition space analysis, the most careful estimate will only be accurate within

a. 0.5 mm
b. 2 mm
c. 4 mm
d. 6 mm

Ans b.

Among the existing mixed dentition space analysis, the most careful estimate will be accurate within 2 mm.

24. The band and loop space maintainer is classified as

a. Bilateral, fixed and functional
b. Unilateral, fixed and functional
c. Unilateral, fixed and nonfunctional
d. Unilateral, removable and nonfunctional

Ans c.

The answer is self-explanatory. Refer to the explanation of Q. Nos. 6 and 19.

25. A mixed dentition analysis determines

a. Intercanine width
b. Skeletal growth pattern
c. Discrepancies in jaw size
d. Space available versus space required.

Ans d.

In a mixed dentition analysis, the permanent mandibular anterior teeth are used as standards for prediction of the sizes of unerupted permanent teeth. This gives the space available and the space required.

26. When dealing with decayed primary teeth, the best space maintainer is a

a. Lingual arch
b. Band and loop
c. Properly restored primary tooth
d. Functional removable space maintainer

Ans c.

Natural teeth are the best space maintainers. Hence a properly restored primary tooth is the best space maintainer of all.

27. A patient, aged 10 years, has lost a maxillary permanent central incisor. The correct treatment is to

a. Construct a suitable space maintainer immediately
b. Delay treatment until a fixed bridge can be constructed
c. Allow complete healing before constructing a replacement
d. Observe

Ans a.

The loss of anterior permanent teeth requires immediate treatment by the dentist if inter- or intra-arch changes are to be prevented. Within a few days after the loss of a tooth as a result of trauma or the extraction of a severely traumatized tooth, the teeth adjacent to the space will begin to drift, and often within a few weeks several millimetres of space will be lost. The temporary appliance is constructed and inserted as soon as possible after the loss to prevent space closure. If any degree of space closure has occurred, the space should be regained if possible, before the construction of a space maintainer. After the space is regained, a tooth may be added or a new retainer with a replacement tooth can be used until a fixed replacement is made. Fixed restorative or implant solutions are usually done around the age of 16 years when the growth is complete.

28. Following extraction of the mandibular primary second molar in a 3½-year-old child, the treatment of choice is to

a. Place a removable appliance to replace the tooth
b. Allow the permanent first molar to erupt and then maintain the space for the premolar
c. Place a fixed appliance to guide the eruption of the first permanent molar
d. Place a removable appliance to replace the extracted tooth and prevent elongation of opposing primary molar

Ans c.

Distal shoe appliance or eruption guiding appliance is used to maintain the space of a primary second molar that has been lost before the eruption of the permanent first molar. An unerupted permanent first molar drifts mesially within the alveolar bone if the primary second molar is lost prematurely which will result in loss of arch length and possible impaction of the second premolar. The main objective of the distal shoe space maintainer is to retain and guide the permanent first molar into normal eruptive position. Also refer to Q. No. 15.

29. The treatment of choice for a normal girl whose dental age is 10 years and who has lost a mandibular primary first molar unilaterally would be

a. A steel crown and loop space maintainer

b. An acrylic unilateral partial denture
c. A temporary three unit bridge
d. No treatment

Ans d.

Premature loss of the primary molar at an age near the time of normal eruption of the succedaneous teeth may actually accelerate the eruption of the permanent tooth and make the space maintenance unnecessary. The premolar will tend to erupt earlier than normal if the primary molar is lost after age 8.

30. The band and crib space maintainer is classified as

a. Bilateral, fixed and functional
b. Unilateral, fixed and functional
c. Unilateral, fixed and nonfunctional
d. Unilateral, removable and nonfunctional

Ans c.

Band and crib space maintainer is one of the fixed space maintainers effectively used for unilateral loss of single primary tooth in buccal segment before or after the eruption of first permanent molar. One of the disadvantages is that it does not restore the chewing function.

31. Which of the following is the best method of preserving arch length?

a. Restoring the carious teeth
b. Placing a lingual arch
c. Placing a cast gold retainer
d. Placing an acrylic removable maintainer

Ans a.

Space maintenance begins with good restorative dentistry. The dentist should strive for ideal restoration of all interproximal contours. Early restoration of interproximal caries ensures that no space loss occurs. In some instances, however, large carious lesions may make ideal restorations of the tooth impossible and space loss is inevitable. Even if pulp tissues have been compromised, pulp therapy should be initiated and the tooth maintained, if at all possible, because the natural tooth is still superior to the best space maintainer available; it is functional, is of the correct size and exfoliates naturally (refer to the explanation of Q. No. 26).

32. Following the loss of a permanent mandibular first molar at age 8, one could expect which of the following changes to occur in that quadrant over a period of time?

a. No premolar movement but mesial drift of the second molar

b. Mesial drift of both second premolar and the permanent second molar
c. Distal drift of the second premolar and mesial drift of the second molar
d. Neither tooth will shift appreciably

Ans c.

Loss of interproximal contact as a result of decay, extraction or ankylosis of an adjacent tooth results in space loss because of mesial and occlusal drift of the tooth distal to the newly created space. There is also evidence that the tooth mesial to the affected molar will drift distally into the space. Therefore, loss of space or arch length can occur from both directions.

33. A 10-year-old girl with clinically normal occlusion reports for examination immediately after losing a primary mandibular second molar. The dentist should

a. Keep the patient under observation
b. Place a lingual arch space maintainer
c. Place a functional space maintainer
d. Place a removable partial denture
e. Base his choice of treatment upon radiographic findings

Ans e.

Accurate method of determining delayed or accelerated eruption of permanent teeth is to examine the amount of root development and alveolar bone overlying the unerupted permanent tooth from panoramic or periapical films. The succedaneous tooth begins to actively erupt when root development is approximately one-half to two-third completed. In terms of alveolar bone coverage, roughly 6 months should be anticipated for every millimetre of bone that covers the permanent tooth.

34. An 8-year-old patient has a permanent maxillary first molar extracted because of caries. The best approach to prevent malocclusion is

a. Place a space maintainer
b. Wait for the second molar to erupt and bodily drift mesially into the space
c. Extract the mandibular first molar to equalize the tooth size
d. Extract the contralateral maxillary first molar to maintain arch symmetry

Ans b.

The second permanent molars, even if unerupted, start to drift mesially after the loss of the first permanent molar. A greater degree of movement will occur in children in the age group of 8–10 years ; in older children, if the loss of first permanent molar occurs after the eruption of the second permanent molar, only tipping of this tooth can be expected.

35. When the primary canines are lost prematurely, the permanent incisors may drift

a. Labially
b. Lingually
c. Mesially
d. Distally
e. None of the above

Ans d.

The permanent incisors moves into the available space (distally).

36. When primary mandibular right first and second molars are lost in an 8-year-old patient, space is best maintained by constructing and placing

a. Multiple space maintainers
b. Bands on the remaining teeth
c. A functional removable appliance
d. A bilateral nonfunctional space maintainer

Ans d.

Unilateral multiple tooth loss in the mandible is an indication for bilateral nonfunctional space maintainer.

37. Mesioangular ectopic eruption of a permanent maxillary first molar causing resorption of distal surfaces of the roots of the primary second molar should be treated by

a. Extracting the primary second molar
b. Disking the distal surface of the primary second molar
c. Tipping the permanent first molar distally using a separating device
d. Removing the soft tissue overlying the occlusal surface of the permanent molar

Ans c.

The goal of the treatment is to move the ectopically erupting tooth away from the tooth which is resorbing, allow it to erupt and retain the second molar. If a small amount of movement is needed and little or none of the permanent molar is clinically visible, a piece of brass wire can be passed around the contact between the permanent molar and the primary second molar. When the wire is tightened, the molar is forced distally until it can slip pass the primary molar and facilitate eruption. A second method of moving the permanent molar distally is to band the primary second molar and apply a distal force to the permanent molar through a helical spring.

38. Mesial drift of a permanent mandibular first molar after premature extraction of the primary mandibular second molar is an example of

a. Pathologic tooth movement
b. Physiologic tooth movement
c. Functional force displacement
d. Collagenous fiber tension movement
e. None of the above

Ans b.

The answer is self-explanatory.

39. Which of the following is not a space maintainer?

a. Lingual arch
b. Nance holding arch
c. Class III restoration
d. Stainless steel crown
e. Palatal expansion appliance

Ans e.

Lingual arch and Nance holding arch are bilateral nonfunctional space maintainers. Class III restoration and stainless steel crown prevent proximal space loss and can be considered as space maintainers.

40. Of the following, a space maintainer is least indicated for premature loss of a

a. Primary maxillary first molar
b. Primary mandibular first molar
c. Primary maxillary central incisor
d. Permanent maxillary central incisor

Ans c.

Some dentists believe that space closure rarely occurs in the anterior part of the mouth but this is not true; if the anterior primary teeth were in contact before the loss or there is evidence of an arch length inadequacy in the anterior region, a collapse in the arch after the loss of one of the primary incisor is almost certain. However, in the maxillary anterior segment, space maintainers are not usually necessary, even with the drifting of the contiguous teeth, since normal growth and developmental processes usually increase the intercanine width to accommodate the larger permanent successors.

41. Space closure is least likely to occur after loss of which of the following teeth?

a. Primary mandibular canines
b. Primary mandibular second molars
c. Primary maxillary first molars
d. Primary maxillary central incisors
e. Permanent maxillary central incisors

Ans d.

Refer to the explanation of Q. No. 40.

42. In which of the following situations is space maintenance most difficult to manage?

a. 9½-year-old patient with loss of a permanent maxillary first molar
b. 5-year-old patient with loss of a primary maxillary central incisor
c. 6-year-old patient with loss of a primary mandibular first molar
d. 7-year-old patient with loss of a primary maxillary second molar
e. 5-year-old patient with loss of a primary mandibular second molar

Ans e.

Mesial movement and migration of the first permanent molar occur before the eruption in instances of premature loss of a second primary molar. This is one of the most difficult problems of the developing dentition to confront the pediatric dentist. Use of a space maintainer (distal shoe) that will guide the first permanent molar into its normal position is indicated. Distal shoe space maintainer contains crown and band appliance with a distal intragingival extension and uses the first primary molar as abutment.

43. A distal shoe space maintainer is indicated when a primary

a. Incisor is avulsed
b. First molar is prematurely lost
c. Second molar is lost after eruption of a permanent first molar
d. Second molar is lost before eruption of a permanent first molar

Ans d.

Refer to the explanation for Q. Nos. 15 and 28.

44. A mandibular lingual arch appliance used to maintain space maintenance should be designed to contact the

a. Lingual aspect of most anterior teeth in the arch
b. Lowest aspect of the cingula of anterior teeth

c. Incisal third of the lingual surface of anterior teeth
d. Gingival tissue 2 mm below the cingula of anterior teeth
e. Both (a) and (b)

Ans e.

Stainless steel lingual arch wire is adapted carefully to the cast so that the wire itself is well adapted to the lingual side where the unerupted teeth are expected to make their clinical entry. The "U" shaped portion of the lingual arch wire should rest on the cingulum of each mandibular incisor, if possible, to prevent the mesial tipping of the mandibular first permanent molar and lingual retrusion of the incisors themselves.

45. The passive soldered lingual arch appliance should be removed

a. At once and no further treatment instituted
b. At once and placed with an active lingual arch appliance to regain space
c. At once and replaced with individual space maintainers from first premolar to molars
d. When premolars have almost reached the occlusal plane

Ans d.

Usually, space maintainers are removed once the permanent tooth erupts into the oral cavity.

46. When a patient has a severe arch space insufficiency (greater than 10 mm) in the permanent dentition, proper alignment of teeth will

a. Require extraction of some permanent dental units
b. Require use of a myofunctional appliance
c. Be achieved without extraction if started at an early age
d. Be achieved without extraction if an arch-developing appliance is used

Ans a.

If the crowding approaches (space deficiency) 10 mm per arch, extraction of permanent teeth is inevitable. Usually premolars are extracted. The average width of a premolar is approximately 7 mm ; therefore, the extraction of two premolars would effectively result in a gain of 14 mm of arch length.

47. A 7-year-old child shows premature loss of primary mandibular canines. He has no caries in his remaining teeth. This situation strongly suggests

a. Caries
b. Lack of dental care

c. Insufficient arch length
d. A developing Class III malocclusion

Ans c.

Early loss of primary canines is more common due to erupting permanent lateral incisors resorbing the roots of primary canines rather than caries. Early loss of primary canines leads to arch length deficiency by closure of space by the mesial movement of the posterior teeth or by lingual displacement of the anterior incisors.

48. After clinically identifying mild, anterior crowding in a patient with an early mixed dentition, which of the following is indicated?

a. Extract primary canines
b. Perform a space analysis
c. Regain space in the arch
d. Strip proximal contacts of incisors
e. Strip proximal contacts of primary canines

Ans b.

The first sign of crowding in the mixed dentition coincides with eruption of the permanent incisors. Arch length insufficiency may manifest in several ways ranging from slight incisor rotation and irregularity to gross incisor malalignment. The first step should be to perform a space analysis and determine the extent of the arch length inadequacy.

49. Of the following, the most common cause of malocclusion is

a. Congenitally missing permanent teeth
b. Trauma at birth or in later years of development
c. Habit pattern of the primary or mixed dentition period
d. Inadequate space management following early loss of primary teeth

Ans d.

The children who had a premature loss of one or more primary canines or molars more commonly received orthodontic treatment for the permanent dentition. The frequency of orthodontic treatment in children who had lost one or more primary teeth through 9 years of age was more than three times higher than in the control group. Also refer to the explanation of Q. No. 7.

50. Mesial drift may occur as a result of

a. Interproximal caries
b. Interproximal attrition
c. Premature loss of primary molars
d. All of the above

Ans d.

The answer is self-explanatory.

51. Amount of space closure after premature extraction of primary teeth is

a. More in mandible
b. More in maxilla
c. Equal in both arches
d. 4–5 mm in maxilla and 5–7 mm in mandible

Ans b.

Maxillary spaces have a higher average rate of closure than mandibular extraction spaces. Space loss after premature loss of maxillary second molar is greater than premature loss of first primary molar. However, the space closure is fairly constant with a slight tendency for closure rate to slow after first year.

52. According to Gron, the tooth starts erupting after

a. One-fourth of the root is formed
b. One-half of the root is formed
c. Three-fourth of the root is formed
d. The entire root is formed

Ans c.

Gron studied the emergence of permanent teeth based on the root development of premolars. She found that the tooth erupts when three-fourth of the root is completed regardless of the chronologic age.

53. It is observed that loss of primary molar before the age of 7 years will lead to delayed eruption of succedaneous tooth whereas the loss after 7 years lead to an early emergence of succedaneous tooth.

a. Both the statements are true
b. Both the statements are false
c. First statement is true and the second is false
d. First statement is false and the second is true

Ans a.

Premature loss of a primary molar at a very early age delays the eruption of the permanent tooth. On the other hand, premature loss of a primary molar at an age near the time of normal eruption of the succedaneous tooth may actually accelerate the eruption of the permanent tooth and make the space maintenance unnecessary. In general, eruption of the premolar will be delayed if the primary molar is lost before the age of 7, whereas the premolar will tend to erupt earlier than normal if the primary molar is lost after age of 7.

54. After premature removal of a primary tooth, the maximum amount of space closure occurs in the first

a. 1 month
b. 6 months
c. 12 months
d. 18 months

Ans b.

Space loss usually occurs within the first 6 months after the premature extraction of primary molar. Space maintenance should be undertaken unless the tooth is expected to erupt within 6 months or unless there is enough space in the arch that a 1 or 2 mm space reduction will not compromise eruption of the permanent tooth.

55. An unerupted premolar usually takes __________ months to travel through 1 mm of bone.

a. 1–2 months
b. 2–3 months
c. 4–5 months
d. 8–10 months

Ans c.

Refer to the explanation of Q. No. 33.

56. Transpalatal arch space maintainer was introduced by

a. Moyers
b. Nance
c. Robert A. Goshgarian
d. Williams

Ans c.

The answer is self-explanatory.

57. The depth of the distal shoe into the gingiva to guide the unerupted first permanent molar should be

a. 3 mm below the mesial marginal ridge of the first molar
b. 4 mm below the mesial marginal ridge of the first molar
c. 5 mm below the mesial marginal ridge of the first molar
d. 1 mm below the mesial marginal ridge of the first molar

Ans d.

Determination made in constructing the appliance is the intra-alveolar depth of the gingival extension. If the extension is left too long, there may be a possible harm to the developing second premolar. If the extension is too short, the first permanent molar could erupt underneath the appliance. The gingival extension of the appliance should be constructed to extend about 1 mm below the mesial marginal ridge of the first permanent molar or just sufficient to "capture" its mesial surface.

58. One of the following is not a fixed space regainer

a. Open coil

b. Gerber

c. Hotz

d. Split saddle

Ans d.

Split saddle is a removable space regainer.

Chapter 30

Oral Habits

1. The method of choice to correct thumb sucking with posterior crossbite in a patient aged 7 years is

a. Fixed appliance with cribs
b. Removable appliance with rakes
c. Quadhelix appliance
d. Kentucky appliance

Ans c.

The quadhelix is a fixed appliance used to expand a constricted maxillary arch. The anterior helices also discourage a sucking habit by reminding the child not to place a finger in the mouth. This appliance is often used in children in whom there is an active sucking habit and a posterior crossbite.

2. "Nonnutritive sucking is an adaptive response" is based on which of the following theory?

a. Learning theory
b. Psychosexual theory
c. Psychosocial theory
d. Classical conditioning

Ans a.

The learning theory states that nonnutritive sucking is an adaptive response. This theory assumes no underlying psychologic cause to prolonged non-nutritive sucking. It views that the response was continuously rewarded and eventually became a learnt habit.

3. When the breast is brought into contact with the infant's cheek he or she seeks the nipple. This is

a. Moro's reflex
b. Rooting reflex
c. Grasp reflex
d. Sucking reflex

Ans b.

Rooting reflex. Rooting reflex is when the breast is brought into contact with the infant's cheek; he or she seeks the nipple.

Sucking reflex. When a well-defined area around the mouth is touched by an object, an infant turns the head toward the object and opens the mouth. In other words, it is the movement of an infant's head and tongue towards a stimulus touching the infant's cheek.

Grasp reflex. When the baby's palm is stroked with the examiner's index finger, the baby's fingers close on it and grasp it. As the examiner lifts his or her index finger, the flexor muscles of the infant's forearm become tight.

Moro's reflex. The supine infant's hands are grasped and shoulders lifted a few centimetres while keeping the back of the head on the bed. A positive response consists of sudden abduction of the arms at the shoulder and extension arms at the elbow; this is followed by adduction of the arms and flexion of the forearm. There is complete opening of hands in the first phase.

4. **One of the following is a form of nutritive sucking**
   a. Thumb sucking, finger sucking
   b. Pacifier sucking
   c. Bottle-feeding

Ans c.

Sucking can be divided into two types:

a. Nutritive sucking. Breastfeeding, bottle-feeding—this provides essential nutrients to the individual.

b. Nonnutritive sucking. Thumb sucking, finger sucking, etc.—this provides a feeling of well being, warmth and a sense of security.

5. **Bruxism is a type of**
   a. Dyssomnia
   b. Parasomnia
   c. REM disturbance
   d. Insomnia

Ans b.

Parasomnias are dysfunctions or episodic events occurring with sleep, sleep stages and partial arousals. Bruxism or tooth grinding occurring in stage 3 or 4 of non-rapid eye movement (NREM) sleep is a classical example of parasomnia.

6. **One of the following is not a type of mouth breathing**
   a. Anatomic
   b. Physiologic
   c. Habitual
   d. Obstructive

Ans b.

There is no entity as physiologic mouth breathing.

7. Masochistic habits are associated with one of the following syndrome

a. Guillain-Barre syndrome
b. Lesch-Nyhan syndrome
c. Stevens-Johnson syndrome
d. Paterson-Kelly syndrome

Ans b.

The answer is self-explanatory.

8. Onychophagia is the

a. Other name for finger biting habit
b. Other name for nail biting habit
c. Other name for mouth breathing habit
d. Developmental disorder involving the nails

Ans b.

Nail biting is observed in children older than 6 years. It may serve the need of oral gratification. This habit also manifests itself as response to stress.

9. The only reliable method for determining the mode of respiratory function is

a. Butterfly test
b. Water test
c. Plethysmography
d. Halimeter

Ans c.

Plethysmography and nasal transducers are used to ascertain total nasal and oral airflow.

10. Adenoid facies is associated with

a. Brachycephalic face
b. Long narrow face
c. Mesoprosopic face
d. Mesomorphic individual

Ans b.

Adenoid facies is a term used to describe a particular type of facial configuration frequently associated with mouth breathing habit. Adenoid facies is characterized by long narrow face with accompanying narrow nose and nasal passages, flaccid lips with upper lip being short, and dolichofacial skeletal patterns.

11. Atypical activity of the orbicularis oris muscle is suggestive of

a. Bruxism
b. Nail biting
c. Thumb sucking
d. Tongue thrusting

Ans d.

In patients who continue to exhibit a tongue thrusting pattern of swallowing, the swallow is marked by, contraction of the circumoral musculature (orbicularis oris), separation of the maxillary and mandibular posterior teeth, and protrusion of the tongue between the incisors.

12. Asymmetrical anterior open bite with normal posterior occlusion is characteristic of

a. Thumb sucking
b. Mouth breathing
c. Abnormal swallowing habits
d. None of the above

Ans a.

Anterior open bite or the lack of vertical overlap of the upper and lower incisors when the teeth are in occlusion, develops because the digit rests directly on the incisors. This prevents complete or continued eruption of the incisors, whereas the posterior teeth are free to erupt.

13. A 7-year-old child has localized gingival recession between two teeth only. The most probable cause of the condition is

a. An oral habit
b. A chronic disease
c. A hereditary factor
d. Poor eating habits

Ans a.

The loss of attachment and recession that occurs with a labially malpositioned tooth is sometimes called stripping. Other factors that may contribute to recession are the use of smokeless tobacco and habit-related self-induced injury.

14. Which of the following is least likely to result from persistent long term thumb sucking?

a. A deep overbite
b. Protrusion of maxillary incisors
c. Constriction of maxillary arch
d. Rotation of maxillary lateral incisors

Ans a.

Persistent long term thumb sucking can lead to anterior open bite, facial movement of maxillary incisors, rotation of lateral incisors, lingual movement of mandibular incisors and maxillary constriction and not deep overbite.

15. The parents of a 4-year-old girl are distressed because her thumb-sucking habit has resulted in an anterior open bite of approximately 3 mm. Most authorities agree that the parents should be advised to

a. Stop worrying about the habit
b. Do their best to break the child's habit, even if considerable unpleasantness is involved
c. Have their dentist construct an appliance to stop the habit
d. Consult a psychologist or a psychiatrist, because thumb sucking at this age is a symptom of serious psychological disturbance

Ans a.

The prevalence of thumb-sucking habit decreases with age and most children give up this activity by 3.5 to 4 years of age. Most often, the treatment considerations are delayed until this age. If the habit is arrested before the eruption of maxillary permanent incisors there is no effect on the alignment or eruption of the permanent teeth.

Section IX

Children with Special Health Care Needs and Medical Emergencies

Chapter 31

Dental Care for Children with Special Health Care Needs

1. Which of the following is not an indication for the use of physical restraints?

a. A patient who requires diagnosis or treatment and cannot cooperate because of lack of maturity

b. A patient who requires diagnosis or treatment and cannot cooperate because of mental or physical disabilities

c. A patient who requires diagnosis or treatment and does not cooperate before and other behavior management techniques failed

d. When the safety of the patient or practitioner would be at risk without the protective use of restraint

Ans c.

Option (c) is not an indication for physical restraint. Physical restraint should be used in a patient who requires diagnosis or treatment and does not cooperate only after the other behavior management techniques have failed. All the other options are indications for using physical restraints.

2. Which of the following is not an aid in maintaining the mouth in an open position?

a. Padded tongue blade

b. Molt mouth prop

c. McKesson mouth prop

d. Towel and tape

Ans d.

Common mechanical aids for maintaining the mouth in open position are wrapped tongue blades, open wide disposable mouth props, molt mouth prop and McKesson bite blocks. Padded and wrapped tongue blades are easy to use, disposable and inexpensive. Open wide mouth props are also easy to use but are slightly more expensive than the wrapped blades. They are available in two sizes. Molt mouth prop is used in the management of difficult patients for prolonged periods. It is available in adult and child sizes and it gives accessibility to the opposite side of the mouth. It has the disadvantage of causing lip and palatal ulcerations and luxation of teeth if not used correctly.

Rubber bite blocks available in various sizes can be used to stabilize the mouth in the open position. Always remember that the patient's mouth should not be forcibly stretched because it may cause further resistance and airway compromise.

3. Which of the following physical restraints is not used to control body position?

a. Papoose board
b. Pedi wrap
c. Safety belt
d. Posey straps

Ans d.

Refer the following table:

S. No.	Body part	Restraints
1.	Body	Papoose board Triangular sheet Pedi wrap Beanbag dental chair insert Safety belt Extra assistant
2.	Extremities	Posey straps Velcro straps Towel and tape Extra assistant
3.	Head	Forearm body support Head positioner Plastic bowl Extra assistant

Posey straps are used to control extremities whereas all the other three are used to control body position on the dental chair. The Papoose board is available in different sizes to hold large and small children. It is simple to use and store and has attached head stabilizers. An extremely resistant patient may develop hyperthermia if immobilized for too long. The Pedi wrap does not have head straps or back board. It is made up of mesh fabric which permits better ventilation and lessens the chances of hyperthermia. The bean bag dental chair insert comfortably accommodates hypotonic and spastic children who need more support and less immobilization. It actually encourages relaxation and allows the dental work to be done more efficiently.

4. All of the following physical restraints are used to control extremities except

a. Posey straps
b. Velcro straps
c. Towel and tape
d. Triangular sheet

Ans d.

Triangular sheet is not used to restrict the extremities. The child's arms and legs can be immobilized with Posey straps, a towel and adhesive tape, velcro straps or with the help of an extra assistant. Refer to the explanation of Q. No. 3.

5. Which one of the following restraints was developed to help comfortably accommodate the hypotonic and severely spastic persons?

a. Bean bag dental chair insert
b. Pedi wrap
c. Papoose board
d. Posey straps

Ans a.

The beanbag dental chair insert was developed to help comfortably accommodate the hypotonic and severely spastic persons as they need more support and less immobilization on a dental chair. They also relax in this type of setting.

6. Autism is a severely incapacitating disturbance of mental and emotional development that causes problems in learning, communication and relating to others. This lifelong developmental disability manifests itself during the first 3 years of life, is difficult to diagnose and has no cure.

a. Both the statements are true
b. Both the statements are false
c. The first statement is true and the second is false
d. The first statement is false and the second is true

Ans a.

The answer is self-explanatory. Autism occurs approximately in 5 out of every 10,000 births and is more common in boys. These children have multiple medical and behavioral problems, which make their dental treatment difficult.

7. Which of the following is true of autism?

a. Children with autism look like normal children and have normal life spans but they have limited capacity to communicate, socialize and learn

b. Children with autism have poor muscle tone, poor coordination, drooling, a hyperactive knee jerk, strabismus and some children eventually develop epilepsy
c. Children with autism have strict routines and prefer soft food and sweetened foods. Because of poor tongue coordination, they tend to pouch food instead of swallowing
d. All of the above

Ans d.

All the above statements regarding autism are true. These children apart from having a tendency to pouch food instead of swallowing also have an increased desire for sweets. This leads to increased caries susceptibility.

8. The disability involved in patients with cerebral palsy can be

a. Muscle weakness
b. Paralysis or stiffness
c. Poor balance or irregular gait
d. Uncoordinated or involuntary movements
e. Any of the above

Ans e.

Cerebral palsy is one of the primary handicapping conditions of childhood with an incidence of 1 in 200 live births approximately. The disability in these children includes any of the four options above.

9. Cerebral palsy is classified based on the neuromuscular dysfunction and the extent of anatomic involvement. The cause for one-third of cerebral palsy cases is not known.

a. Both the statements are true
b. Both the statements are false
c. The first statement is true and the second is false
d. The first statement is false and the second is true

Ans a.

The answer is self-explanatory.

10. The most common type of cerebral palsy is

a. Dyskinetic
b. Ataxic
c. Spastic
d. Mixed

Ans c.

The most common type is spastic type (approximately 70% of cases).

S. No.	Type	Percentage of cases (approximately)
1.	Spastic	70%
2.	Dyskinetic	15%
3.	Ataxic	5%
4.	Mixed	10%

11. Bruxism is most commonly seen in ____________ type of cerebral palsy.

a. Dyskinetic
b. Ataxic
c. Spastic
d. Mixed

Ans a.

Bruxism is most commonly seen in dyskinetic type of cerebral palsy. Severe occlusal attrition of the primary and permanent dentition is noticed. *Temporomandibular* joint disorders may be a sequelae of this condition noticed in adult patients.

12. Limping gait and circumduction of affected leg are characteristic features in

a. Hemiplegia
b. Quadriplegia
c. Monoplegia
d. Paraplegia

Ans a.

In spastic hemiplegia, the hand and arm are flexed and held against the trunk. The foot and leg may be flexed and rotated internally resulting in a limping gait with circumduction of the affected leg.

S. No.	Type	Description
1.	Monoplegia	Involvement of one limb only
2.	Hemiplegia	Involvement of one side of the body
3.	Paraplegia	Involvement of both legs only
4.	Diplegia	Involvement of both legs with minimum involvement of both arms
5.	Quadriplegia	Involvement of all four limbs

13. Some of the neonatal reflexes persist long after the age in which they normally disappear in cerebral palsy patients. Which of the following reflexes is retained?

a. Asymmetric tonic neck reflex
b. Tonic labyrinthine reflex
c. Startle reflex
d. All of the above

Ans d.

In patients with cerebral palsy, certain neonatal reflexes may persist long after the age at which they normally disappear. These primitive reflexes are usually modified or are progressively replaced as the subcortical dominance of the infant's behavior is suppressed by the higher centers of the maturing central nervous system. Three such reflexes are mentioned in the following table.

S. No.	Reflex	Description
1.	Asymmetric tonic neck reflex	If the patient's head is suddenly turned to one side, the arm and leg on the side to which the face is turned will extend and stiffen. The limbs on the opposite side will flex.
2.	Tonic labyrinthine reflex	If the patient's head suddenly falls backwards while the patient is supine, the back may assume the position known as postural extension; the legs and arms will straighten out and the neck and back will arch.
3.	Startle reflex	Sudden, involuntary and forceful bodily movements are produced when the patient is surprised by stimuli such as sudden noises or unexpected movements by other people.

14. If a patient's (cerebral palsy) head suddenly falls backward while the patient is in supine position, legs and arms straighten out and the neck and back will arch. Which reflex is this?

a. Asymmetric tonic neck reflex
b. Tonic labyrinthine reflex
c. Startle reflex
d. All of the above

Ans b.

Refer to the explanation of Q. No. 13.

15. Which of the following is considered to be one of the approaches in handling children with cerebral palsy in the dental office?

a. Providing dental treatment in the wheel chair
b. Use of mouth props and finger splints
c. Avoidance of abrupt stimuli which will initiate the startle reflex
d. All of the above

Ans d.

All the above-mentioned approaches are to be used in the dental office while handling a child with cerebral palsy.

16. Difficulty in grasping objects is characteristic of which type of cerebral palsy?

a. Dyskinetic
b. Ataxic
c. Spastic
d. Mixed

Ans b.

Poor sense of balance and uncoordinated voluntary movements (e.g. stumbling or staggering gait or difficulty in grasping objects) is characteristic of ataxic type of cerebral palsy.

17. The touch taste smell method (instead of TSD) is usually used in children who are affected by

a. Deafness
b. Blindness
c. Cerebral palsy
d. Down syndrome

Ans b.

The touch taste smell method is used in children affected with blindness, as these senses are acute in these children.

18. Which of the following factors are to be considered while treating a child who has hearing impairment?

a. Determining the mode of communication
b. Usage of visual aids and allowing the patient to see the instruments
c. Adjusting the hearing aids
d. All of the above

Ans d.

All the above factors must be considered while treating a child who has hearing impairment.

19. Which of the following factors are to be considered while treating a child who is blind?

a. Reassuring physical contacts
b. Detailed description of the office and the instruments to be used
c. Do not move, grab or stop the patient without verbal warning
d. Usage of audio cassettes and Braille pamphlets
e. All of the above

Ans d.

All the above factors are to be considered while treating a child who is blind. Making physical contact like holding the patient's hand often promotes relaxation.

20. All of the following are physical restraints for the body except

a. Triangular sheet
b. Papoose board
c. Pedi wrap
d. Posey straps

Ans d.

Physical restraints involving an extra personnel like an assistant, hygienist or parents are called active physical restraints. Passive physical restraints include the use of devices.

Part immobilized	Name of passive physical restraint
Body	Triangular sheet, Papoose board, Pedi wrap, beanbag dental chair insert, safety belt
Extremities	Posey straps, velcro straps, towel and tape
Head	Forearm body support, head positioner, plastic bowl
Intraoral	Molt mouth prop, McKesson bite blocks, wrapped tongue blades

21. Which of the following are the other names of autism?

a. Kanner's syndrome
b. Infantile psychosis
c. Childhood schizophrenia
d. All of the above

Ans d.

The term "autism" is derived from the Greek word "autos" meaning self. These children show profound withdrawal from people and social environment. It is also called *early infantile autism.*

22. Learning disability is otherwise called

a. Dyslexia
b. Developmental aphasia
c. Minimal brain dysfunction
d. Any of the above

Ans d.

Learning disability may be manifested in disorders of listening, thinking, reading, talking, writing or spelling. It includes dyslexia, developmental aphasia, brain injury and minimal brain dysfunction.

23. Feingold diet is associated with treatment of

a. Autism
b. Hyperactivity
c. Mental retardation
d. Porphyria

Ans b.

The Feingold diet is a food elimination program developed by Ben F Feingold to treat hyperactivity. It eliminates a number of artificial colors, artificial flavors, aspartame, three petroleum-based preservatives and (at least initially) certain salicylates. There has been much debate about the efficacy of this program.

24. The IQ of children in profound mental retardation category ranges from

a. 60 to 70
b. 40 to 50
c. 50 to 60
d. less than 39

Ans d.

Mild retardation IQ score ranges from 52 to 69. Moderate retardation score is 36 to 54 and for severe or profound retardation, the score is less than 35 to 39.

25. The word "autism" is derived from a Greek word "autos" meaning

a. Others
b. Self
c. Spontaneous
d. Predictable

Ans b.

Refer the explanation of Q. No. 21.

26. One of the following is not a restraint for extremities

a. Posey straps
b. Velcro straps
c. Towel and tape
d. Pedi wrap

Ans d.

Refer to the explanation of Q. No. 3.

27. Parrot-like repetitious speech is associated with

a. Dyslexia
b. Autism
c. Minimal brain dysfunction
d. Cerebral palsy

Ans b.

Kopel (1977) has described 12 behavioral characteristics seen in children with autism. These include: extreme aloneness, language disturbances, mutism, parrot-like repetitious speech, difficulty with the concept of "yes", confusion in the use of personal pronouns, obsessive desire for the maintenance of sameness, pouching food preferably soft food, intrigue with spinning objects, self-stimulatory behavior, hyperactivity and seizure disorder.

28. Athetosis and choreoathetosis are associated with which of the following types of cerebral palsy?

a. Dyskinetic
b. Ataxic
c. Mixed
d. Spastic

Ans a.

Cerebral palsy is classified according to the type of neuromuscular dysfunction: spasticity, dyskinetic, ataxic and mixed. Athetosis (slow, twisting and writhing involuntary muscles) and choreoathetosis (sudden jerky movements) are included in the dyskinetic group.

29. A 6-year-old child who has been diagnosed with hyperkinesis appears at your office in an obvious state of anxiety at the impending treatment. Upon interview, his mother relates that he is taking 30 mg of methylphenidate (Ritalin) daily. Which of the following should you do in planning to make the child more manageable?

a. Double the daily dose of Ritalin 1 hour before the dental appointment
b. Ask the mother to discontinue medication on the day of the dental visit
c. Balance the medication with 65 mg Phenobarbital
d. Call the child's physician and discuss with him the child's drug regimen

Ans d.

Methylphenidate is a psychostimulant drug used for the treatment of attention-deficit hyperactivity disorder. It is always better to check with the child's physician before any dental treatment is attempted.

30. Which of the following is least likely to be effective in attempting to communicate with a mentally challenged patient?

a. Verbal rationalization of the patient's fears and anxieties
b. Rewarding appropriate behavior with verbal praise
c. Expressing verbal disapproval of negative behavior
d. Utilizing the parents as models, if they are cooperative

Ans a.

A mentally challenged child is one who has no or less communicative abilities and verbal rationalization would not suit them.

31. A well developed 8-year-old boy is referred by a pediatric neurologist to you for dental treatment. His mother narrates the following history: At present he is receiving daily dose of an amphetamine. His teacher complains that he never pays attention. He is left-handed and a bit clumsy. The most probable behavior disorder this patient demonstrates is

a. Autism
b. Epilepsy
c. Hyperkinesis
d. Mental retardation

Ans c.

Hyperkinesis or hyperkinesia is a state of overactive restlessness (e.g. hyperactivity), particularly in children. Typical symptoms include: extreme excess of motor activity (the children flits from activity to activity); restlessness; oscillating mood swings (he is fine one day, a terror the next); clumsiness; aggressive-like behavior; in school he cannot sit still, cannot comply with rules, has low frustration levels; frequently there may be sleeping problems and acquisition of speech may be delayed.

32. A mother and her 4-year-old son are seated alone in a reception area with the child staring off into space and constantly twisting a strand of hair about his fingers. Upon entry of another person, the child begins to beat his fist against the side of his face and behaves as though he does not hear his mother speaking to him. This behavior is most characteristic of

a. Child with autism

b. An overprotected child

c. A mentally retarded child

d. First dental appointment anxieties of a 4-year-old child

Ans a.

Refer to the explanation of Q. No. 27 for features shown by children with autism.

Chapter 32

Management of Medically Compromised Children

1. In which of the following clinical situations, does the dietary intake of the child include restriction of specific foods or total caloric consumption?

a. Phenylketonuria

b. Diabetes

c. Prader-Willi syndrome

d. All of the above

Ans d.

Patients with metabolic disturbances or syndromes like phenylketonuria, diabetes and Prader-Willi syndrome have diets that restrict specific foods or caloric consumption. The dietary recommendations should be made individually after proper consultation with the patient's primary physician or dietician.

2. Which of the medical conditions increase the mortality of infants and children with Down syndrome?

a. Cardiac defects

b. Increased incidence of leukemia

c. Increased incidence of upper respiratory infections

d. All of the above

Ans d.

All the above-mentioned medical conditions are responsible for increased mortality of infants and children with Down syndrome or Trisomy 21. The incidence of cardiac defects is about 40%. These children also have a 10- to 20-fold increase in the incidence of leukemia when compared to the general population. There is also a high incidence of rapid destructive periodontal disease noticed in these children.

3. Fragile X syndrome is a common inherited form of mental retardation and autism. It accounts for 30–50% of cases of X-linked mental retardation.

a. Both the statements are true
b. Both the statements are false
c. The first statement is true and the second is false
d. The first statement is false and the second is true

Ans a.

The answer is self-explanatory. The defect in this syndrome is the presence of an abnormal gene on the terminal portion of the long arm of X chromosome. Males are more vulnerable as they have only one X chromosome and are also more significantly affected than females.

4. In which of the following conditions is there a high incidence of dental and skeletal malocclusions?

a. Prader-Willi syndrome
b. Fragile X syndrome
c. Fetal alcohol Syndrome
d. Autism

Ans c.

Most of the dental problems associated with FAS (fetal alcohol syndrome) children are related to the high incidence of dental and skeletal malocclusions. The consumption of one to three drinks per day during the first 2 months of pregnancy can result in significant damage to the developing baby. Other complications in such babies include neurologic abnormalities, cardiac defects, growth retardation and cognitive defects.

5. In a patient with cardiac disease (susceptible to infective endocarditis), pulp therapy of primary teeth is not recommended. In permanent dentition, endodontic therapy may be undertaken after a careful evaluation and case selection.

a. Both the statements are true
b. Both the statements are false
c. The first statement is true and the second is false
d. The first statement is false and the second is true

Ans a.

Pulp therapy for primary teeth with poor prognosis is not recommended because of the high incidence of associated chronic infection. Extraction of such teeth and appropriate fixed space maintainers are preferred. Endodontic therapy in the permanent dentition can usually be accomplished successfully if the teeth are carefully selected and endodontic therapy is adequately performed.

6. **Rheumatic fever is common in which of the following age groups?**
   a. Less than 6 years
   b. 6–15 years
   c. 15–30 years
   d. More than 30 years

Ans b.

Rheumatic fever appears most commonly between 6 and 15 years of age. It is rare in infancy. It is most prevalent in temperate zones, high altitudes and is more common and severe in children who live in substandard conditions.

7. **The acute form of bacterial endocarditis is a fulminating disease that usually occurs as a result of microorganisms of high pathogenicity attacking a normal heart, causing erosive destruction of valves. Subacute bacterial endocarditis usually develops in a person with pre-existing congenital cardiac disease or rheumatic valvular lesions.**
   a. Both the statements are true
   b. Both the statements are false
   c. The first statement is true and the second is false
   d. The first statement is false and the second is true

Ans a.

The acute form is caused by Staphylococcus, Group A Streptococcus and Pneumococcus whereas the subacute form is caused by *Streptococci viridans.*

8. **Which of the following is correct regarding the agent and dosage used for antibiotic prophylaxis?**
   a. Amoxicillin; adults 2 g and children 50 mg/kg one hour prior to the procedure
   b. Clindamycin; adults 600 mg and children 20 mg/kg one hour prior to the procedure
   c. Azithromycin or clarithromycin; adults 500 mg and children 15 mg/kg one hour prior to the procedure
   d. Any of the above

Ans d.

Any dental patient with a history of congenital heart disease or rheumatic heart disease or who has a prosthetic valve should be considered susceptible. With only one large dose of antibiotics, routine restorative and surgical dental procedures, which are known to precipitate transient bacteremia, can be safely completed. All the above regimens can be used as antibiotic prophylaxis for dental, oral, respiratory tract or esophageal procedures.

9. Which of the following factors are correct regarding hemophilia A?

a. It is caused by a deficiency of factor VIII
b. It is inherited as X-linked recessive trait
c. Males are affected and females are carriers
d. All of the above

Ans d.

All the above-mentioned factors are correct regarding hemophilia. If a normal male has children with a female carrier of hemophilia, there is a 50% chance that hemophilia will occur in each male offspring and a 50% chance that each female offspring will be a carrier. If a male hemophiliac has children with a normal female, all male offsprings will be normal and all female offsprings will be carriers.

10. Christmas disease is

a. Hemophilia A
b. Hemophilia B
c. Hemophilia C
d. Von Willebrand's disease

Ans b.

Christmas disease is otherwise called hemophilia B. It is caused by deficiency of factor IX (plasma thromboplastin component).

11. Impaired formation of platelet plug in von Willebrand's disease may result in bleeding from the skin and mucosa, bruising, epistaxis, prolonged bleeding after surgical procedures and menorrhagia. This is in contrast to factors VIII and IX deficient hemophilia in which bleeding tends to involve muscles and joints.

a. Both the statements are true
b. Both the statements are false
c. The first statement is true and the second is false
d. The first statement is false and the second is true

Ans a.

The answer is self-explanatory.

12. Which of the following agents are used for treatment of hemophilia?

a. Factor VIII concentrate
b. Synthetic analog of vasopressin (1-deamino-8-D-arginine vasopressin)

c. Epsilon-amino caproic acid

d. Tranexamic acid

e. All of the above

Ans **e.**

The mainstay of therapy for Hemophilia is replacement of the deficient coagulation factor either by the use of purified concentrate made from blood plasma or through recombinant technology. DDAVP (1-deamino-8-D-arginine vasopressin) is a synthetic analogue of vasopressin and can be used for minor hemorrhagic episodes to achieve hemostasis. Antifibrinolytics are adjunctive therapies for dental management of patients with bleeding disorders. These agents include epsilon-amino caproic acid or tranexamic acid. They prevent the lysis of loose friable clots that a Hemophiliac forms within the oral cavity.

13. Periodontal ligament injections are contraindicated in Hemophiliac patients. Inferior alveolar nerve block and posterior superior alveolar nerve block predispose to the development of hematoma, which can lead to airway obstruction.

a. Both the statements are true

b. Both the statements are false

c. The first statement is true and the second is false

d. The first statement is false and the second is true

Ans **d.**

In the absence of factor replacement, periodontal ligament (PDL) injections may be used. The anesthetic is administered along the four axial surfaces of the tooth by placement of the needle into the gingival sulcus and the periodontal ligament space. The loose connective, nonfibrous and highly vascularized tissue at the sites of inferior alveolar injection and posterior superior alveolar injections are predisposed to the development of a dissecting hematoma, which has the potential of obstructing the airway and of creating a life-threatening bleeding episode.

14. A pulpotomy or pulpectomy is preferable to extraction in Hemophiliac patients. Rubber dam clamp retainers with sub-gingival extensions (8A or 14A) should be avoided.

a. Both the statements are true

b. Both the statements are false

c. The first statement is true and the second is false

d. The first statement is false and the second is true

Ans a.

The extraction of a tooth in an individual with Hemophilia implies more complicated treatment and expense to the patient. Hemorrhage from the pulp chamber does not present a significant problem if readily controlled with pressure from cotton pledgets.

15. Acute hepatitis classically presents with lethargy, loss of appetite, nausea, vomiting, abdominal pain and ultimately jaundice. In children the disease is usually more benign and jaundice is uncommon.

a. Both the statements are true
b. Both the statements are false
c. The first statement is true and the second is false
d. The first statement is false and the second is true

Ans a.

16. The most frequent cause of death in AIDS patients is

a. Non-Hodgkin's lymphoma
b. Kaposi's sarcoma
c. Pneumocystis carinii pneumonia
d. Herpes virus infection

Ans c.

The answer is self-explanatory.

17. The most frequently seen neoplasm in AIDS patients is

a. Non-Hodgkin's lymphoma
b. Hodgkin's lymphoma
c. Kaposi's sarcoma
d. Burkitt's lymphoma

Ans c.

Often, the first lesions of Kaposi sarcoma appear in the oral cavity. The most common oral site is the hard palate. The lesions may be red, blue or purple, flat or raised and solitary or multiple.

18. The leading cause of death in children is

a. Accidents
b. Malignancy
c. Heart disease
d. Respiratory disorders

Ans a.

Malignancy is second only to accidents as the leading cause of death in children.

19. Leukemia is a malignancy of the hematopoietic tissues in which there is a disseminated proliferation of abnormal leukocytes in the bone marrow. These immature appearing undifferentiated blast cells replace normal cells in bone marrow and accumulate in other tissues and organs of the body.

a. Both the statements are true
b. Both the statements are false
c. The first statement is true and the second is false
d. The first statement is false and the second is true

Ans a.

The answer is self-explanatory.

20. The commonest type of leukemia affecting children is

a. Acute lymphocytic leukemia
b. Acute myelocytic leukemia
c. Chronic lymphocytic leukemia
d. Chronic myelocytic leukemia

Ans a.

Acute leukemia is the most common malignancy in children. It accounts for about one-third of all childhood malignancies; of these, approximately 80% are lymphocytic (acute lymphocytic leukemia). Chronic leukemia is rare in children accounting for less than 2% of all cases.

21. In a leukemic child whose first remission has not been obtained or one who is in relapse, all elective dental procedures should be deferred. Pulp therapy in primary and permanent teeth are contraindicated in leukemic children.

a. Both the statements are true
b. Both the statements are false
c. The first statement is true and the second is false
d. The first statement is false and the second is true

Ans a.

Both the statements are true. However, it is essential that potential sources of systemic infection within the oral cavity be controlled or eradicated whenever they are recognized (e.g. immediate extraction of carious primary teeth with pulpal involvement). Endodontic treatment for permanent teeth is not recommended for any patient with leukemia. Even with the most exacting technique, an area of chronic inflammatory tissue may remain in the periapical region, which in an immunosuppressed neutropenic patient can act as an anachoretic focus with devastating sequelae.

22. The minimum platelet level required to perform most dental procedures is

a. 50,000–100,000/mm^3
b. 200,000–300,000/mm^3
c. 400,000–500,000/mm^3
d. 20,000–50,000/mm^3

Ans a.

A platelet level of 100,000/mm^3 is adequate for most of the dental procedures.

S. No.	Counts	Significance
1.	1,50,000–400,000	Normal
2.	50,000–100,000	Bleeding time is prolonged, but patient would tolerate most routine procedures
3.	20,000–50,000	At moderate risk of bleeding; defer elective surgery procedures
4.	<20,000	At significant risk for bleeding

23. Infection is the primary cause of death in approximately 80% of children with Leukemia. Bleeding is the second most common cause.

a. Both the statements are true
b. Both the statements are false
c. The first statement is true and the second is false
d. The first statement is false and the second is true

Ans a.

The answer is self-explanatory. Hence, the primary objective of dental treatment in a child with leukemia should be the prevention, control and eradication of oral inflammation, hemorrhage and infection.

24. Which of the following diseases in children needs bone marrow transplantation?

a. Aplastic anemia
b. Leukemia
c. Myelofibrosis
d. All of the above

Ans d.

The answer is self-explanatory.

25. The most common cause of failure of bone marrow transplantation is

a. Infection due to endogenous opportunistic microorganisms
b. Infection due to extraneous viruses and bacteria
c. Postoperative hemorrhage
d. Any of the above

Ans a.

In almost all organ transplant procedures, host rejection of the transplanted organ and infection are the prime reasons for treatment failure.

26. Which of the following are oral complications of total body irradiation?

a. Mucositis
b. Transient salivary gland dysfunction
c. Oral ulceration
d. Gingival bleeding
e. Any of the above

Ans e.

Oral ulceration, mucositis and transient salivary gland dysfunction are frequent consequences of somatotoxic chemotherapy and total body irradiation. Minor trauma to atrophic mucous membranes often results in self-induced ulceration of the buccal mucosa, lips and the tongue. Thrombocytopenic gingival bleeding and bleeding from oral ulcerations are also frequently encountered.

27. As a pretransplant preparation, which of the following can be undertaken by a patient to maintain good oral hygiene?

a. Daily brushing and flossing
b. Daily use of self-applied topical fluoride gel
c. Chlorhexidine mouth rinse every 12 hours
d. All of the above

Ans d.

The answer is self-explanatory. The integrity of the oral cavity is maintained by keeping the oral structures both hard and soft tissues clean, moist and free of infection. The resultant decrease in septic episodes in the oral cavity should diminish the patient's morbidity and mortality since the mouth is the most common source of infection in these patients.

28. Which of the following malignant diseases is common in childhood?

a. Wilm's tumor
b. Osteosarcoma
c. Rhabdomyosarcoma
d. Neuroblastoma
e. All of the above

Ans e.

The answer is self-explanatory. Solid tumors account for approximately half of the cases of childhood malignancy. Dental management of patients with solid tumors is similar to that of patients with acute leukemia.

29. The most common genetic disease of Caucasians is

a. Bronchial asthma
b. Fragile X syndrome
c. Fetal alcohol syndrome
d. Cystic fibrosis

Ans d.

Cystic fibrosis is considered as the most common genetic disease of Caucasians with 1 in 20 people considered to be carriers. It is transmitted as an autosomal recessive trait.

30. Dose of amoxicillin given intraorally for infectious endocarditis prophylaxis is

a. 50 mg/kg
b. 15 mg/kg
c. 2 g/kg
d. 10 mg/kg

Ans a.

For children, amoxicillin is given 50 mg/kg orally 1 hour before the dental procedure. Postoperative antibiotic coverage is not required.

Type	Drugs
Standard general prophylaxis for patients at risk	Amoxicillin: Adults – 2 g (children — 50 mg/kg) given orally one hour before the procedure
Unable to take oral medications	Ampicillin: Adults – 2 g (children — 50 mg/kg) given IM or IV within 30 minutes before the procedure

Amoxicillin/ ampicillin/penicillin allergic patients	Clindamycin: Adults – 600 mg (children –20 mg/kg) given orally one hour before the procedure OR Cephalexin or cefadroxil: Adults – 2 g (children – 50 mg/kg) orally one hour before procedure OR Azithromycin or clarithromycin: Adults 500 mg (children 15 mg/kg) orally one hour before the procedure
Amoxicillin/ ampicillin/penicillin allergic patients unable to take oral medications	Clindamycin: Adults – 600 mg (children – 20 mg/kg IV) within 30 minutes before the procedure OR Cefazolin: Adults – 1 g (children – 25 mg/kg) IM or IV within 30 minutes before procuedure

Antibiotic prophylaxis regimen for dental, oral, respiratory tract or esophageal procedures (follow-up dose after the procedure no longer recommended).

31. One of the following procedures does need endocarditis prophylaxis

a. Replantation of avulsed tooth
b. Placement of rubber dams
c. Postoperative suture removal
d. Impression making

Prophylaxis recommended	Prophylaxis not recommended
1. Dental extractions 2. Periodontal procedures including scaling, root planning, probing and surgery 3. Dental implant placement and replantation of an avulsed tooth 4. Endodontic surgery or instrumentation beyond the apex 5. Subgingival placement of antibiotic fibers or strips	1. Restorative dentistry with or without retraction cord 2. Local anesthetic injections (nonintraligamentary) 3. Intracanal endodontic treatment; postplacement and composite build-up 4. Placement of rubber dams 5. Postoperative suture removal 6. Impression taking

6. Initial placement of orthodontic bands but not brackets 7. Intraligamentary local anesthetic injections 8. Prophylactic cleaning of teeth or implants where bleeding is anticipated	7. Fluoride treatment 8. Orthodontic appliance adjustment 9. Shedding of primary teeth 10. Placement of removable appliances

Ans a.

Refer the following table .

Recommendation of endocarditis prophylaxis based on type of dental procedures

32. Febrile seizures tend to occur in preschool children when fever rises above

a. 100°F
b. 101°F
c. 102°F
d. 104°F

Ans d.

Febrile seizures occur in preschool children who develop sudden fever above 104°F. Most of these children do not have subsequent episodes.

33. Chipmunk facies is seen in

a. Sickle cell anemia
b. Megaloblastic anemia
c. β Thalassemia
d. Iron deficiency anemia

Ans c.

β Thalassemia is an autosomal recessive disorder where there is a deficiency in the β chains of hemoglobin. The most common oral manifestation is the enlargement of maxilla and continuous increase in the marrow spaces leading to "chicken-wire" appearance radiographically and "chipmunk facies" clinically.

34. Which of the following diseases occurs because of defective second chromosome?

a. Sickle cell anemia

b. Megaloblastic anemia
c. β Thalassemia
d. Iron deficiency anemia

Ans a.

Defective second chromosome leads to production of impaired erythrocytes that can block the blood vessels. Normal HbA is replaced by HbS which has decreased oxygen carrying capacity.

35. Which of the following is true about hemophilia?

a. Prolonged partial thromboblastin time
b. Prolonged bleeding time
c. Prolonged prothrombin time
d. Prolonged thrombin time

Ans a.

Diagnosis of hemophilia is made when the partial thromboplastin time is prolonged with normal bleeding time, platelet count, prothrombin time and thrombin time.

36. Which of the following factor is closely associated with platelet plug formation?

a. Factor VIII
b. Factor IX
c. Factor VII
d. Factor XIII

Ans a.

von Willebrand factor and factor VIII circulate together and help in the formation of the primary platelet plug. They help in platelet adhesion to the subendothelium via collagen.

37. Presence of fetal hemoglobin protects the infant from sickle cell anemia up to

a. 12 months
b. 18–24 months
c. 4 years
d. 6 years

Ans b.

High levels of fetal hemoglobin protect the infant from sickling in the infancy period. Most of the fetal hemoglobin is replaced in the middle of the second year of life after which the child may get affected.

38. In a child with a suspected diagnosis of leukemia and with a badly infected primary tooth, the procedure of choice would be to

a. Administer antibiotics and refer the patient to a physician
b. Obtain consultation before determining the course of action
c. Obtain a blood count, admit the child to a hospital for extraction
d. Provide palliative treatment only

Ans b.

Consultation with the child's physician, hematologist and oncologist is a must to determine the course of the treatment. Infection is the primary cause of death in these children followed by bleeding. Special care should be taken to carry out a completely sterile and least traumatic dental procedure.

39. Examination of a mixed dentition malocclusion reveals an abnormal resorption pattern in primary teeth, delayed eruption of permanent teeth, incompletely formed roots of permanent teeth and a large tongue. Which of the following would be suspected to be an etiologic factor?

a. Hypothyroidism
b. Addison disease
c. Von Recklinghausen disease
d. History of severe febrile disease

Ans a.

Hypothyroidism is characterized by delayed development, mental retardation and above dental anomalies.

40. A serious complication that can develop as a result of juvenile diabetes mellitus is

a. Ataxia
b. Aphasiac
c. Deafness
d. Blindness

Ans d.

Juvenile diabetes mellitus is now more commonly called *Type 1 diabetes.* It is a syndrome with disordered metabolism and inappropriately high blood glucose levels due to a deficiency of insulin secretion in the pancreas. If juvenile diabetes is left unmanaged, it can damage the eyes leading to diabetic retinopathy and possible blindness.

41. How is tooth development affected by severe congenital heart disease?

a. Tooth development is delayed
b. Tooth development is advanced
c. Cyst formation is likely, but the effect is unpredictable
d. Development of posterior teeth is advanced; development of anterior teeth is delayed

Ans a.

The answer is self-explanatory.

42. Referral of a 6-year-old child with a speech problem to a speech pathologist is

a. Needed only if the patient is having great difficulty in being understood
b. Not particularly important until the child reaches the age of 10
c. Not needed if a myofunctional therapist is a member of the dental team
d. Helpful because both patient and parents are likely to benefit from counseling

Ans d.

The answer is self-explanatory.

43. Dental management of a child with minimal brain dysfunction syndrome should include

a. General anesthesia
b. Adequate premedication
c. Full coverage when caries occurs
d. The tell-show-do technique
e. A comprehensive preventive program

Ans e.

Minimal brain dysfunction was formally defined in 1966 by Samuel Clements as a combination of average or above average intelligence with certain mild to severe learning or behavioral disabilities characterizing deviant functioning of the central nervous system. It can involve impairments in visual or auditory perception, conceptualization, language and memory and difficulty in controlling. The term is often used either in connection (or interchangeably) with hyperactivity and/or attention deficit disorder.

44. A 12-year-old child is 30 inches tall and has excellent body proportions. Laboratory studies are likely to reveal which of the following conditions?

a. Hypothyroidism

b. Hypopituitarism

c. Malabsorption syndrome

d. Adrenogenital syndrome

Ans b.

Hypopituitarism is the decreased secretion of one or more of the eight hormones normally produced by the pituitary gland at the base of the brain. Growth hormone deficiency leads to a decrease in muscle mass, central obesity and impaired attention and memory. Children experience growth retardation and short stature.

Chapter 33

Cleft Lip and Palate Management

1. The most frequently used classification of cleft lip was given by

a. Veau

b. Kernahan and Starke

c. Classification of Cleft Palate Association

d. Classification of American Association of Cleft Lip and Palate

Ans a.

Veau's classification of cleft lip is as follows:

Class I—Unilateral notching of vermilion not extending to the lip.

Class II—Unilateral notching of vermilion border with cleft extending into the lip but not including the floor of the nose.

Class III—Unilateral clefting of the vermilion border of the lip extending into the floor of the nose.

Class IV—Any bilateral clefting of the lip whether this is incomplete notching or complete clefting.

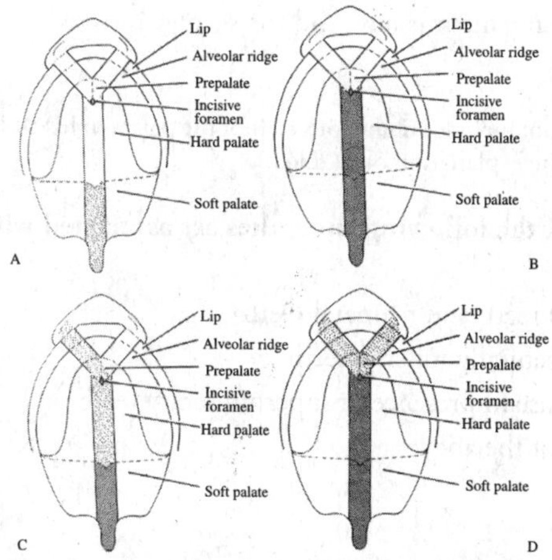

Fig. 33.1 Patient with crowding of lower anterior tooth.

2. **Which of the following regarding Veau's classification of cleft palate is incorrect?**
   a. Class I—Cleft of soft palate
   b. Class II—Cleft of soft and hard palate with alveolar process
   c. Class III—Cleft of soft and hard palate and alveolar process on one side of premaxillary area
   d. Class IV—Involves soft palate and continues through alveolus on both sides of premaxilla leaving it free and often mobile

Ans b.

Veau's classification of cleft palate is as follows:

Class I—Cleft of soft palate.

Class II—Cleft of soft and hard palate without involvement of the alveolar process.

Class III—Cleft of soft and hard palate and the alveolar process on one side of the premaxillary area.

Class IV—Involves the soft palate and continues through the alveolus on both sides of the premaxilla, leaving it free and often mobile.

3. **Veau included the submucous cleft of the palate in his classification system. Submucous clefts may be frequently diagnosed by the presence of bifid uvula, palpable notch at the posterior portion of hard palate and Zona pellucida (thin translucent membrane).**
   a. Both the statements are false
   b. Both the statements are true
   c. First statement is true and the second is false
   d. First statement is false and the second is true

Ans d.

Veau did not include submucous cleft of the palate in his classification system. Refer to the explanation of Q. No. 2.

4. **Which of the following anomalies are associated with cleft lip and palate?**
   a. Natal teeth and neonatal teeth
   b. Congenitally missing teeth
   c. Increase in presence of supernumerary teeth
   d. Any of the above

Ans d.

All the above-mentioned features are associated with cleft lip and palate.

Natal teeth (teeth found at birth) and neonatal teeth (teeth erupted within first 30 days after birth) are usually maxillary central incisors observed in patients with a complete unilateral or bilateral cleft palate. There is high incidence of congenitally missing teeth especially the primary or permanent lateral incisors (adjacent to the cleft) and premolars. Supernumerary teeth are often seen in patients with complete unilateral or bilateral clefts.

5. With a complete cleft of the palate and alveolus there is no longer a contiguous maxillary arch. External forces applied to muscles of mastication or the contraction of scar tissue subsequent to surgical repair of cleft palate can result in medial collapse of posterior segments causing posterior crossbite.

a. Both the statements are false
b. Both the statements are true
c. First statement is true and the second is false
d. First statement is false and the second is true

Ans b.

The answer is self-explanatory.

6. The initial surgical closure of cleft lip is done at

a. 6 months
b. 3 months
c. 1 year and 6 months
d. 2 years

Ans b.

Surgical closure of cleft lip is usually accomplished at 10 weeks of age (3 months).

7. The rule of tens used in determining optimal timing of surgical lip closure considers which of the following

a. Age
b. Weight
c. Hemoglobin
d. All of the above

Ans d.

Rule of tens says that the child should be of 10 weeks of age, weighing 10 pounds and having 10 g of hemoglobin to undergo any surgical procedure.

8. Which of the following statements regarding palatoplasty is/are true?

a. Palatoplasty (surgical closure of palate) is usually accomplished between 12 months and 2 years of age
b. The primary purpose of palatal closure by 2 years of age is to facilitate the acquisition of normal speech
c. The procedure may also improve hearing and swallowing by aligning the cleft palatal musculature
d. All of the above

Ans d.

The answer is self-explanatory.

9. Lefort I maxillary advancement is not technically feasible until the patient has a full complement of permanent dentition. The horizontal cuts to free the maxilla must necessarily be made above the apices of permanent dentition; hence unerupted cuspids or bicuspids would make the procedure impractical.

a. Both the statements are false
b. Both the statements are true
c. First statement is true and the second is false
d. First statement is false and the second is true

Ans b.

The answer is self-explanatory.

10. Speech may be observed as the ordered utterance of language. It is controlled by four basic processes called respiration, phonation, resonance and articulation.

a. Both the statements are false
b. Both the statements are true
c. First statement is true and the second is false
d. First statement is false and the second is true

Ans b.

The answer is self-explanatory.

11. All of the following statements regarding speech sounds are true except

a. Two major categories of speech sounds in the English language are vowels and consonants
b. Consonants are the first speech sounds to be fully mastered.

c. Vowels are produced with minimal constriction of vocal tract (by open vocal tract)
d. Consonants are produced by constriction or obstruction of vocal tract (closed vocal tract)

Ans b.

Vowels are the first speech sounds to be fully mastered. Most children articulate vowels by 3–3½ years. Consonant sounds require more time to master. Consonant sound maturation remains incomplete even at 8 years.

12. Impairment of velopharyngeal motion has been demonstrated in which of the following conditions?

a. Cleft palate
b. Poliomyelitis
c. Myasthenia gravis
d. Muscular dystrophy
e. All of the above

Ans e.

All the above-mentioned conditions affect the muscular function. Hence impairment of velopharyngeal motion is seen in all the above-mentioned conditions.

13. Stuttering typically begins in childhood between 2.5 and 4 years of age. Stuttering is characterized by breakdowns (repetitions, prolongations and hesitations) in the rhythm or fluency of speech.

a. Both the statements are false
b. Both the statements are true
c. First statement is true and the second is false
d. First statement is false and the second is true

Ans b.

The answer is self-explanatory.

14. Cleft lip occurs due to nonunion of

a. Maxillary and frontonasal processes
b. Maxillary and mandibular process
c. Maxillary process and palatine process
d. Medial nasal process and maxillary process

Ans d.

The answer is self-explanatory.

15. A submucous cleft of the palate is best detected by

a. Occlusal laminograph
b. Periapical laminograph
c. Cephalometric laminograph
d. Ultraviolet fiber optics
e. Palpation

Ans e.

The diagnosis of submucous cleft palate is made by identification on physical examination.

16. The proposed mode of inheritance of cleft lip and palate is

a. Multifactorial
b. Autosomal dominant
c. Autosomal recessive
d. X-linked recessive

Ans a.

Cleft lip and palate (CLAP) was initially thought to be inherited as an autosomal recessive trait. But it is now considered to have a multifactorial inheritance pattern where susceptible genes may be present in an individual requiring exposure to adverse environmental stimuli conducive for the formation of the defect.

17. A cleft palate deformity occurs during which trimester of pregnancy?

a. First
b. Second
c. Third

Ans a.

Cleft palate occurs due to failure of the fusion of the palatine shelves. This occurs in the first trimester of pregnancy.

18. Speech problems associated with cleft palate are usually the results of

a. Poor tongue control that produces lisping
b. Poor lip musculature or heavy scars in the lip that limit production of vowel sounds
c. Inability of the tongue to close airflow from the epiglottis
d. Inability of the soft palate to close air from the nasopharynx
e. Missing teeth that make the formation of articulation sounds by the tongue difficult

Ans d.

The answer is self explanatory.

19. Which of the following is the most common orofacial malformation that produces malocclusion?

a. Cleft palate
b. Ectodermal dysplasia
c. Pierre Robin syndrome
d. Osteogenesis imperfecta
e. Cleidocranial dysostosis

Ans a.

The answer is self explanatory.

20. Which of the following dental anomalies are associated with cleft lip and palate?

a. Supernumerary tooth
b. Missing tooth
c. Peg laterals or conical-shaped tooth
d. All of the above

Ans d.

The answer is self-explanatory.

21. Cheiloplasty is

a. Surgical closure of alveolus
b. Surgical closure of lip
c. Surgical closure of palate
d. Surgical closure of fistula

Ans b.

Refer to the explanation of Q. No. 22.

22. Millard flap technique is carried out for

a. Closure of lip
b. Closure of palate
c. Closure of oroantral fistula
d. Closure of velopharyngeal opening

Ans a.

The surgical closure of lip is carried out at approximately 3 months of age. Two most commonly employed techniques are the Tennison and Millard flaps. These techniques involve the preparation of flaps which are rotated over the cleft and united.

23. The primary objective of closure of palate at 18 months is to

a. Facilitate normal speech pattern
b. Improve esthetics
c. Facilitate eating habits
d. Improve breathing

Ans a.

The main objective of this surgical closure is to facilitate normal speech pattern. If the palate is not closed, speech is irreversibly damaged. Repair is carried out by elevating flaps from lateral and posterior regions of the cleft.

24. A preliminary speech assessment for a child with cleft lip and palate should be carried out by

a. 2 years
b. 4 years
c. 6 years
d. 6 months

Ans a.

Treatment schedule for patients with CLAP is provided in the following table.

Treatment schedule for patient with cleft lip and palate.

Age	Treatment
Birth	1. Construction of feeding plate 2. Referral to a center where a multidisciplinary team exists 3. Primary care advice about weight gain for fitness to surgery 4. Infant oral care measures
3 months	1. Surgical repair of the lip
6 months	1. Preventive oral care measures 2. Discussion of anticipatory guidance protocol with pediatric dentist 3. Reinforcement of infant oral care measures and importance of preventive dentistry

12–18 months	1. Surgical repair of cleft palate 2. Preliminary speech assessment
2 years	1. Initial assessment by orthodontist, ENT surgeon, speech therapist 2. Assessment of surgical result by plastic surgeon or oral and maxillofacial surgeon
3 years	1. Quarterly dental check-ups 2. Parental education of effective oral hygiene measures
4 years	1. ENT assessment 2. Beginning of speech therapy
7 years	1. Early correction of crossbite 2. Orthodontist's assessment on early orthodontic treatment
9 years	1. Esthetic surgery — lip and nose revision 2. Growth modification treatment 3. Early orthodontic treatment
12 years	1. Correction of malalignment begins 2. Creation of space for replacement of missing teeth
16 years	1. Esthetic surgery to improve appearance 2. Any major orthognathic surgeries 3. Fixed and permanent replacement of missing teeth 4. Regular restorative care

25. The earliest description of presurgical orthopedics in literature is by

a. Veau in 1901
b. Kernahan in 1898
c. Fogh-Anderson in 1858
d. Hoffman in 1686

Ans d.

The earliest description of presurgical orthopedics was given by Hoffman where he used maxillary strap to reposition the maxilla.

26. Striped "Y" classification is given by

a. Veau

b. Starke

c. Fogh-Anderson

d. Kernahan

Ans d.

The classification uses the letter "Y" to represent the areas in which the clefts are found. The two upper arms represent the lip, alveolus and hard palate as far as the incisive foramen. The single lower arm represents the hard and soft palate. When a defect is present, the appropriate area is shaded.

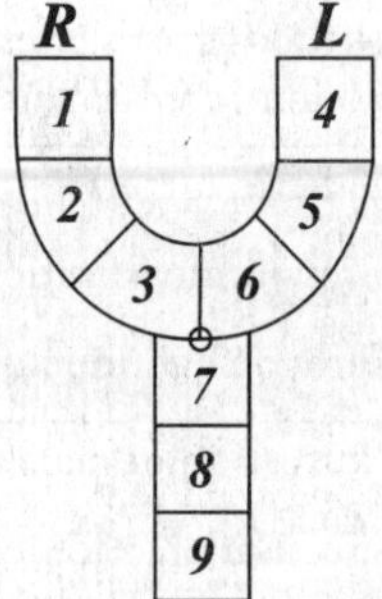

Fig. 33.2 Kernahan classification of cleft palate.

Chapter 34

Medical Emergencies

1. A 9-year-old epileptic patient has a petit mal seizure in the office. No other member of the office staff is available to render assistance. The proper course of management is to

a. Administer oxygen
b. Inject a barbiturate
c. Wait until the episode passes
d. Inject epinephrine subcutaneously
e. Call the local emergency code for assistance

Ans c.

A petit mal seizure is the term commonly given to a staring spell, most commonly called an "absence seizure". It is a brief (usually less than 15 seconds) disturbance of brain function due to abnormal electrical activity in the brain. Petit mal seizures occur most commonly in children aged 6 to 12 years.

2. Labored breathing is an indication of

a. Completely obstructed airway
b. Partially obstructed airway
c. Presence of foreign body in the lungs at the alveoli level
d. Circulatory insufficiency

Ans b.

Labored breathing is the presence of abnormal high-pitched sound heard when the airway is blocked. It is an indication of respiratory insufficiency caused by the obstruction of the airway.

3. Which of the following is true regarding mouth-to-mouth breathing?

a. Most commonly used method of artificial ventilation
b. Rescuer places himself at the side of the patient while performing this method

c. Rescuer blows into the victim's mouth once in every 3 seconds.
d. All of the above

Ans d.

The rescuer takes a deep breath, makes a tight seal with his mouth around the victim's mouth and blows into the victim's mouth. The victim is allowed to exhale passively; falling of the chest wall can be observed. The disadvantage is that the exhaled air from the rescuer's lung contains a maximum of only 15–18% oxygen.

4. Which of the following is sign of adequate ventilation during mouth-to-mouth breathing?

a. Observing the rise and fall of victim's chest
b. Feeling of the resistance and compliance of the victim's lungs in his or her (the rescuer) own airway as they expand
c. Hearing and feeling the air escape during exhalation
d. All of the above

Ans d.

The answer is self explanatory.

5. External cardiac compression (ECC) can produce

a. Systolic pressure of 100 mm Hg and diastolic of 0 mm Hg
b. Systolic pressure of 0 mm Hg and diastolic of 100 mm Hg
c. Systolic pressure of 40 mm Hg and diastolic of 20 mm Hg
d. Systolic pressure of 20 mm Hg and diastolic of 40 mm Hg

Ans a.

ECC comprises of rhythmic application of pressure over the lower half of the sternum. The intermittent pressure applied compresses the heart and produces a pulsatile artificial circulation. It should be done on a firm surface and requires a pressure application which can depress the sternum by 1 to 2 inches.

6. Effective external cardiac compression requires sufficient pressure to depress a child's sternum by a minimum of

a. 1 inch
b. 1 to 2 inches
c. 2 to 3 inches
d. 3 to 4 inches

Ans b.

Refer to the explanation of Q. No. 5.

7. **The dosage of Diazepam to be given during convulsions is**
   a. 0.9 mg/kg body weight
   b. 0.3 mg/kg body weight
   c. 0.6 mg/kg body weight
   d. 1.3 mg/kg body weight

Ans b.

Diazepam is given 0.3 mg/kg intravenously without dilution over 1–2 minutes. If the seizure persists it can be repeated after 30 minutes. The maximum dose that can be given is 10 mg.

8. **Which of the following is Heimlich's maneuver?**
   a. Delivering sharp back blows
   b. Abdominal thrusts
   c. Finger sweep motion to retrieve a foreign body from pharynx
   d. Performing a cricothyrotomy

Ans b.

Heimlich's maneuver is done in conscious patients with foreign body obstruction when back blows are not successful. The rescuer stands behind the victim, places one fist below the xiphoid process and clenches with the other hand and pulls up and back forcefully. This pushes the diaphragm up and increases the intrathoracic pressure. This expels air through the larynx dislodging the foreign body. Usually four thrusts are carried out in succession.

9. **Most rapid, convenient and accurate method of assessing circulation is**
   a. Checking the radial pulse
   b. Palpation of carotid pulse
   c. Pupillary dilatation
   d. Color of the tongue

Ans b.

Lack of tactile perception of a pulse in large arteries like carotid artery indicates circulatory insufficiency.

10. **Most common cause of loss of consciousness in dental office is due to**
    a. Syncope
    b. Allergic reaction
    c. Angioneurotic edema
    d. Hypoglycemia

Ans a.

Syncope or simple faint is the most common cause for loss of consciousness in the dental office. Anxiety in the dental office usually triggers the sympathetic nervous system resulting in the release of epinephrine and norepinephrine. This causes peripheral pooling of the blood in skeletal muscles and less blood supply to the brain, making the patient dizzy.

11. The dosage of Epinephrine (1:1000) used in management of anaphylaxis in children is

a. 0.01 mg/kg
b. 0.001 mg/kg
c. 0.2 mg/kg
d. 0.002 mg/kg

Ans a.

Epinephrine is administered 0.1 mg/kg or 0.3 mg/m^2. A single pediatric dose should not exceed 0.5 mL (0.5 mg).

Section X
Interdisciplinary Pediatric Dentistry

Chapter 35

Oral Surgical Considerations and Local Anesthesia

1. **The most effective topical anesthetic is**
   a. Lignocaine
   b. Tetracaine
   c. Ethyl amino benzoate (benzocaine)
   d. Dyclonine

Ans c.

Benzocaine is the most effective topical anesthetic. It is otherwise known as ethyl amino benzoate. It has a rapid onset and longer duration of anesthesia than the other topical agents.

2. **Jet injection was introduced by**
   a. Figge and Scherer (1947)
   b. Schroeder (1948)
   c. McKay (1952)
   d. Frank (1966)

Ans a.

The jet injection is based on the principle that small quantities of liquids forced through very small openings under high pressure can penetrate mucous membrane or skin without causing excessive trauma.

3. **All of the following are true regarding jet injection (Syrijet) except**
   a. It is based on the principle that small quantities of liquids forced through very small openings under high pressure can penetrate mucous membrane or skin without causing excessive trauma
   b. It produces surface anesthesia instantly
   c. It can be used for obtaining gingival anesthesia before rubber dam placement
   d. It cannot be employed in the place of needle injection for nasopalatine and long buccal nerve blocks

Ans d.

Jet injection (Syrijet) can be used in the place of needle injection for nasopalatine and long buccal nerve blocks.

4. **Mandibular foramen is situated at a level lower than the occlusal plane of primary teeth of the pediatric patient. Therefore the injection must be made slightly higher and more anteriorly than that for an adult patient.**
   a. Both the statements are false
   b. Both the statements are true
   c. First statement is true and the second is false
   d. First statement is false and the second is true

Ans c.

Mandibular foramen is situated at a level lower than the occlusal plane of primary teeth of the pediatric patient. Therefore the injection must be made slightly lower and more posteriorly than that for an adult patient.

5. **Long buccal nerve block is needed for placement of a rubber dam clamp in molars. To obtain long buccal nerve block small quantity of solution is deposited in the mucobuccal fold at a point distal and buccal to the indicated tooth.**
   a. Both the statements are false
   b. Both the statements are true
   c. First statement is true and the second is false
   d. First statement is false and the second is true

Ans b.

The answer is self-explanatory.

6. **Gow Gates mandibular block technique anesthetizes all except**
   a. Mandibular molars
   b. Mylohyoid
   c. Premolars
   d. Mandibular incisors

Ans d.

This single injection anesthetizes the entire right or left half of the mandibular teeth and soft tissues except the incisors which may receive partial innervation from the incisive nerves of the opposite side.

7. **In a child with only primary dentition erupted, the injection for greater palatine block should be made approximately 30 mm**

posterior to the distal surface of the second primary molar. The innervation of soft tissue of posterior two-third of palate is derived from the greater and lesser palatine nerves.

a. Both the statements are false
b. Both the statements are true
c. First statement is true and the second is false
d. First statement is false and the second is true

Ans d.

The injection for greater palatine block should be given 10 mm posterior to the distal surface of the second primary molar.

8. The preferred block for a surgical removal of impacted canines in a child is

a. Supra periosteal injection
b. Posterior and middle superior nerve block
c. Infra orbital nerve block
d. Mental nerve block

Ans c.

Infra orbital nerve block anesthetizes anterior and middle superior alveolar nerves. It also affects innervation of the soft tissues below the eye, half of the nose and the oral musculature of the upper lip on the injected side of the face.

9. In intraligamentary injection, the needle is placed in the gingival sulcus usually on the mesial surface and advanced along the root surface until resistance is met. Then 0.2 mL of solution is deposited into the periodontal ligament.

a. Both the statements are false
b. Both the statements are true
c. First statement is true and th second is false
d. First statement is false and the second is true

Ans b.

The question explains the technique of intraligamentary injection. For multirooted teeth, injections are made both mesially and distally. This technique is useful in patients with bleeding disorders that contradict other injections.

10. Which of the following are advantages of intraligament injection technique?

a. Provides reliable pain control rapidly and easily

b. It provides pulpal anesthesia for 30–45 minutes
c. It may be useful in patients with bleeding disorders that contraindicate other injection
d. It may be useful in young or disabled patients in whom the problems of postoperative trauma to the lips or tongue is a concern
e. All of the above

Ans e.

The answer is self-explanatory.

11. The British-styled extraction forceps differ from American-designed forceps, especially those for the lower teeth. The British system of exodontia usually employs a stand up posture and the force is applied via the whole forearm whereas in the American system it is via wrist action.

a. Both the statements are true
b. Both the statements are false
c. First statement is true and the second is false
d. First statement is false and the second is true

Ans a.

The answer is self-explanatory.

12. All of the following are amide group of local anesthetic agents except

a. Lignocaine
b. Mepivacaine
c. Bupivacaine
d. Procaine

Ans d.

The answer is self-explanatory. Procaine is an ester type of local anesthetic agent.

13. The maximum dose of lignocaine which can be administered is

a. 4.4 mg/kg body weight
b. 2 mg/kg body weight
c. 6.4 mg/kg body weight
d. 2 g/kg body weight

Ans a.

The answer is self-explanatory.

14. All of the following local anesthetic agents are vasodilators except

a. Lignocaine
b. Bupivacaine
c. Mepivacaine
d. Cocaine

Ans d.

Cocaine is the only local anesthetic that consistently produces vasoconstriction. The initial action of cocaine is vasodilation, which is followed by an intense and prolonged vasoconstriction.

15. Which of the following are used in a traditional local anesthetic solution?

a. Vehicle
b. Fungicide
c. Preservative
d. All of the above

Ans d.

The fungicide used in local anesthetic solution is thymol and the preservative is methylparaben. The vehicle is usually water.

16. Centbucridine is a local anesthetic agent categorized as

a. Amides
b. Esters of benzoic acid
c. Esters of para-amino benzoic acid
d. Quinoline derivative

Ans d.

The answer is self-explanatory.

17. Onset of action of lidocaine is

a. 1–2 minutes
b. 2–3 minutes
c. 3–5 minutes
d. 5–6 minutes

Ans c.

Lidocaine is the commonly used LA agent. Once the LA is given, it is better to wait for a minimum of 3 minutes before any procedure is done. This is often forgotten and children undergo pain if a procedure is attempted immediately after LA.

18. For nerve block anesthesia in young and difficult children, ________ needle length is preferred.

a. ½ inch
b. ⅝ inch
c. 1 inch
d. 1¼ inch

Ans c.

A short 1 inch (25 mm) length needle is preferred. An extra-short ⅝ inch (16 mm) needle is used for infiltration and intraligamentary injections.

19. TeDiE technique is

a. Distraction using teddy bear toys
b. Technique of removing impacted teeth
c. Technique integrating tell-show-do, distraction and euphemism for administering local anesthesia
d. Technique for impression making and pouring casts

Ans c.

The technique integrates three basic principles of behavior management to make administration of LA easy and was proposed by MS Muthu (the author).

20. The most common local complication seen in children following the administration of LA is

a. Cheek bite
b. Hematoma
c. Trismus
d. Allergy

Ans a.

The most common complication is cheek bite and it occurs because of masticatory trauma. As the anesthetic effect lingers even after the procedure, children and parents should be instructed properly of the existing numbness.

21. Maxillary premolars are supplied by

a. Anterior superior alveolar nerve
b. Middle superior alveolar nerve
c. Posterior superior alveolar nerve
d. Nasopalatine nerves

Ans b.

Middle superior alveolar nerve which arises from the infra orbital nerve supplies the maxillary molars, premolars and the mesiobuccal root of the permanent first molars. It appears as a differentiated entity 30% of the times. Otherwise, the superior alveolar nerves blend and form the superior alveolar dental plexus and supply the maxillary teeth.

22. Buccal soft tissues near the mandibular primary molars are supplied by

a. Long buccal nerve
b. Lingual nerve
c. Inferior alveolar nerve
d. Mental nerve

Ans a.

The long buccal nerve is the first branch of the inferior alveolar nerve and it supplies the buccal mucosa over the second premolars and molars.

23. While giving a nerve block, a dentist should take at least __________ seconds to deposit 1.8 mL (cartridge) of local anesthetic solution into the tissues.

a. 15
b. 60
c. 90
d. 120

Ans b.

The rate of injection of LA solution should ideally be 1 mL per minute. But practically it might not be possible. Deposition of 2 mL of LA solution should take at least 1 minute.

24. One of the following is NOT an indication for extraction of primary tooth

a. Unrestorable decayed teeth
b. Submerged tooth interfering with permanent tooth eruption
c. If the retained primary tooth is interfering with permanent tooth eruption
d. Retained second primary molar at the age of 13

Ans d.

Retained deciduous teeth by itself is not an indication for extraction. The presence of second premolar should be ascertained before removal.

25. In one of the following techniques, local anesthetic solution is to be deposited against resistance. Which one is that?

a. WAND
b. EDA
c. Intrapulpal and intraligamentary
d. Inferior alveolar nerve block

Ans c.

0.2 mL of ŁA solution should be deposited against resistance for intrapulpal and intraligamentary injections. Adequate anesthesia will not be obtained if not given against resistance.

26. Which one of the following is needle less anesthesia?

a. EDA
b. WAND
c. Jet injection
d. Peri-Press

Ans a.

EDA is electronic dental anesthesia where an attempt is made to deliver LA without needles. However, the effectiveness of anesthesia is not consistently reliable when compared with the conventional techniques.

27. Which type of anesthesia does not require vasoconstrictors?

a. WAND
b. Jet injection
c. Peri-Press
d. Inferior alveolar nerve block

Ans c.

In intraligamentary injections, the LA solution is injected into the confined area of the periodontal ligament. The use of vasoconstrictors is not warranted here. Peri-Press syringes are of two types: gun-like and pen-like.

Chapter 36

Prosthodontic Considerations for Children and Adolescents

1. The most important step in making a successful impression is

a. Selection of appropriate impression material
b. Proper seating of the tray
c. Tray selection
d. Consistency of the impression material

Ans c.

Regardless of the type of impression being made, tray is the most important part of the impression-making procedure. If the tray selection goes wrong, then all the other parameters like tray placement, consistency of the material, etc. will not be of any use. The proper recognition of the shape and size of the arch and appropriate tray selection is the most important step in making an impression and maximum time should be spent on this to avoid failures. This holds good for adults as well as children.

2. Which of the following is not a distraction technique for children while making impressions?

a. Ask the child to hold breath for a while and concentrate
b. Asking the child to bend forward and breathe through mouth and pant like a dog
c. Place unset material on the child's thumb and ask him to raise the thumb once it sets
d. Raise legs alternatively

Ans a.

The various distraction techniques followed for children are:

1. Asking the child to raise his or her finger or thumb as specified, e.g. show me the right little finger or left thumb or left middle finger, etc.

2. Asking the child to lean forward and breathe through the mouth and "pant like a puppy dog."

3. After placing a small dab of alginate over the child's thumb or finger and asking the child to raise the hand once it sets.

4. Asking the patient to breathe rapidly.

5. Asking the patient to raise the legs alternatively and point the toe towards the roof.

6. Asking the patient to count within himself until 30 or 50.

3. The axial reduction, width of margin, lingual reduction for occlusal clearance and incisal reduction, in that order, for an all-ceramic restoration in children are

a. 1.8 mm, 0.8 mm, 1.0 mm, 1.5–2.0 mm respectively
b. 0.8 mm, 0.08 mm, 1.0 mm, 1.5–2.0 mm respectively
c. 1.5 mm, 0.8 mm, 1.0 mm, 1.5–2.0 mm respectively
d. 0.8 mm, 0.8 mm, 1.0 mm, 1.5–2.0 mm respectively

Ans d.

The finish line for all ceramic restorations should be 0.8 mm in width and the axial walls should be reduced to a thickness of 0.8 mm to provide adequate bulk of the material. Incisal reduction for anterior occlusal clearance should be 1.0 mm and incisal reduction should be 1.5–2.0 mm. A shoulder margin is preferable for all-ceramic restorations.

4. The ideal contact position of mandibular anterior teeth opposing maxillary all-ceramic crowns is

a. Cervical to the cingulum of maxillary crowns
b. Concave lingual portion, incisal to the cingulum
c. Edge-to-edge contact
d. Just below the margin of the preparation

Ans b.

Placement of the contact at the margin or cervical to it will produce undue stress on the restoration and will lead to fracture of the crown.

5. Which of the following is not true about a "wing" in a metal-ceramic preparation?

a. Results from a lingual shoulder and labial chamfer
b. Improves retention and resistance
c. Conserves tooth structure
d. Aids in structural durability

Ans a.

Preparing a labial shoulder and lingual chamfer margin will result in a ledge of tooth structure known as the "wing". This provides retention, resistance, structural durability and conserves tooth structure.

6. **A clinician plans to restore an anterior tooth with a ceramic crown for a child. He finds that in his clinic he has only zinc phosphate cement for luting the restoration. Which type of margin is most preferable for the success of restoration?**
   a. Chamfer is most preferred as the cement since it has the least film thickness
   b. Shoulder is most preferred for optimal strength
   c. Both margins can be used but the consistency of the cement while luting is most important
   d. Both margins can be used but the control of film thickness of the cement is most important

Ans b.

Resin cements have the advantage of bonding to the tooth structure, which improves the crown strength. So while using resin cements, either a shoulder or chamfer finish line can be used without compromising the restoration. When zinc phosphate or glass ionomer cements are used, a shoulder finish line is preferred for optimal strength.

7. **A "collarless design" in a metal ceramic restoration refers to**
   a. Facial margin is eliminated to enhance esthetics
   b. The facial collar is placed subgingivally to enhance esthetics
   c. Facial shoulder with a bevel which merges into the adjacent tooth structure
   d. Metal framework not covering the facial shoulder

Ans d.

A collarless metal ceramic restoration is one that eliminates metal framework covering the facial shoulder. It does not mean that there is no margin prepared. This design prevents visibility of marginal metal on the facial aspect and thus enhances esthetics. In a collarless design, the metal framework does not cover the shoulder finish line.

8. **A 12-year-old boy, who is an athlete, broke his upper right incisor during a practice session 2 days back. Almost half of the clinical crown is fractured. Which of the following is the least preferred treatment for this patient?**
   a. Pulpectomy and obturation, wait and watch
   b. Pulpectomy, obturation and post and core to restore the crown
   c. Pulpectomy, obturation followed by stainless steel crown with window
   d. None of the above

Ans b.

It is important that teeth in accident-prone adolescents or those in whom athletic trauma has previously occurred be restored without using a post, if possible. This practice helps to avoid irreparable damage in the form of root fracture, should the restored tooth be subjected to trauma again.

9. Which of the following is the first choice of treatment for replacing a missing maxillary left lateral incisor with normal and healthy abutments in an adolescent?

a. A three unit metal-ceramic crown
b. A cantilever metal-ceramic crown
c. Maryland bridge
d. Implant and crown

Ans c.

The first choice of treatment for replacing a single missing tooth is by using a resin-bonded retainer. This has the advantage of conservation of tooth structure, pulpal protection and good periodontal health. Use of implants in children and adolescent is still controversial as the position of the implant is subjected to change with growth.

10. Which of the following is not a resin-bonded fixed partial denture?

a. Maryland bridge
b. Virginia bridge
c. Cast mesh fixed partial denture
d. Andrew's bridge

Ans d.

The various types of resin-bonded fixed partial dentures are: Rochette bridge (1973), Maryland bridge, Virginia bridge and cast mesh fixed partial denture. The Andrew bridge system is also a fixed partial denture which has fixed retainers with a removable pontic component. Thus, it is a modified removable fixed partial denture.

11. Which marginal configuration is used while preparing a tooth for a resin-bonded fixed partial denture?

a. Chamfer
b. Light chamfer
c. Knife edge
d. No margin needed

Ans b.

Though the preparation for a resin-bonded fixed partial denture is minimal, it does not mean that a margin is not necessary. The preferred marginal configuration is small peripheral chamfer made with a round end diamond.

12. A dentist notices a rash on a child's wrist while treating a fractured tooth. Upon enquiry the child says that he was wearing a metal bracelet in that region. Which type of crown should he use for restoring this tooth?

a. Procera All Ceram
b. Porcelain fused to metal
c. Stainless steel crown
d. Resin-bonded FPD

Ans a.

This patient is most likely to be suffering from allergy to nickel from metals. Nickel, among all the metal is the most common allergen. So it is best to avoid any restoration containing metal, is the most common allergen. Thus, an all-ceramic crown such as the Procera would be a good alternative.

13. All are true about "lingual ledges" except

a. Part of tooth preparation for a resin-bonder retainer
b. Increases the retention and resistance form
c. Decreases the casting rigidity
d. Aids in orientation of the casting during cementation

Ans c.

Lingual ledges are small horizontal grooves placed on the lingual aspect while preparing a tooth for resin-bonded retainers. These increase the retention and resistance forms, increase casting rigidity and aid in orienting the casting while cementation of the prosthesis.

14. An adolescent had malaligned teeth in the maxillary anterior region due to a congenitally missing left lateral incisor. Treatment with a fixed prosthesis was planned after orthodontic repositioning and de-rotation of the teeth. Which restoration is least preferred?

a. Metal ceramic crown
b. All-ceramic crown
c. Cantilever pontic
d. Resin-bonded prosthesis

Ans c.

A cantilever design should not be used in case of mal aligned teeth and mobile teeth. It is indicated only in the presence of stable arch forms. Recent orthodontic treatment involving significant de-rotation is also a contraindication for the use of cantilever pontic because the position of the pontic is subject to change with relapse.

15. Which of the following is not true about Adam's clasp for use in a removable partial denture in children?

a. Is a valuable aid for retention
b. Can be easily adjusted
c. Interferes with occlusion
d. It is an excellent all around clasp

Ans c.

Adam's clasp is used in a removable partial denture for added retention. It is an excellent all around clasp, does not interfere with occlusion (due to spaced dentition in children) and can be easily adjusted. Adam's clasp is mostly preferred because it engages both mesiobuccal and distobuccal undercuts and can be used with short clinical crowns seen in children.

16. The thickness of the wire used for fabrication of retentive clasps for partial dentures is

a. 0.020 to 0.030 inch
b. 0.022 to 0.032 inch
c. 0.028 to 0.030 inch
d. 0.030 to 0.032 inch

Ans c.

The answer is self-explanatory.

17. Which of the following is false about use of articulators in children and adolescents?

a. While using a semiadjustable articulator a face-bow transfer is required
b. Use of semiadjustable articulators minimizes the occlusal errors
c. Semiadjustable articulators can be used for young children with minor discrepancies
d. The semiadjustable articulators are not designed to simulate the jaws of young and adolescent

Ans c.

The geometry of semiadjustable articulators is based on values obtained from adults. Though these values do not simulate the values of patients in whom growth is incomplete, their use in teenagers and adolescents will be useful in obtaining prosthesis with less occlusal errors. But in case of young children, there exists a large discrepancy between the articulator values and patient values. So their use in young children has no rationale. A simple hinge articulator can be used in these patients, just to have a static record.

18. The depth of undercut for use of wrought clasp is

a. 0.25 to 0.30 mm

b. 0.5 to 0.75 mm

c. 0.30 to 0.50 mm

d. 0.75 to 0.80 mm

Ans b.

Cobalt–chromium clasp (cast) is used when the undercut is 0.25 mm and wrought clasp is used when the undercut is 0.5–0.75 mm, to provide more flexibility.

19. Which of the following will pose a problem in removable partial denture design in children?

a. Retention

b. Stability

c. Support

d. Esthetics

Ans a.

The clinical crowns for children are often short and adequate undercuts or guiding planes cannot be found for retention of the prosthesis. This can be overcome by recontouring the crowns using composite resin to achieve adequate undercuts.

20. Which of the following cannot be used for making edentulous impressions in a very young child (preschooler)?

a. Bent, soft steel wire

b. Mouth mirror

c. Trimmed plastic stock trays

d. Metal stock trays

Ans d.

The metal stock trays available are often too large for making edentulous impressions in very small children. A plastic stock tray can be used after it has been trimmed to suit the arches. The other alternatives are using a bent soft steel wire, shaped to support the mandibular compound impression or using a mouth mirror to support a maxillary compound impression.

21. Which of the following is incorrect regarding the use of complete dentures in children?

a. Improves masticatory efficiency
b. It is a preventive procedure
c. Restricts growth along midpalatine suture
d. Is a treatment modality for ectodermal dysplasia

Ans c.

Though it may seem that an appliance crossing the midpalatine suture would restrict the growth of the maxilla, it is not true in the case of complete dentures. Instead of restricting the growth, the dentures become increasingly difficult to insert until a time when insertion is no longer possible. Complete dentures in this case would prevent the development of harmful habits and loss of bone.

22. Which of the following would be the least important reason for replacing an anterior tooth in a child?

a. Restoration of appearance
b. Prevention of psychological trauma
c. Prevention of speech abnormalities
d. Prevention of development of harmful habits

Ans c.

The question says replacing "an anterior tooth", meaning a single missing anterior tooth in a child. Speech will not be affected much in this case. Speech problems do develop in case of loss of all incisors or complete absence of teeth. In case a speech pathology is detected, a speech therapist should be consulted for proper diagnosis.

23. A wrap around design for a posterior resin-bonded fixed partial denture should cover the tooth by

a. 120°
b. 180°
c. 360°
d. 220°

Ans b.

A wrap around design is advocated by Livaditis and Thompson for resin-bonded prosthesis in the posterior region and should cover the tooth by 180° for good retention.

24. Which radiograph will be more appropriate to determine the course of action for replacing missing teeth in children?

a. Lateral cephalogram
b. OPG
c. Periapical radiograph
d. Occlusal view

Ans b.

A panoramic radiograph is more desirable as it provides us details about different stages of development of the succedaneous teeth.

25. A removable appliance with a clasp on the primary maxillary canine was used to replace missing posterior teeth in a child when he was 4 years old. Approximately at what age of the child should this clasp be removed from the primary canine?

a. 5 years
b. 7 years
c. 9 years
d. 11 years

Ans b.

During the time of eruption of the permanent maxillary incisors, the primary canine should be allowed to freely migrate distally and laterally to accommodate the erupting incisors. If the clasp continues to be on the canine, then this migration will be prevented and there would be crowding of the incisors. So the clasp has to be removed at approximately 7 years of age when the incisors begin to erupt.

26. Which of the following is not an indication for the use of removable partial denture in children?

a. 1-year-old child with missing maxillary lateral incisor
b. Premature loss of primary molar
c. Loss of maxillary anteriors due to trauma
d. Congenital absence of tooth

Ans a.

Lindahl recommends a mental age of 2½ years for the use of a removable partial denture in children. All the other options mentioned are indications for use of partial dentures.

27. In designing a removable partial denture for children, which of the following would be a wrong design?

a. Using an acrylic denture base for a maxillary partial denture with clasps
b. Using clasps on maxillary canines for better retention of the prosthesis

c. Lingual bar in a mandibular denture should be closely adapted to the soft tissues

d. Placing occlusal rests on permanent mandibular molars in the central fossa through a lingual approach

Ans c.

The lingual bar in case of mandibular denture should be away from the soft tissues (by at least 2 mm), in order to accommodate for the lingual bulges of the succedaneous permanent incisors.

Chapter 37

Pediatric Oral and Maxillofacial Pathology and Treatment Considerations

1. **Oral warts are caused by**
   a. Human papilloma virus
   b. Pox virus
   c. Hepatitis B virus
   d. Rota virus

Ans a.

Oral verruca vulgaris or oral warts are exophytic papillomatous lesions indistinguishable clinically from oral squamous cell papillomas. They are caused by human papilloma virus. This virus could be an etiological agent in cervical cancer of uterus.

2. **The most common benign soft tissue tumor found in the oral cavity is**
   a. Verruca vulgaris
   b. Squamous papilloma
   c. Fibroma
   d. Pyogenic granuloma

Ans c.

Fibroma is a dome-shaped lesion with a sessile base and a smooth surface that usually has the color of the surrounding mucosa.

3. **Which of the following are true about oral verruca vulgaris or oral warts?**
   a. They are exophytic papillomatous lesions indistinguishable clinically from oral squamous cell neoplasms
   b. They are caused by human papilloma virus
   c. They can spread to the oral cavity in children through autoinoculation by finger or thumb sucking
   d. Complete surgical excision including the base is the treatment of choice
   e. All of the above

Ans e.

The answer is self-explanatory.

4. Which of the following is/are true about pyogenic granuloma?

a. Soft tissue tumor arises from fibrous connective tissue or mucous membranes
b. Surface may have a smooth, lobulated or occasionally warty appearance that is erythematous and often ulcerated
c. Because of the pronounced vascularity, these lesions often bleed easily when probed
d. Commonly occurring sites are maxillary anterior labial gingiva, lips, tongue, buccal mucosa, palate, mucolabial or mucobuccal fold
e. All of the above

Ans e.

The answer is self-explanatory.

5. Ranula is the clinical term for a mucocele occurring on the floor of the mouth after trauma to components of the submandibular glands. Two varieties of ranula exist: cystic (mucous retention cyst) and pseudocystic (mucous retention phenomenon or mucocele).

a. Both the statements are false
b. Both the statements are true
c. First statement is true and the second is false
d. First statement is false and the second is true

Ans d.

Ranula is the clinical term for a mucocele occurring on the floor of the mouth after trauma to components of the sublingual glands.

6. In the cystic type of mucocele, there is partial obstruction of the distal end of a sublingual gland duct that results in a small epithelial lined cyst usually less than 1 cm in diameter. The most common variety of ranula (which is pseudocystic), however, forms as a result of extravasation of mucous into the fibrous connective tissue after a tear in the sublingual gland duct.

a. Both the statements are false
b. Both the statements are true
c. First statement is true and the second is false
d. First statement is false and the second is true

Ans b.

The answer is self-explanatory.

7. Mucoceles are rarely seen in

a. Upper lip
b. Lower lip
c. Buccal mucosa
d. Floor of the mouth

Ans a.

Mucoceles are noted to occur most commonly on the lower lip, with the floor of the mouth and buccal mucosa being the next most frequent sites of involvement. They are rarely seen on the upper lip, retromolar pad or palate.

8. The commonest site of occurrence of congenital epulis of newborn is

a. Mandibular anterior alveolar ridge
b. Maxillary anterior alveolar ridge
c. Maxillary posterior alveolar ridge
d. Mandibular posterior alveolar ridge

Ans b.

Congenital epulis of newborn is a rare lesion of uncertain histogenesis that occurs exclusively in newborn infants chiefly on the maxillary anterior alveolar ridge and less commonly on the mandibular anterior alveolar ridge. Usually they are solitary lesions but they may be multiple also, often affecting both the maxilla and mandible. At birth it presents as pink, smooth to lobulated, pedunculated mass that may vary in size from a few millimetres to greater than 7 cm in diameter. More than 90% of cases occur in females.

9. Neurofibroma is a benign neural neoplasm of Schwann cell origin for which several clinical forms are recognized. It is an autosomal recessive inherited disease.

a. Both the statements are false
b. Both the statements are true
c. First statement is true and the second is false
d. First statement is false and the second is true

Ans c.

Neurofibroma is inherited as an autosomal dominant disease.

10. Which of the following conditions exist in neurofibromatosis?

a. Café-au-lait spots
b. Lisch nodules

c. Pigmented iris hamartomas

d. All of the above

Ans d.

Café—Coffee, Lait—Milk (when coffee is mixed with milk the resulting color is brown). Hence it is called café-au-lait spots. They are light brown macules with smooth borders and often located over nerve trunks. This is seen in Type I neurofibromatosis (von Recklinghausen's disease). Lisch nodules—Pigmented hamartomas in the iris present in more than 94% of patients who are 6 years old or older. They do not produce any symptoms but are helpful in establishing the diagnosis.

11. The most frequent intraoral location for neurofibromatosis is palate or floor of the mouth. Occasionally, intraosseous lesion occurs in the posterior part of the mandible.

a. Both the statements are false

b. Both the statements are true

c. First statement is true and the second is false

d. First statement is false and the second is true

Ans d.

The most frequent intraoral location for neurofibromatosis is tongue or buccal mucosa.

12. Lymphangiomas are thought to arise as benign hamartomatous proliferations of sequestrated lymphatic rests. They form along tissue planes or penetrating adjacent tissue; they become canalized and in the congenital absence of venous drainage accumulate fluid.

a. Both the statements are false

b. Both the statements are true

c. First statement is true and the second is false

d. First statement is false and the second is true

Ans b.

The answer is self-explanatory. Lymphangiomas are classified into three types: Capillary lymphangiomas, cavernous lymphangiomas and cystic hygroma.

13. Hemangioma is a benign vasoformative tumor that frequently occurs in the head and neck in children. Most hemangiomas develop when the child is 5–8 years of age.

a. Both the statements are false

b. Both the statements are true

c. First statement is true and the second is false
d. First statement is false and the second is true

Ans c.

Most hemangiomas are either present at birth or develop within the first year of life.

14. Hemangiomas in the oral soft tissues commonly affect palate and floor of the mouth. Their histologic classification is based on the type of the blood vessels involved.

a. Both the statements are false
b. Both the statements are true
c. First statement is true and the second is false
d. First statement is false and the second is true

Ans a.

Hemangiomas in the oral soft tissues commonly affect tongue, lips and buccal mucosa. Their histologic classification is based on the size of the vascular spaces.

They are classified as capillary, cavernous, central and cellular hemangiomas.

15. The fibro-osseous lesions of the jaws include a diverse group of lesions sharing a common denominator, the replacement of normal bone architecture by a benign fibro cellular stroma. Because of their histomorphology, diagnosis is made on the basis of distinguishing clinical and radiographic features.

a. Both the statements are false
b. Both the statements are true
c. First statement is true and the second is false
d. First statement is false and the second is true

Ans b.

The answer is self-explanatory. Fibrous dysplasia and the ossifying fibroma are the common fibro-osseous lesions in children.

16. All of the following statements are true regarding fibrous dysplasia except

a. It is a neoplastic developmental lesion of the bone
b. Two forms exist: rare polyostotic form and common monostotic form
c. Maxillary involvement is a more serious form of disease
d. Radiographically they show a ground glass appearance

Ans a.

Fibrous dysplasia is a nonneoplastic lesion of the bone. The other three statements are true regarding fibrous dysplasia.

17. Which of the following is/are true regarding monostotic fibrous dysplasia?

a. Slow growing and painless
b. Progressive enlargement of bone whose growth pattern stabilizes with time frequently after the onset of puberty
c. The margins are ill defined and blend into normal bone necessitating conservative therapy
d. All of the above

Ans d.

The answer is self-explanatory. Surgery in the form of osseous recontouring should be considered only in those cases where there is functional or significant cosmetic deformity and usually after stabilization of the disease process.

18. Which of the following fibro-osseous lesions is of periodontal ligament origin?

a. Fibrous dysplasia
b. Ossifying fibroma
c. Central giant cell granuloma
d. Peripheral giant cell granuloma

Ans b.

The ossifying fibroma is a benign fibro-osseous neoplasm of periodontal ligament origin included in the broad category of benign fibro-osseous lesions of the jaws. It is characterized histologically by benign fibro cellular stroma, with the formation of variable amounts of woven bone, lamellar bone and spherical to annular to amorphous cementum like calcifications. When the predominant calcified component is bone, it is known as ossifying fibroma. On the other hand, if cementum or cementum-like calcifications predominate, it is known as cementifying fibroma.

19. Which of the following is true regarding central giant cell granuloma?

a. 50% of the patients are less than 16 years of age
b. Occurs more often in females than in males
c. Mandible is involved more than maxilla
d. All of the above

Ans d.

The answer is self-explanatory. Majority of the lesions occur in the anterior portion of the maxilla (anterior to first permanent molar).

20. The cyst formed by cystic degeneration of enamel organ is

a. Dentigerous cyst
b. Primordial cyst
c. Odontogenic keratocyst
d. Eruption cyst

Ans b.

Cyst formed by the cystic degeneration of the enamel organ before the formation of enamel or dentin is known as primordial cyst.

21. A patient aged 12 years reports with a swelling in the left mandibular premolar region. Radio graphically there is a well circumscribed, unilocular radiolucent lesion where the first premolar failed to develop and there was no history of extraction before. The probable diagnosis is

a. Dentigerous cyst
b. Primordial cyst
c. Odontogenic keratocyst
d. Eruption cyst

Ans b.

Refer to the explanation of Q. No. 20.

22. The cyst which is associated with erupting primary and permanent tooth in its soft tissue phase after erupting through bone is

a. Dentigerous cyst
b. Primordial cyst
c. Odontogenic keratocyst
d. Eruption cyst

Ans d.

Eruption cyst is usually a translucent, smooth, painless swelling over the erupting tooth. If bleeding occurs into the cystic space, it may appear blue to blue-black and it is then called an eruption hematoma.

23. The cyst which is associated with the crown of an impacted, embedded or unerupted tooth is

a. Dentigerous cyst
b. Primordial cyst
c. Odontogenic keratocyst
d. Eruption cyst

Ans a.

Dentigerous cysts are usually large, destructive and expansile lesions of bone. The radiographic appearance may be unilocular or multilocular.

24. All of the following are true about odontogenic keratocyst except

a. It has a high rate of recurrence
b. Peak incidence is in second and third decades of life
c. Maxilla is involved twice as frequently as the mandible
d. Histologically it has a thin uniform lining epithelium with palisading of basal layer of cells and a corrugated surface

Ans c.

Odontogenic keratocyst involves mandible twice as frequently as the maxilla.

25. Ameloblastoma found in children is usually the polycystic variety. The most common histopathologic picture found in Ameloblastoma in children is plexiform variety.

a. Both the statements are false
b. Both the statements are true
c. First statement is true and the second is false
d. First statement is false and the second is true

Ans d.

Ameloblastoma found in children is usually the unicystic variety.

26. The most common site for ameloblastoma in children is

a. Mandibular anterior region
b. Mandibular molar ramus area
c. Maxillary antrum
d. Maxillary posterior region

Ans b.

The answer is self-explanatory.

27. All of the following are true about adenomatoid odontogenic tumor except

a. Otherwise known as adenoameloblastoma
b. Classified as intraosseous (follicular and extrafollicular) and extraosseous variants
c. Occurs most commonly in the second decade of life

d. Occurs most commonly in the mandibular incisor and canine region

Ans d.

Adenomatoid odontogenic tumor occurs nearly twice as frequently in the maxilla as in the mandible, with a noticeable predilection for occurrence in the canine and incisor regions.

28. The most common and least severe form of Histiocytosis X, when the disease is confined to bone is known as

a. Hand-Schuller-Christian disease
b. Eosinophilic granuloma
c. Letterer-Siwe disease
d. Histiocytosis Y

Ans b.

Eosinophilic granuloma is the most common and least severe form of LCH, if that form of the disease is confined to bone. Langerhans cell histiocytosis is the current term replacing the term Histiocytosis X introduced by Lichtenstein in 1953 as a unifying term for several previous eponyms including Letterer-Siwe disease, Hand-Schuller-Christian disease and eosinophilic granuloma.

29. All of the following are true regarding eosinophilic granuloma except

a. Characterized by single or multiple well-defined radiolucent bony lesions and occasionally accompanied by pain and swelling
b. Older children and young adults are most commonly affected
c. Mandible, skull, femur, humerus, ribs and pelvis are frequently involved
d. Skin and visceral involvement is common

Ans d.

Skin and visceral involvement are absent (similar to Hand-Schuller-Christian disease and Letterer-Siwe disease).

30. Which of the following is the chronic disseminated form of Histiocytosis X?

a. Hand-Schuller-Christian disease
b. Eosinophilic granuloma
c. Letterer-Siwe disease
d. Histiocytosis Y

Ans a.

The term Hand-Schuller-Christian disease is used to describe the chronic, disseminated form of LCH and is characterized by the development of multifocal eosinophilic granulomas of bone, lymphadenopathy and visceral involvement especially hepatosplenomegaly.

31. The classical triad of multiple punched out radiolucent lesions of membranous bones, exophthalmos and diabetes insipidus is characteristic of

a. Hand-Schuller-Christian disease
b. Eosinophilic granuloma
c. Letterer-Siwe disease
d. Histiocytosis Y

Ans a.

The answer is self-explanatory.

32. Which of the following is characterized initially by a development of a scaly erythematous skin rash?

a. Hand-Schuller-Christian disease
b. Eosinophilic granuloma
c. Letterer-Siwe disease
d. Histiocytosis Y

Ans c.

This scaly rash is initially prominent on the trunk but progressing to involve the scalp and extremities. This is accompanied by a persistent low-grade fever, anemia, thrombocytopenia, hepatosplenomegaly and lymphadenopathy.

33. Which of the following is true regarding Ewing's sarcoma?

a. It usually affects the skull, mandible and the maxilla in the head and neck region
b. Localized pain and swelling are the most frequent complaints at the time of presentation
c. Soft tissue overlying the swelling may be erythematous and warm to touch suggestive of an inflammatory process than a neoplasm
d. Any of the above

Ans d.

The answer is self-explanatory. Following osteosarcoma, the Ewing's family of tumors is the second most common primary malignancy of bone in children and adolescence.

34. Sun ray appearance in the radiograph is characteristic of

a. Osteogenic sarcoma

b. Ewing's sarcoma
c. Hand-Schuller-Christain disease
d. Rhabdomyosarcoma

Ans a.

A frequently described radiographic feature of osteogenic sarcoma is a sun-ray appearance, with delicate, hair-like trabeculae radiating in a sunburst fashion away from the peripheral surface of the lesion.

35. All of the following are true regarding rhabdomyosarcoma except

a. A benign neoplasm of skeletal muscle origin
b. Most common soft tissue sarcoma in children
c. 2–6 years and adolescence are the commonly affected age group
d. Primary site of involvement in children is the head and neck region

Ans a.

Rhabdomyosarcoma is a malignant neoplasm of skeletal muscle origin.

36. Presence of Reed-Sternberg cells is characteristic of

a. Non-Hodgkin's lymphoma
b. Hodgkin's lymphoma
c. Burkitt's lymphoma
d. Rhabdomyosarcoma

Ans b.

Hodgkin's disease is a malignant neoplasm of lymphoreticular origin distinguished from non-Hodgkin's lymphoma by diverse but distinctive morphologic features with one common denominator, the presence of Reed-Sternberg cells which are widely accepted as the neoplastic cells in this disease.

37. Geographic tongue may require

a. No treatment
b. Excision of discrete lesion
c. Application of nystatin
d. Penicillin

Ans a.

No treatment is indicated. Since etiology is unknown and the condition is a benign one there should be no need for concern or treatment other than to reassure the patient.

38. A purulent lesion in the facial vestibule of an 8-year-old patient is (most likely)

a. A pyogenic granuloma

b. An odontogenic fistula

c. An infected aphthous ulcer

d. An isolated herpetic lesion

Ans b.

A purulent lesion in the facial vestibule of an 8-year-old patient is most likely an odontogenic fistula. The fistula is usually associated with an untreated decayed primary molar which has a deep carious lesion or a proximal caries lesion with pulpal involvement. Purulent exudate is not a characteristic feature of pyogenic granuloma or an aphthous ulcer. In herpetic lesions, inflammation of the site precedes the formation of vesicles which ruptures to form ulcers by several days.

39. In a 10-year-old girl, a large radiolucent area was detected radiographically in the apical region of the permanent mandibular incisors. They tested vital. The lesion was asymptomatic. When the lesion was explored surgically it revealed a large, nonlined, hollow space containing a few cobweb-like fibers and a small pool of dark reddish fluid. Most probably the diagnosis is

a. Central fibroma

b. A ranula

c. Hand-Schuller-Christian disease

d. A chronic periapical abscess

e. A traumatic or a hemorrhagic cyst

Ans e.

Traumatic or hemorrhagic cysts are usually asymptomatic and patients seek treatment only when expansion of jaw occurs. The associated teeth are generally vital. The cavity is not lined by epithelium but contains small amounts of straw colored fluid, shreds of necrotic blood clot, fragments of fibrous connective tissue or nothing. Mandible is more affected than maxilla. Central fibroma is comprised of fibrous connective tissue with scattered islands of odontogenic epithelium. It occurs in relation to unerupted teeth and shows multilocular radiolucency. Ranula occurs in the floor of the mouth in association with ducts of sublingual and submaxillary glands. Hand-Schuller-Christian disease is characterized by widespread skeletal and extraskeletal lesions and a chronic clinical course. Chronic periapical abscess is symptomatic and shows thickening of the periodontal membrane.

40. Treatment of severe intraoral infection in children differs from that in adults because

a. Leucocytopenia develops more frequently in children than in adults
b. The incidence of bleeding diathesis is greater in children than in adults
c. Dehydration occurs more rapidly and severely than in adult
d. More children are allergic to penicillin than adults are

Ans c.

Dehydration is the loss of water and salts that are essential for normal body function. Children need more water than adults because they expend more energy and most children who drink when they are thirsty get as much water as their systems require. Dehydration in children usually results from losing large amounts of fluid and not drinking enough water to replace the loss.

41. In a 7-year-old child small, irregular, bright red spots on the buccal mucosa, with bluish-white specks in the centers, may be seen at the onset of

a. Mumps
b. Herpes
c. Leukemia
d. Rubella
e. Rubeola

Ans e.

The question gives the description of Koplik's spots in measles. Rubella does not show Koplik's spots and the buccal mucosa is not involved. Mumps is an acute contagious viral infection characterized by swelling of salivary glands. In herpetic lesions, inflammation of the site precedes the formation of vesicles which ruptures to form ulcers by several days. Leukemia is characterized by progressive over production of WBCs.

42. An aphthous ulcer should be treated by

a. Palliation and patience or no treatment
b. Tetracycline
c. Penicillin V
d. Mycostatin topical application

Ans a.

There is no specific treatment for aphthous ulcer as the exact etiology is unknown.

43. A light bluish, dome-shaped lesion on the inside lip of 2-year-old child is most likely a

a. Melanoma

b. Hematoma
c. Mucocele
d. Hemangioma

Ans c.

Mucocele is a superficial lesion that appears as a raised circumscribed vesicle several millimetres to centimetres in diameter with a bluish translucent cast. Melanoma is an uncommon neoplasm of the oral mucosa and usually appears as a deeply pigmented area, at times ulcerated and hemorrhagic which tends to increase progressively in size. Hemangioma appears as a flatter raised lesion of the mucosa, usually deep red or bluish red and is seldom well circumscribed. Common sites involved are lip, tongue, buccal mucosa and palate. Hematoma appears as a circumscribed fluctuant often translucent swelling of the alveolar ridge over the site of the erupting tooth. It contains blood and appears purple or deep blue. Also refer Q. Nos. 6 and 7.

44. Odontogenic infection spreading into the lymphatic chain of the neck is detected by

a. Hematologic examinations
b. Biopsy of cervical nodes
c. Palpation
d. Radiographs

Ans c.

The answer is self-explanatory.

45. A tender, somewhat painful, unilateral or bilateral swelling of the salivary glands is characteristic feature of

a. Fibrous dysplasia
b. Tumor of the gland
c. Parotitis
d. Maxillary sinus infection

Ans c.

Parotitis is usually preceded by the onset of headache, chills, moderate fever, vomiting and pain in the preauricular region. These symptoms are followed by rubbery or elastic swelling of the glands. It produces pain on sighting food and or mastication. Fibrous dysplasia is one of the most perplexing disease of the osseous tissue. It is a lesion of unknown etiology and certain pathogenesis and diverse histopathology. Maxillary sinus infection can be an acute or chronic inflammation of the sinus and is often due to direct extension of dental infection but also originates from infectious diseases such as common cold, influenza and exanthematous disease.

46. In a child, a combination of malnutrition, steatorrhea, chronic respiratory infections, thyroid deficiency, a great salt loss through

skin and functional disturbances in secretory mechanisms of various glands is indicative of

a. Cystic fibrosis
b. Pierre Robin syndrome
c. Hereditary fructose intolerance
d. Immune deficiency syndrome

Ans a.

Cystic fibrosis is basically an inborn error of metabolism with generalized dysfunction of the exocrine glands and is characterized by chronic airway obstruction. Pierre Robin syndrome consists of cleft palate, micrognathia and glossoptosis. Due to breakdown in the immune system of the body, patients may first develop unexplained fever, weight loss and lymphadenopathy. Hereditary fructose intolerance is an autosomal recessive trait and is manifested by hypoglycemia and vomiting after ingestion of fructose containing foods. It results from a deficiency in fructose 1-phosphate aldolase. Affected individuals acquire an intense aversion to all sweets and fruits.

47. Transillumination of soft tissues is useful in detecting which of the following problems in a child?

a. Koplik's spots
b. Sialolithiasis
c. Aortic stenosis
d. Sickle cell disease

Ans b.

Transillumination is the technique of sample illumination by transmission of light through the sample. Koplik's spots are small, irregular, bright red spots on the buccal mucosa, with bluish-white specks in the centers. Transillumination has no role in diagnosis of aortic stenosis, sickle cell disease or Koplik's spots.

48. An occluded submandibular duct is best demonstrated by

a. Palpation
b. Thermography
c. Transillumination
d. Sialograms

Ans d.

An occluded submandibular duct is best demonstrated by sialograms. Sialography is a retrograde injection of a radiopaque material into the duct system of a salivary gland and the study of its distribution by roentgenogram.

49. A nystatin rinse is effective in controlling which of the following oral infections?

a. Cellulitis
b. Candidiasis
c. Recurrent aphthous ulcers
d. Necrotizing ulcerative gingivitis

Ans b.

Rinse or suspension of nystatin held in contact with the oral lesions have been successfully used even in chronic cases and severe cases of candidiasis. Cellulitis is treated by administration of antibiotics and by removal of the cause of the infection. Recurrent aphthous ulcer has no specific treatment. Treatment of necrotizing ulcerative gingivitis varies extremely.

50. A left mandibular swelling with an external drainage under the body of the mandible in a 4-year-old child should be evaluated for

a. Tuberculosis
b. Actinomycosis
c. Dental infection
d. All of the above

Ans d.

Tuberculosis infection of submandibular and cervical lymph nodes or scrofula (tuberculous lymphadenitis) may progress to a formation of an actual abscess or remain as a typical granulomatous lesion. They are painful and often show inflammation of skin, when an actual abscess exists, typically perforate and discharge pus. In cervicofacial actinomycosis, the organisms may enter the tissues, through the oral mucous membrane and may either remain localized in the subjacent soft tissues or spread to involve salivary glands, bones, and skin of face and neck, producing swelling and induration of the tissues. The swellings in these soft tissues eventually develop into one or more abscesses which tend to discharge upon a skin surface liberating pus containing the typical sulfur granules. In the sequelae of dental caries, the long standing periapical cyst may undergo an acute exacerbation of the inflammatory process and rapidly develop into an abscess that may ultimately drain or discharge through the surface of the skin.

51. Premature exfoliation of teeth is associated with

a. Hypophosphatasia
b. Hyperparathyroidism
c. Rickets
d. All of the above

Ans a.

Hypophosphatasia is an autosomal recessive hereditary disease characterized by deficiency of alkaline phosphatase. Premature exfoliation and loosening of primary teeth is a characteristic feature and is associated with absence of cementum and lack of sound periodontal fibers in the histologic picture.

52. Ground glass radiographic appearance is associated with

a. Rickets
b. Hyperparathyroidism
c. Osteomyelitis
d. Ameloblastoma

Ans b.

Primary hyperparathyroidism is a disease in which the parathyroid glands secrete an excessive quantity of parathyroid hormone. It is a rare disease and is three times more common in women than men. It usually affects people of middle age, but it may occur in childhood or in later life. Malocclusion caused by sudden drifting with definite spacing of teeth may be the first sign of the disease. In the radiographs of the jaws, the bone tends to show a ground glass appearance, with loss of lamina dura around the teeth.

53. The common site of compound odontoma is

a. Incisor region
b. Molar region
c. Premolar region
d. Third molar region

Ans a.

Compound odontoma is an agglomeration of various numbers of denticles. It is a miniature of a tooth and occurs most commonly in the incisor region.

54. One of the sclerosing agent used in treatment of lymphangioma is

a. IK 234
b. OK-432
c. Heparin sulphate
d. Bismuth

Ans b.

Recently a sclerosing agent called OK-432 is used as intralesional sclerosant. Also refer to Q. No. 12.

55. Tetany and carpopedal spasm is associated with

a. Hypothyroidism
b. Hypoparathyroidism

c. Hypopituitarism

d. Hypoadrenalism

Ans b.

Hypoparathyroidism is characterized by an increased excretion of calcium with low blood levels of calcium and a high concentration of phosphorus. If the serum levels fall to 5–6 mg/dL, tetany and the characteristic carpopedal spasms are apparent.

56. The cyst which develops in the place of a tooth is

a. Dentigerous cyst

b. Primordial cyst

c. Globulomaxillary cyst

d. Nasopalatine cyst

Ans b.

Refer to the explanation of Q. Nos. 20 and 21.

Chapter 38

Gingival and Periodontal Diseases in Children

1. Which of the following is true about gingiva?

a. Gingiva is that part of oral mucous membrane that covers the alveolar processes and the cervical portions of the teeth
b. Free gingiva is the tissue coronal to the bottom of the gingival sulcus
c. Attached gingiva is the tissue which extends apically from where the free gingiva ends up to the mucogingival junction
d. All of the above

Ans d.

The above-mentioned options define gingiva, free gingiva and attached gingiva respectively.

2. The color of the gingiva is determined by

a. Complexion of the person
b. Thickness of the tissue
c. Degree of keratinization
d. All of the above

Ans d.

The gingival tissues are normally light pink in color. But the color is usually related to any of the above-mentioned factors. In a healthy adult, the marginal gingiva has a sharp knife-like edge; during the period of eruption in the child, however, the gingiva is thicker and has rounded margins.

3. Gingivitis is an inflammation involving only the gingival tissues next to the tooth. Microscopically, it is characterized by the presence of inflammatory exudates and edema, some destruction of collagenous gingival fibers and ulceration and proliferation of the epithelium facing the tooth and attaching the gingiva to it.

a. Both the statements are false
b. Both the statements are true

c. First statement is true and the second is false
d. First statement is false and the second is true

Ans b.

The answer is self-explanatory.

4. All of the following about plaque are true except

a. It is a complex entity
b. Metabolically interconnected, highly disorganized bacterial system
c. It consists of dense masses of microorganisms
d. It also has an intermicrobial matrix

Ans b.

Plaque is considered to be a complex, metabolically interconnected, highly organized bacterial system consisting of dense masses of microorganisms embedded in an intermicrobial matrix.

5. Plaque begins to form on tooth surface after brushing in

a. 4 hours
b. 6 hours
c. 8 hours
d. 2 hours

Ans d.

Plaque begins to form within 2 hours after the teeth are brushed. Coccus bacteria form on the pellicle first. Within 5 hours, plaque microcolonies develop by cell division. Between 6 and 12 hours, the covering material becomes thinner and is reduced to small-scattered areas. Rod-shaped bacteria appears for the first time in 24 hours old plaque. Within 48 hours, rods and filaments cover the surface of the plaque.

6. Supragingival calculus occurs as soft, firmly adherent masses on the crowns of teeth. Subgingival calculus is found as a concretion on the tooth in the confines of the periodontal pocket.

a. Both the statements are false
b. Both the statements are true
c. First statement is true and the second is false
d. First statement is false and the second is true

Ans d.

Supragingival calculus occurs as hard, firmly adherent masses on the crowns of the teeth.

7. **All of the following are true regarding eruption gingivitis except**
   a. It is not seen during the eruption of primary teeth
   b. It is usually seen during the eruption of first and second permanent molars
   c. It can lead to pericoronitis or a pericoronal abscess
   d. It occurs because the gingival margin receives no protection from the coronal contour of the tooth during the early stages of active eruption. Also the continual impingement of food on the gingiva causes the inflammatory process

Ans **a.**

It is often observed in young children when the primary teeth are erupting. This gingivitis often associated with difficult eruption subsides after the teeth emerge into the oral cavity. The greatest increase in the incidence of gingivitis in children is again seen in the 6–7 years age group when the permanent teeth begin to erupt.

8. **Which of the following is true of acute herpetic gingivostomatitis?**
   a. It is caused by HSV 1
   b. 99% of all primary infections are of subclinical type
   c. It usually affects preschool children
   d. All of the above

Ans **d.**

The answer is self-explanatory.

9. **The active symptoms of acute herpetic gingivostomatitis are**
   a. Malaise, irritability, headache
   b. Pain associated with intake of food and liquids
   c. Presence of yellow or white liquid-filled vesicles
   d. All of the above

Ans **d.**

The active symptoms can occur in children with clean mouth and healthy oral tissues. These children are as susceptible as those with poor oral hygiene. All the above-mentioned symptoms develop suddenly.

10. **Acute herpetic gingivostomatitis in children runs a course of 10–14 days. Treatment should be directed towards the relief of the acute symptoms so that fluid and nutritional intake can be maintained.**
    a. Both the statements are false
    b. Both the statements are true

c. First statement is true and the second is false
d. First statement is false and the second is true

Ans b.

The answer is self-explanatory.

11. Which of the following is a treatment for acute herpetic gingivostomatitis?

a. Application of topical anesthetics like dyclonine hydrochloride (0.5%)
b. Application of a mixture of diphenhydramine elixir and kaopectate
c. Lidocaine topical application
d. Any of the above

Ans d.

Application of a mild topical anesthetic like dyclonine hydrochloride before mealtime will temporarily relieve the pain and allow the child to take a soft diet. Diphenhydramine has mild analgesic and anti-inflammatory properties whereas kaopectate coats the lesions.

12. All of the following are true about recurrent herpes labialis (RHL) except

a. HSV 1 virus remains in the sensory ganglia and reappears later as RHL
b. The sore essentially occurs in the lips
c. Emotional stress and lowered tissue resistance are not related to this condition
d. It can appear after dental treatment and may be related to irritation from rubber dam.

Ans c.

The recurrent form of disease is often related to conditions of emotional stress and lowered tissue resistance resulting from various types of trauma. Excessive exposure to sunlight, irritation from rubber dam during dental treatment can also precipitate recurrent herpes labialis.

13. Recurrent aphthous ulcer is otherwise called

a. Canker sore
b. Cold sore
c. Recurrent herpes labialis
d. Recurrent herpetic infection

Ans a.

Recurrent aphthous ulcer is otherwise called canker sore or recurrent aphthous stomatitis. Recurrent aphthous stomatitis is characterized by recurrent ulcerations on the moist mucous membranes of the mouth in which both discrete and confluent lesions are found rapidly in certain sites and they feature a round to oval crateriform base, raised reddened margins with pain.

14. In a review of aphthous ulcer, it is suggested that the precipitating factor accountable for as much as 75% of episodes is minor trauma. Nutritional deficiencies are found in 20% of persons with aphthous ulcer.

a. Both the statements are true
b. Both the statements are false
c. The first statement is true and the second is false
d. The first statement is false and the second is true

Ans a.

Injuries caused by cheek biting and minor facial irritations are probably the most common precipitating factors. The clinically detectable nutritional deficiencies include iron, vitamin B_{12} and folic acid. Stress may also prove to be an important precipitating factor particularly in stress-prone group such as students in professional schools and military personnel.

15. Which of the following is true regarding ANUG?

a. It is characterized by the involvement of interproximal gingiva and the presence of a pseudomembranous necrotic covering over the marginal tissue
b. It is caused by *Borrelia vincentii* and fusiform bacilli referred to as spirochetal organisms
c. Fever, malaise, fetid odour, painful bleeding gingival tissues and poor appetite are other features
d. The disease responds within 24–48 hours to subgingival curettage , debridement and the use of mild oxidizing solutions
e. All of the above

Ans e.

All of the above-mentioned facts are true regarding ANUG.

16. The enlargement of the gingival tissues in puberty gingivitis is confined to the anterior segment and may be present in only one arch. The lingual gingival tissue generally remains unaffected.

a. Both the statements are true
b. Both the statements are false

c. The first statement is true and the second is false
d. The first statement is false and the second is true

Ans a.

Puberty gingivitis occasionally develops in children in the prepubertal and pubertal period. Treatment of puberty gingivitis should be improved oral hygiene, removal of all local irritants, restoration of carious teeth and dietary recommendations necessary to ensure an adequate nutritional status.

17. In elephantiasis gingivae, the gingival tissues appear normal at birth but begin to enlarge with the eruption of the primary teeth. During surgical removal of the enlarged gingiva excessive hemorrhage is seen.

a. Both the statements are true
b. Both the statements are false
c. The first statement is true and the second is false
d. The first statement is false and the second is true

Ans a.

Elephantiasis gingivae or hereditary hyperplasia of the gums is a rare type of gingivitis. Though the enlarged gingiva appears pale and firm, the surgical procedure is accompanied by excessive hemorrhage.

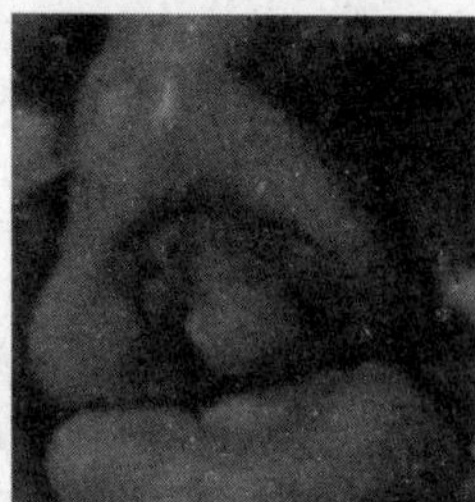

Fig. 38.1 Elephantiasis gingivae.

18. Phenytoin-induced gingival enlargement begins to appear as early as

a. 2–3 days
b. 2–3 weeks
c. 2–3 months
d. 24–48 hours

Ans b.

Phenytoin was first introduced as anticonvulsant in 1938 by Merrit and Putnam. Kimball first described gingival hyperplasia as a side effect of this drug in 1939. Phenytoin-induced gingival overgrowth (PIGO) or dilantin hyperplasia begins to appear as early as 2–3 weeks after initiation of phenytoin therapy and peaks at 18–24 months.

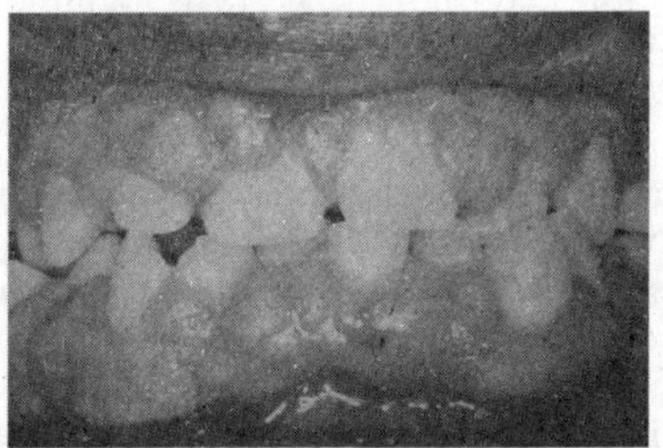

Fig. 38.2 Phenytoin-induced gingival overgrowth.

19. The initial clinical appearance of phenytoin-induced gingival enlargement is painless enlargement of interproximal gingiva in which buccal and anterior segment are more affected than the lingual and posterior segments. Unless secondary inflammation is present, the gingiva appears firm and does not bleed easily upon probing.

a. Both the statements are true
b. Both the statements are false
c. The first statement is true and the second is false
d. The first statement is false and the second is true

Ans a.

The answer is self-explanatory.

20. Which of the following gingival enlargement is primarily a capillary disease (in which the endothelium swells and degenerates)?

a. Scorbutic gingivitis
b. Phenytoin-induced gingival enlargement
c. Fibromatosis gingivae
d. Puberty gingivitis

Ans a.

Gingivitis associated with vitamin C deficiency is called scorbutic gingivitis. The child usually complains of severe pain and spontaneous hemorrhage will be evident on the gingivae.

21. Which of the following microorganisms is/are involved in juvenile periodontitis?

a. *Porphyromonas gingivalis*
b. *Bacteroides melaninogenicus*

c. *Fusobacterium nucleatum*
d. *Actinobacillus actinomycetemcomitans*
e. All of the above

Ans e.

Localized juvenile periodontitis is associated with Bacteroides melaninogenicus and *Actinobacillus actinomycetemcomitans* whereas generalized juvenile periodontitis is associated with *Porphyromonas gingivalis* and *Actinobacillus actinomycetemcomitans.*

22. Frenectomy involves complete excision of the frenum and its periosteal attachment. A frenotomy involves incision of the periosteal fiber attachment and possibly suturing of the frenum to the periosteum at the base of the mandible.

a. Both the statements are true
b. Both the statements are false
c. The first statement is true and the second is false
d. The first statement is false and the second is true

Ans a.

A frenum is a membranous fold that joins two parts and restricts the individual movements of each. The question defines frenectomy and frenotomy procedures.

23. A mandibular frenum that inhibits the tongue from touching the maxillary central incisor would interfere with the child's ability to make 't', 'd', 'l' sounds. As long as the child has enough range of motion to raise the tongue to the roof of the mouth, no surgery would be indicated.

a. Both the statements are true
b. Both the statements are false
c. The first statement is true and the second is false
d. The first statement is false and the second is true

Ans a.

Some commonly observed locations of frenums in the child are on the facial gingival surface of the anterior midline of the maxilla, on the facial and lingual gingival surfaces of the anterior midline of the mandible and on the mandibular and maxillary premolar facial area.

24. PMA index assesses

a. The amount of calculus
b. Gingivitis

c. Periodontal status
d. The marginal gingiva specifically

Ans b.
The answer is self-explanatory.

25. The teeth usually examined in the simplified oral hygiene index are

a. Molars and premolars
b. Molars and incisors
c. Premolars and incisors
d. Incisors and canines

Ans b.
Molars and incisors are usually examined in simplified oral hygiene index.

26. PMA index was given by

a. Greene and Vermilion
b. Massler and Schour
c. Moore
d. Russell

Ans b.
Massler and Schour introduced the PMA index (papillary marginal and attached gingival index). Russell introduced the periodontal index.

27. Papillon–Lefevre syndrome is associated with

a. Palmar keratosis
b. Plantar keratosis
c. Periodontitis
d. All of the above

Ans d.
This syndrome was described by Papillon and Lefevre in 1924. It is a rare autosomal recessive genetic disease characterized by severe periodontitis and hyperkeratosis of the skin.

28. Keyes technique of management of aggressive periodontitis involves the use of

a. Amoxicillin for 14 days
b. Tetracycline for 14 days
c. Minocycline for 14 days
d. Doxycycline for 14 days

Ans b.

The Keyes technique for treating LJP recommends meticulous scaling and root planing of all teeth, with concomitant irrigation to probing depth of saturated inorganic solutions and 1% chlormaine T. In addition to this, the Keyes technique advocates use of systemic tetracycline for 14 days.

29. Herpetic gingivostomatitis is caused by

a. HSV 1
b. HSV 2
c. HSV 3
d. HSV 4

Ans a.

HSV 1—Herpes Simplex Virus 1. A fourfold elevation of antibodies to HSV 1 is a laboratory diagnostic criterion in children with herpetic gingivostomatitis

30. The periodontal ligament is wider and has fewer fibers in children. Alveolar mucosa is redder in color because of the absence of keratin in children.

a. Both the statements are true
b. Both the statements are false
c. The first statement is true and the second is false
d. The first statement is false and the second is true

Ans a.

The answer is self-explanatory.

31. All of the following drugs cause gingival enlargement except

a. Cyclosporine
b. Phenytoin
c. Nifedipine
d. Rifampicin

Ans d.

Phenytoin, a major drug used as an anticonvulsant agent, causes varying degrees of gingival overgrowth. Cyclosporine, calcium channel blockers (Nifedipine), valproic acid and phenobarbital are reported to cause gingival enlargement.

32. Floating teeth appearance in radiographs is seen in

a. Langerhans cell histiocytosis
b. Cyclic neutropenia
c. Papillon–Lefevre syndrome
d. Down syndrome

Ans a.

Due to destruction of alveolar bone, the teeth in radiographs show a "floating teeth" appearance.

33. All of the following conditions are involved with premature exfoliation of teeth except

a. Cyclic neutropenia
b. Hypophosphatasia
c. Chediak-Higashi syndrome
d. ANUG

Ans d.

The answer is self-explanatory.

34. Green stains are commonly seen in

a. Posterior teeth buccal surface
b. Posterior teeth lingual surface
c. Gingival third of the labial surface of maxillary anterior teeth
d. Gingival third of mandibular anterior teeth

Ans c.

Green stains collect on the gingival third of the labial surface of maxillary anterior teeth.

Chromogenic bacteria and stains.

S. No.	Stain	Features
1	Green stain	Seen in young people Cause unknown (may be due to chromogenic bacteria) Seen in gingival third of labial surface of maxillary anterior teeth Commonly seen in labial surface of mouth breathers Enamel beneath the stain might have undergone initial demineralization
2	Orange stain	Occurs less frequently than green stain Cause unknown Often seen in gingival third of the tooth and is associated with poor oral hygiene
3	Black stain	Less common than orange and green stain Seen as a line following gingival contour or it may be generalized (usually on rough and pitted areas) Children with black stains are usually caries free

35. For a patient with generalized acute herpetic stomatitis, the dentist should

a. Refer the patient to a physician for treatment with diluted chickenpox vaccines
b. Debride the mouth, sustain oral hygiene and treat the elevated temperature
c. Use bacterial cultures to rule out acute necrotizing ulcerative gingivitis
d. Prescribe 300,000 units of penicillin orally

Ans 35.b.

Treatment of primary herpetic gingivostomatitis is aimed towards relief of acute symptoms so that fluid and nutritional intake can be maintained.

36. Six months after removal of bands placed to correct alignment of anterior teeth in a 12-year-old girl, heavy fibrotic gingival margins persist. The proper treatment is

a. Gingivectomy
b. Gingivoplasty
c. Deep scaling and curettage
d. Toothbrushing instruction

Ans b.

Gingivoplasty is reshaping of the gingiva to create physiologic contours, with the sole purpose of recontouring the gingiva in the absence of pockets. Gingivectomy is performed to eliminate periodontal pockets and includes reshaping as part of the technique.

37. Localized gingival recession in the region of erupting mandibular incisor teeth is associated with

a. Keratotic melanoplasia
b. Idiopathic cementosis
c. Abnormal frenum attachment
d. Increased spacing of teeth
e. Dilantin therapy

Ans c.

Gingival recession is often seen in children frequently caused by any one of the following predisposing factors:

1. Presence of a narrow band of attached gingiva
2. Presence of a tooth in anterior crossbite
3. Bony dehiscence
4. Toothbrush trauma
5. Prominence of tooth in the arch

6. Oral habits (dummy or pacifier sucking)

7. High frenal attachment

38. The most common cause of generalized acute gingival inflammation in a preschool child is

a. Vitamin B deficiency
b. Vitamin C deficiency
c. Acute herpetic gingivostomatitis
d. Necrotizing ulcerative gingivitis
e. Acute Streptococcus mutans gingivostomatitis

Ans c.

Type 1 herpes simplex virus is responsible for most of the oropharyngeal infections including acute herpetic gingivostomatitis. This disease is observed in young adolescents and children but has its highest incidence in infants and children younger than 6 years of age.

39. In examining a child patient, normal gingiva is diagnosed on the basis of all of the following except

a. Contour
b. Stippling
c. Sulcus depth
d. Depth of the vestibule

Ans d.

The gingiva is part of the oral mucosa that covers the alveolar processes of the jaws and surrounds the necks of the teeth.

40. An 8-year-old girl is admitted to the hospital for treatment of "swollen gums" of three weeks' duration. Oral examination reveals markedly edematous and erythematous gingivae. Her parents state that the child has been well although, in the past month, some malaise, anorexia and occasional fever were noted. The most appropriate course of action is to

a. Refer the child to a periodontist
b. Request a hematologic consultation
c. Scale and curette the affected areas and prescribe mild rinses
d. Prescribe a 10-day course of oral penicillin(1 million units per day)
e. Enroll the child in an active prevention program that emphasizes adequate home care

Ans b.

In young children, swollen gums or spontaneous bleeding can be an indicator of hematologic disorder. Hence any unexplained gum disease needs a routine blood investigation.

41. A 3 ½-year-old child has acute fever, diarrhoea, oral vesicular lesions and gingival tenderness. The most likely diagnosis is

a. Thrush
b. Drug allergy
c. Aphthous ulcerations
d. Acute herpetic stomatitis
e. Necrotizing ulcerative gingivitis

Ans d.

Course of herpetic gingivostomatitis runs for 7 to 10 days. In its initial stage, it is characterized by the presence of discrete spherical grey vesicle, which may occur on the gingiva, labial and buccal mucosa, soft palate, pharynx, sublingual mucosa and tongue. After approximately 24 hours, the vesicles rupture and form a painful, depressed, yellowish or grayish white central portion. These occur either in widely separated areas or in clusters, where confluence occurs.

42. Gingival stripping in the incisor region of a child is best treated by

a. Gingivectomy
b. Alveolectomy
c. Deep lingual frenectomy
d. Decreasing the amount of attached gingiva
e. Increasing the amount of attached gingiva

Ans e.

Increasing the gingival width improves the oral hygiene and esthetics.

43. Which of the following medications shortens the recovery period of primary herpetic gingivostomatitis?

a. Aspirin
b. Penicillin
c. Kenolog in Orobase
d. None of the above

Ans d.

Treatment of primary herpetic gingivostomatitis is aimed towards relief of acute symptoms so that fluid and nutritional intake can be maintained. The application of a mild topical anesthetic such as Dyclomine Hydrochloride (0.5%) before meal time will temporarily relieve the pain and allow the child to take a soft diet. Lidocaine can be prescribed for the child who can hold one teaspoon of the anesthetic in the mouth for 2–3 minutes and then expectorate the solution. Equal parts of Diphenhydramine (Anti-inflammatory) and Kaolin Pectin compound (coats the lesion) is an useful alternative. However, none of the drugs shorten the recovery period.

Chapter 39

Forensic Odontology

1. **Who proposed that there are 1.8×10^{19} possible combinations of 32 teeth being intact, decayed, missing or filled?**
   a. Acharya
   b. Keiser-Nelson
   c. Fellingham
   d. Mac Donald

Ans c.

The number of combinations of 16 (one arch) missing or filled teeth can produce 600 million combinations. Every tooth has five surfaces, and if these surfaces were taken into account the variations produced will be astronomic. Fellingham and coworkers have calculated that there are 1.8×10^{19} possible combinations of 32 teeth being intact, decayed, missing or filled.

2. **Cheiloscopy is the analysis of**
   a. Rugae
   b. Teeth marks
   c. Lip prints
   d. Finger prints

Ans c.

Wrinkles and grooves visible on the lips are referred as sulci labiorum rubrorum by Tsuchihashi. The imprints produced by these grooves are termed lip prints and the examination of them is termed *cheiloscopy.* These grooves are heritable and are supposed to be individualistic.

3. **Impression of human bite marks are taken by**
   a. Alginate
   b. Vinyl polysiloxane
   c. Impression compound
   d. Plaster of paris

Ans b.

The answer is self-explanatory.

4. All of the following are classifications of bite marks except

a. Acharya and Taylor classification
b. MacDonald's classification
c. Cameron and Sims classification
d. Webster's classification

Ans a.

MacDonald's Classification of Bite Marks

This is the most cited of all classifications. This is more specifically applied to human bite marks.

Tooth pressure marks. Marks produced on tissue as a result of 'direct application of pressure by teeth'. These are generally produced by the incisal or occlusal surfaces.

Tongue pressure marks. When sufficient amount of tissue is taken into the mouth, the tongue presses it against rigid areas such as the lingual surfaces of teeth and palatal rugae. The marks thus left on the skin are called suckling as there is a combination of sucking and tongue thrusting involved.

Tooth scrape marks. These are marks caused by the scraping of teeth across the bitten material. They are usually caused by anterior teeth and present as scratches or superficial abrasions.

Cameron and Sims Classification

This is based on the agent producing the bite mark and the material exhibiting it.

Agents

1. Human
2. Animal

Materials

1. Skin or body tissue
2. Food stuff
3. Other materials

Webster's Classification

This is based on the materials which exhibit the marks. this is especially in cases of robbery, etc.

Type I. The tooth item fractures readily with limited depth of tooth penetration (e.g. hard chocolate).

Type II. Fracture of fragment of food item with considerable penetration of teeth (e.g. bite marks on apple).

Type III. Complete or near complete penetration of the food item with slide marks (e.g. cheese).

5. All of the following are included under MacDonald's classification of bite marks except

a. Tooth pressure marks
b. Tongue pressure marks
c. Tooth scrape marks
d. Lip pressure marks

Ans d.

Refer to the explanation of Q. No. 4.

Section XI

Miscellaneous

Chapter 40

Dental Materials Used in Pediatric Dentistry

1. All of the following are advantages of glass ionomer cements except

a. Fluoride release
b. Chemical adhesion to tooth structure
c. Mechanical bonding with tooth structure
d. Tooth colored restorative material

Ans c.

Glass ionomer cements have chemical bonding with tooth structure and mechanical bonding is for composites.

2. While mixing zinc oxide with eugenol if water comes in contact it will ______________ the setting reaction

a. Accelerate
b. Decelerate
c. Does not have any effect in setting
d. It prevents zinc oxide mixing with eugenol

Ans a.

Water acts as an accelerator in this setting reaction.

3. Bonding agents are unfilled resins. Acid etching provides microporosities for the bonding agent to form resin tags.

a. Both the statements are true
b. Both the statements are false
c. First statement is true and the second is false
d. First statement is false and the second is true

Ans a.

Bonding agents are unfilled resins. They flow through the microporosities and provide mechanical retention.

Chapter 41

Radiology

1. X-rays were discovered by

a. Roentgen
b. Fleming
c. Crooks
d. Craig

Ans a.

Roentgen discovered X-rays in 1895.

2. Discovery of X-rays was made in

a. 1895
b. 1905
c. 1960
d. 1885

Ans a.

Refer to the explanation of Q. No. 1.

3. Dental radiography began

a. 10 weeks after the discovery of X-rays
b. 6 months after the discovery of X-rays
c. 6 weeks after the discovery of X-rays
d. 6 days after the discovery of X-rays

Ans c.

Six weeks after Roentgen's announcement of discovery of X-rays, a dentist attempted to record shadows of oral structures on a film. Although they were crude images, dental radiography had begun.

4. The selection of appropriate radiographs for the pediatric patient depends on

a. The age of the child

b. Size of the oral cavity
c. Level of patient cooperation
d. All of the above

Ans d.

The selection of appropriate radiographs for the pediatric patient depends on all the above-mentioned factors.

5. X-rays cause biologic damage by

a. Immediate cell death
b. Enhancing autolysis or apoptosis
c. Imparting its energy and causing injury to the tissues through which it traverses
d. Stimulating killer T cells

Ans c.

One characteristic feature of X-rays is its ability to impart some of its energy to the matter it traverses. If the matter is a living tissue, then biologic injury may occur.

6. Biologic damage caused by X-rays can be

a. Carcinogenesis
b. Mutagenesis
c. Teratogenesis
d. Any of the above

Ans d.

Carcinogenesis and malformations are the response of somatic tissues and in most instances are believed to have a threshold (that is a certain amount of radiation is necessary for the response to be seen). Mutation may occur as a response of genetic tissue to X-radiation and is believed to have no threshold. In general, younger tissues and organs are more sensitive to radiation (with the sensitivity decreasing from the period before birth until maturity).

7. Natural background radiation normally is

a. 102–120 mrem/year
b. 202–220 mrem/year
c. 92 mrem/year
d. 250–300 mrem/year

Ans a.

The answer is self-explanatory. In millisievert, it is 1.02–1.20.

8. Radiation induced damage most often will result in cancer of the following organs except

a. Skin
b. Breast
c. Thyroid
d. Gonads

Ans d.

In gonads, radiation causes mutations, infertility and fetal malformations whereas in skin, breasts and thyroid it causes cancer.

9. The fastest film speed available for dental radiography is

a. A
b. B
c. E
d. D

Ans c.

Faster film speeds have contributed most significantly to the reduction in radiation to the patient. Film speeds of D and E are currently available for dental radiography.

10. All of the following decrease the radiation exposure to the patient except

a. Using a lead apron and a thyroid collar
b. Using high kilovolt peak
c. Using slow speed film
d. Using filters and diaphragms

Ans c.

Use of slow speed film increases the exposure time thereby increasing the exposure of the patient to the radiation. The lead apron protects the gonads and the chest from the primary beam and scatter radiation whereas the collar shields the thyroid.

11. A 4-year-old child with no apparent abnormalities and open contacts should undergo

a. 4-film survey
b. 8-film survey
c. No radiographic examination
d. 12-film survey

Ans c.

When there are open proximal contacts, one need not undergo radiographic examination.

12. Four-film series consists of all except

a. Anterior occlusal maxillary
b. Anterior occlusal mandibular
c. Bitewings
d. OPG

Ans d.

Refer to the following explanation:

4-film survey	– Maxillary anterior occlusal
	Mandibular anterior occlusal
	Two posterior bitewings
8-film survey	– Maxillary/mandibular anterior occlusal (or periapicals)
	Right, left, maxillary posterior occlusal (or periapicals)
	Right, left, mandibular primary molar periapicals
	Two posterior bitewings
12-film survey	– Four primary molar/premolar periapicals
	Four canine periapicals
	Two incisor periapicals
	Two posterior bitewings
16-film survey	– 12-film survey +
	Four permanent molar periapicals

13. All of the following are correct regarding 12-film survey except

a. Four primary molars/premolar periapicals
b. Four canine periapicals
c. Two incisor periapicals
d. Two molar periapicals

Ans d.

Refer to the explanation of Q. No. 12.

14. The size of the film commonly used for bitewing radiography is

a. 0 and 4
b. 0 and 2
c. 2 and 4
d. 1 and 2

Ans b.

The answer is self-explanatory.

15. During bitewing radiography, the ala-tragus line is

a. Parallel to the floor
b. Perpendicular to the floor
c. The position of the ala-tragus line is not significant
d. Parallel to the occlusal plane

Ans a.

While taking a bitewing radiograph, the head is positioned so that the midsagittal plane is perpendicular and the ala-tragus line is parallel to the floor.

16. Which of the corners of the film is to be folded while taking a bitewing radiograph?

a. Anterosuperior and posteroinferior
b. Posterosuperior and anteroinferior
c. Posterosuperior and posteroinferior
d. Anterosuperior and posteroinferior

Ans b.

Anteroinferior corner is bent to prevent damage to the lingual frenum and posterosuperior corner is bent to prevent gagging.

17. The vertical angulation for bitewing radiography is

a. +8
b. +12
c. –8
d. –12

Ans a.

The vertical angulation for bitewing radiography is +8 to +10 degrees.

18. Bisecting angle and paralleling techniques are used to take

a. Periapical radiographs
b. Bitewing radiographs
c. Occlusal radiographs
d. Mandibular occlusal view

Ans a.

The answer is self-explanatory.

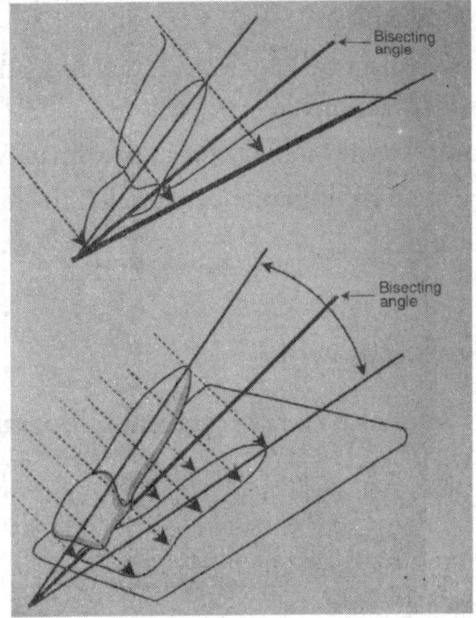

Fig. 41.1 Rule of isometry—bisecting angle technique.

19. In paralleling technique, the film is placed (for maxillary radiography)

a. Close to the object
b. Far from the object
c. Object–film distance is not a criterion
d. None of the above

Ans b.

The paralleling technique requires the object and film to be in parallel in all dimensions. To achieve this, the film packet is placed farther away from the object, particularly in the maxilla.

20. All of the following are true regarding the bisecting angle technique except

a. It is based on rule of isometry
b. The central X-ray is directed perpendicular to the bisector
c. It is used to take periapical radiographs
d. The accuracy is better than that of the paralleling technique

Ans d.

The rule of isometry states that two triangles are equal if they have two equal angles and a common side. Radiographs taken by paralleling technique have better contrast and accuracy than bisecting angle technique.

21. Orthopantomography

a. Uses a mechanism by which the X-ray film and the source move in opposite directions
b. Needs complete immobility for approximately 5–22 seconds
c. Is a supplement for intraoral periapical radiographic series
d. All of the above

Ans d.

The answer is self-explanatory.

22. The normal range of kVp for intraoral radiography is

a. 20–40 kVp
b. 80–120 kVp
c. 60–90 kVp
d. More than 120 kVp

Ans b.

The use of higher kilovolt peak techniques reduces patient exposure to radiation and lowers the contrast thus increasing the number of shades of gray on the film.

23. Bitewing radiographs of a 5-year-old child show interproximal caries just short of DE junction. The dentist should recommend

a. Restoration of the tooth as soon as possible
b. Prophylaxis and topical fluoride application
c. Disking of the affected areas
d. 3 month recall for re-evaluation

Ans a.

Interproximal caries in the primary molars involve the pulp faster. Hence, restoration as soon as it is detected is the treatment of choice.

24. When no new decay is formed, the frequency of repeated bitewing radiographs recommended in permanent dentition is

a. Once in every 18–24 months
b. Once in every 12–18 months
c. Once in 48 months
d. Once a year

Ans a.

If no evidence of caries is found, then X-rays may be taken every 12–18 months if primary teeth are in contact or every 18–24 months if permanent teeth are in contact.

25. **According to buccal object rule, the object that is present in the buccal side**
   a. Moves in the same direction
   b. Moves in the opposite direction
   c. Remains static
   d. None of the above

Ans b.

The object localization technique uses the SLOB rule. It says that if the object is present on the buccal side, it moves in the opposite direction and if it is in the lingual side it moves in the same direction.

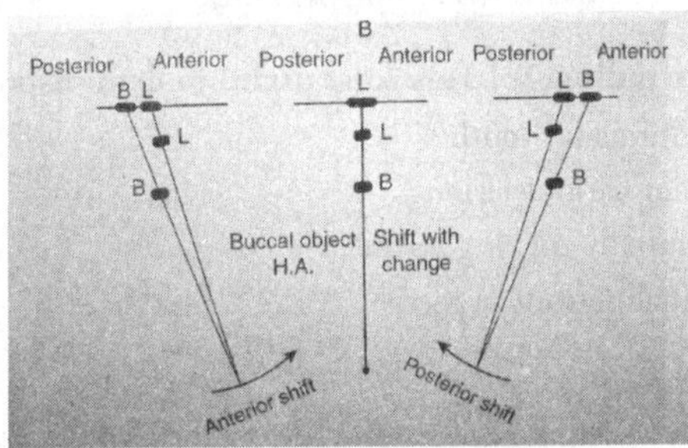

Fig. 41.2 SLOB rule.

26. **For all maxillary films, the ala-tragus line is**
   a. Parallel to the floor
   b. Perpendicular to the floor
   c. Parallel to the occlusal plane
   d. None of the above

Ans a.

The answer is self-explanatory. Refer to the explanation of Q. No. 15.

27. **When a panoramic radiograph is possible, the ideal survey for primary dentition with closed contacts is**
   a. OPG only
   b. OPG and a pair of bitewings
   c. OPG and a pair of bitewings and two periapicals
   d. OPG and two occlusal view

Ans c.

A pair of bitewings evaluates the proximal areas while the two anterior periapicals assess the anterior teeth and the OPG gives the overall status of the dental development.

28. To utilize the buccal object rule for object localization, one has to take

a. One radiograph
b. Two radiographs
c. Three radiographs
d. Four radiographs

Ans b.

Two radiographs have to be taken to utilize the SLOB rule. The first film is taken as a routine radiograph. The second film is placed in the same position. The head position and the vertical angle remains the same but the horizontal angle is shifted either anteriorly or posteriorly.

29. Panoramic radiographs are least useful in demonstrating

a. Supernumerary tooth
b. Incipient carious lesion
c. Congenitally missing tooth
d. Axial inclinations of teeth

Ans b.

Good bitewing radiographs usually detect incipient caries. In OPG, the proximal surfaces are usually overlapped which makes it a poor indicator of proximal caries.

30. Emulsion on the radiographic film is made of

a. Silver bromide grains
b. Polyester terethalate
c. Pure silver grains
d. Carbon-containing compound

Ans a.

Emulsion is one of the two components of the X-ray film. It is sensitive to X-rays and visible light and records the radiographic image. It is made of silver halide (silver bromide) grains which are sensitive to X-radiation and visible light.

31. Speed of the film refers to the amount of radiation required to produce an image of standard density. A fast film requires a relatively low exposure.

a. Both the statements are true
b. Both the statements are false
c. First statement is true and the second is false
d. First statement is false and the second is true

Ans a.

Speed of the film refers to the amount of radiation required to produce an image of standard density. A fast film requires relatively low exposure. The fastest dental film currently available has a speed rating F. Only films with rating D or faster speed rating are appropriate for intraoral radiography.

32. Image sharpness measures how well a boundary between two areas of differing radio density is revealed. Image resolution measures how well a radiograph is able to reveal small objects that are close together.

a. Both the statements are true
b. Both the statements are false
c. First statement is true and the second is false
d. First statement is false and the second is true

Ans a.

Both sharpness and resolution are interdependent, and for better clinical diagnosis, it is desirable to optimize conditions that will result in images with high sharpness and resolution. This can be achieved by use of a small effective focal spot, increasing the distance between the focal spot and the object by using a long open-ended cylinder and by decreasing the distance between the object and the film.

33. The size of the pedo film is

a. 24 × 40
b. 22 × 35
c. 31 × 41
d. 36 × 48

Ans b.

Periapical films come in three sizes.

S. No.	Size	Description
1.	0	For small children (pedo film—22 × 35mm)
2.	1	Relatively narrow and used for anterior teeth (24 × 40 mm)
3.	2	Standard film size used for adults (31 × 41 mm)

34. Foreshortening of image results when the central ray is perpendicular to the film but object is not parallel with the film. Elongation of a radiographic image results when the central ray is perpendicular to the object but not to the film.

a. Both the statements are true
b. Both the statements are false
c. First statement is true and the second is false
d. First statement is false and second is true

Ans a.

Foreshortening results when the central ray is perpendicular and the object is not parallel and elongation results when the central ray is perpendicular to the object and not the film.

35. The size of the pulp chamber can be clearly assessed by

a. Periapical view
b. Cross-sectional occlusal view
c. Bitewing view
d. Panoramic view

Ans c.

To determine pulp chamber configuration, depth of carious lesion and proximity of restoration to pulp space, bitewing view is used.

36. Miller's right angle technique is best for the mandible. In maxilla, the superimposition of features in the anterior part of the skull may obscure the area of interest.

a. Both the statements are true
b. Both the statements are false
c. First statement is true and the second is false
d. First statement is false and the second is true

Ans a.

Occasionally, dentists are encountered with a situation where localizing the object whether they are placed buccally or lingually is critical for a surgical intervention. Instead of a tubeshift technique, Miller's right angle technique is used in the mandible where the cone is shifted vertically upwards or downwards in relation to the mandible.

37. Which of the following is a disadvantage of digital radiography?

a. Any bending or scratching the digital receptor can create permanent artifacts on the receptor
b. It may not be possible to consistently capture the distal surface of the canines in premolar views
c. One should have different size of receptors to capture images in children and adults

d. Children under 4 or 5 years of age may not tolerate the wired sensors, may damage the cables because they do not understand the procedure and may chew on the cable
e. All of the above

Ans e.

All the above-mentioned issues are disadvantages of digital radiography.

38. All of the following are methods to decrease hazards due to radiation except

a. Use films of D or C speed
b. Filter the X-ray beam, use open ended cones
c. Collimate the X-ray beam, rectangular collimators better than round ones
d. Increase the tube to patient distance

Ans a.

Use of E or F speed films decreases the amount of radiation more than D or C speed films. Also refer to the explanation of Q. No. 31.

Chapter 42

Indices Used in Pediatric Dentistry

1. One of the following defines sensitivity of an index

a. Index must measure what it is intended to measure, so it should correspond with clinical stages of the diseases under study at each point

b. An index should be virtually synonymous with reproducibility, the ability of the same or different examiner to interpret and use the index in the same way. It should also measure consistently at different times under a variety of conditions

c. An index should be amenable to statistical analysis, so that the status of a group can be expressed by a number that corresponds to a relative position on a scale from zero to the upper limit

d. Index should be able to detect reasonably small shifts, in either direction in the group conditions

Ans a.

Sensitivity is the ability of the index to identify correctly all those who have the disease, that is "true positive". A 90% sensitivity means that 90% of the diseased people screened by the test will give a "true positive" result and the remaining 10% a "false negative" result.

2. One of the following statements defines reliability of an index

a. Index must measure what it is intended to measure, so it should correspond with clinical stages of the diseases under study at each point

b. An index should be virtually synonymous with reproducibility, the ability of the same or different examiner to interpret and use the index in the same way. It should also measure consistently at different times under a variety of conditions

c. An index should be amenable to statistical analysis, so that the status of a group can be expressed by a number that corresponds to a relative position on a scale from zero to the upper limit

d. Index should be able to detect reasonably small shifts, in either direction in the group conditions

Ans b.

Reliability is the ability to give consistent results when repeated more than once on the same individuals or material, under the same conditions. The reliability of the test depends upon three major factors, namely observer variation, biological variation and errors relating to technical methods.

3. OHI-S index was given by

a. Greene and Vermilion
b. Loe and Silnes
c. WHO
d. Knutson and Palmer

Ans a.

The OHI-S index was developed by John C Greene and Jack R Vermilion in 1964. It is a simple and sensitive method for assessing group or individual oral hygiene quantitatively.

4. Plaque index was given by

a. Greene and Vermilion
b. Silness and Loe
c. WHO
d. Knutson and Palmer

Ans b.

Plaque index was given by Silness P and Loe H in 1964 and 1967. The purpose of the index is to assess the thickness of plaque at the gingival area of the tooth.

5. Massler and Schour introduced the __________ index.

a. PMA index
b. DMFT index
c. deft index
d. Gingival bleeding index

Ans a.

Papillary marginal attachment index was given by Maury, Massler and Schour in 1944. This index measures the severity of gingivitis based on color, consistency and bleeding on probing.

6. Papillary bleeding index was introduced by

a. Loe and Silness

b. Massler and Schour
c. Muhleman HR
d. Palmer and Knutson

Ans c.

Papillary bleeding index (PBI) was given by Muhleman HR in 1977. This index assesses the gingival inflammation.

7. Oral hygiene is said to be excellent when the OHI-S score is

a. 1
b. 2
c. 3
d. 0

Ans d.

The scoring chart for OHI-S index is as follows:

Excellent—0

Good—0.1–1.2

Fair—1.3–3

Poor—3.1–6

8. In deft, "e" stands for

a. Exfoliated tooth
b. Extracted tooth due to caries
c. Tooth indicated for extraction
d. Either (b) or (c)

Ans b.

d—decayed tooth, e—extracted tooth, f—filled tooth, t—tooth. The deft index is used to score primary teeth. DMFT stands for permanent teeth.

9. deft and defs index were introduced by

a. Loe and Silness
b. Massler and Schour
c. Gruebbel
d. Palmer and Knutson

Ans c.

deft and defs index were introduced by Gruebbel in 1944.

Chapter 43

Genetic Aspects of Dental Anomalies

1. **The genetic material, DNA, that controls the production of a single protein (or polypeptide chain) is called a chromosome. There are thousands and thousands of human genes each one regulating the production of a specific polypeptide.**
   a. Both the statements are true
   b. Both the statements are false
   c. First statement is true and the second is false
   d. First statement is false and the second is true

Ans d.
Gene is defined as the genetic material that controls the production of a single protein or polypeptide chain. There are thousands of genes, each regulating the production of specific polypeptide. These genes are grouped into units called chromosomes.

2. **Who demonstrated that the fundamental defect in Down syndrome is the presence of an extra chromosome in the affected individuals' karyotype?**
   a. Le Jeune
   b. Turpin
   c. Gautier
   d. All of the above

Ans d.
In 1959 Le Jeune, Turpin and Gautier demonstrated that the fundamental defect in Down syndrome is the presence of an extra chromosome. They have proved this by karyotyping the chromosomes of the affected individuals.

3. **Match the following structural alterations of chromosomes**
   a. A-2, B-3, C-4, D-1
   b. A-4, B-1, D-2, C-3
   c. A-3, B-4, C-1, D-2
   d. A-3, B-2, C-1, D-4

A	Deletion	1	The attachment of a broken piece from one chromosome to another nonhomologous chromosome
B	Duplication	2	The absence of a segment of a chromosome
C	Inversion	3	The insertion of an extra fragment into a chromosome from its now deficient homolog
D	Translocation	4	The breaking of a chromosome in two places and subsequent rejoining with the middle piece inverted

Ans a.

Humans have 46 chromosomes. Each chromosome has a pair that is referred to as the homolog. Genes on homologs control the same genetic trait and with the single exception of those genes on the sex chromosomes, there are at least two genes that control each inherited trait.

4. **Monosomy of an autosome or a missing autosomal chromosome is not believed to be compatible with life. On the other hand, monosomy of the sex chromosomes does occur and it is compatible with life.**
   a. Both the statements are true
   b. Both the statements are false
   c. First statement is true and the second is false
   d. First statement is false and the second is true

Ans a.

In Turner syndrome, monosomy of X chromosome is seen (45X) and it is compatible with life. But monosomy of an autosome is not compatible with life.

5. **All of the following statements are true regarding traits except**
   a. Monogenic traits are produced and regulated by a single gene
   b. Monogenic traits are usually easy to recognize in families and the transmission of the trait from one family member to the next follows simple Mendelian principles of dominant recessive, autosomal or sex-linked inheritance
   c. Many genes at different loci control polygenic traits
   d. Polygenic traits are common and are illustrated by examples such as albinism, achondroplasia, etc.

Ans d.

Some of the monogenic traits are albinism, achondroplasia and neurofibromatosis. Polygenic traits are hereditary and typically exert control over rather common characteristics such as height, skin pigmentation and intelligence. Genetic control takes place through many gene loci collectively asserting their regulation of the trait.

6. Individuals affected with heritable syndromes involving the face often look more like others with the same disease who are not genetically related than they do their own siblings. Which of the following is an example of this?

a. Down syndrome
b. Hereditary ectodermal dysplasia
c. Infantile hypercalcemia syndrome
d. Stickler syndrome
e. All of the above

Ans e.

Individuals affected with the above-mentioned syndromes have a striking similarity to each other.

7. The term multifactorial inheritance has been employed to describe traits that do not fit simple mendelian inheritance pattern. A multifactorial inheritance disorder is one that is determined by environmental factors only.

a. Both the statements are true
b. Both the statements are false
c. First statement is true and the second is false
d. First statement is false and the second is true

Ans c.

A multifactorial inheritance disorder is one that is determined by a combination of genetic and environmental factors. Dental caries, malocclusion and periodontal disease are examples of diseases with multifactorial etiology. Some of the common systemic disorders which are multifactorial in etiology are diabetes, hypertension, etc.

8. While evaluating genetic traits, the first affected individual in a family who brings that family to attention is referred to as the

a. Proband
b. Propositus
c. Index case
d. Any of the above

Ans d.

The affected individual in a family who first brings that family to the attention of the geneticist is called the proband or propositus. This individual is also known as the index case.

9. The clinical appearance of a given trait for an individual such as eye color or height, is the individual's genotype. The specific genetic make-up that controls that genotype is the phenotype.

a. Both the statements are true
b. Both the statements are false
c. Frst statement is true and the second is false
d. First statement is false and the second is true

Ans b.

The clinical appearance of a given trait for an individual such as eye color or height, is the individual's phenotype whereas the specific genetic make-up that controls the phenotype is the genotype.

10. A gene that expresses a particular phenotype in a single dose is a recessive gene. If the gene must be present in double dose (homozygous) to express a phenotype it is a dominant gene.

a. Both the statements are true
b. Both the statements are false
c. First statement is true and the second is false
d. First statement is false and the second is true

Ans b.

A gene that expresses a particular phenotype in a single dose is a dominant gene. If the gene must be present in double dose (homozygous) to express a phenotype, it is a recessive gene.

11. Which of the following general criteria for making the diagnosis of autosomal dominant inheritance is incorrect?

a. The trait appears in each generation
b. On an average, 100% of the offspring of affected parents will also be affected
c. Unaffected parents do not have an affected offspring. There are two important exceptions: a fresh gene mutation in one of the parental gametes and when the trait shows nonpenetrance
d. The occurrence and transmission of the trait are not affected by sex. Males and females are equally likely to have or transmit the trait

Ans b.

In autosomal dominant inheritance, an average of 50% of the offsprings of affected parents will be affected.

12. Which of the following criteria about autosomal recessive inheritance is true?

a. The trait typically appears only in siblings, not in parents or other relatives
b. On an average, one-fourth of the siblings of an affected individual will be similarly affected
c. The rarer the trait, the more likely that the parental meeting is consanguineous
d. Males and females are equally likely to be affected
e. All of the above

Ans e.

The answer is self-explanatory.

13. Dentinogenesis imperfecta is inherited as an autosomal dominant trait, has practically 100% penetrance, since all individuals who carry that gene shows the phenotype. But osteogenesis imperfecta shows incomplete penetrance since pedigree studies have demonstrated individuals who carry the gene but do not appear to be affected themselves.

a. Both the statements are true
b. Both the statements are false
c. First statement is true and the second is false
d. First statement is false and the second is true

Ans a.

The answer is self-explanatory.

14. Cardinal features of osteogenesis imperfecta is/are

a. Multiple fractures
b. Blue sclera
c. Dentinogenesis imperfecta
d. Otosclerosis
e. All of the above

Ans e.

All the above are characteristic features of osteogenesis imperfecta.

15. Monogenic traits have a low recurrence rate. Multifactorial traits have a very high recurrence rate.

a. Both the statements are true
b. Both the statements are false
c. First statement is true and the second is false
d. First statement is false and the second is true

Ans b.

Monogenic traits have a high recurrence rate. Multifactorial traits have a very low recurrence rate.

16. Monozygotic twins result from a single ovum fertilized by a single sperm. Dizygotic twins result from fertilization of two ova by two sperms.

a. Both the statements are true
b. Both the statements are false
c. First statement is true and the second is false
d. First statement is false and the second is true

Ans a.

The answer is self-explanatory.

17. Which of the following syndromes show periodontal destruction as one of its clinical features?

a. Ehlers–Danlos syndrome Type VIII
b. Histiocytosis X disease
c. Papillon–Lefevre syndrome
d. All of the above

Ans d.

Genetic conditions that predispose to periodontal disease, such as leukocyte adhesion deficiencies, Chediak–Higashi syndrome, cyclic neutropenia and Papillon–Lefevre syndrome have been associated with impaired function of phagocytes or phagocyte adherence to the walls of the blood vessels.

18. In which race (country) is malocclusion virtually nonexistent?

a. Japanese
b. Colored people
c. Filipinos
d. Chinese

Ans c.

Dental anthropologists feel that malocclusion is uncommon in pure racial populations. This could be because of lack of procreation with other populations or a less refined diet often eaten by these typically isolated groups.

19. BRAX-I gene is associated with

a. Dentin formation
b. Enamel formation
c. Cementum formation
d. Alveolar bone formation

Ans b.

The answer is self-explanatory.

20. Proline rich proteins in saliva are associated with

a. 11th chromosome
b. 12th chromosome
c. 4th chromosome
d. 1st chromosome

Ans b.

Proline rich proteins are associated with the genes located in the 12th chromosome in 12p13.2 region.

21. Cleidocranial dysostosis is of interest to the dentist because of

a. Premature loss of teeth
b. Concomitant micrognathia
c. High incidence of cleft
d. Associated high caries risk
e. Multiple supernumerary and unerupted teeth

Ans e.

Dental abnormalities seen in cleidocranial dysplasia may include delayed loss of the primary teeth; delayed appearance of the permanent teeth; unusually shaped, peg-like teeth; malocclusion and supernumerary teeth. It is sometimes accompanied by cysts in the oral cavity.

22. Children with Down syndrome may be described as

a. Affectionate
b. Fearful of quick movements
c. Capable of learning dental procedures
d. All of the above
e. None of the above

Ans d.

Children with Down syndrome (mongoloid child) are very affectionate and friendly. They are capable of learning dental procedures when explained to them. They are scared of sudden jerky movements. The dentist must be careful when changing the dental chair position and switching on the light in the dental chair. They can be managed on the dental chair without the use of pharmacological management.

23. In patients suffering from achondroplasia in which midfacial structures are most affected, one would expect to find which of the following malocclusions?

a. Class I

b. Class II

c. Class III

d. Group 5

Ans c.

Achondroplasia is the most common form of short stature. The facial features include a large head with a prominent forehead. The midface is often small with a flat nasal bridge and narrow nasal passages. The mandible appears to be prominent and occasionally dental crowding can occur since the maxilla is small.

24. In which of the following conditions is oligodontia a significant diagnostic characteristic?

a. Down syndrome

b. Hypothyroidism

c. Ectodermal dysplasia

d. Cleidocranial dysostosis

Ans c.

Ectodermal dysplasias are described as heritable conditions in which there are abnormalities of two or more ectodermal structures such as the hair, teeth, nails, sweat glands, craniofacial structures, digits and other parts of the body. Oligodontia and defective enamel are the most commonly seen dental anomalies.

25. A 4-year-old child has normally shaped, greyish colored teeth that exhibit extensive wear. Radiographic examination shows a normal complement of teeth, but extensive deposits of secondary dentin have almost obliterated pulp chambers and canal. The most probable diagnosis is

a. Tetralogy of Fallot

b. Tetracycline staining

c. Amelogenesis staining
d. Cleidocranial dysostosis
e. Dentinogenesis imperfecta

Ans e.

The extensive deposition of secondary dentin occurs to compensate for the defectively formed dentin. It obliterates the pulp chamber space and since the dentin is defective, the dentinoenamel junction is also weak leading to loss of tooth structure.

26. Radiographic examination of a child reveals several missing primary and permanent teeth. No teeth have been extracted. Medical history indicates practically no perspiration during hot, summer months. These facts suggest a preliminary diagnosis of

a. Achondroplasia
b. Osteogenic imperfect
c. Cleidocranial dysostosis
d. Anhidrotic ectodermal dysplasia

Ans d.

Anhidrotic ectodermal dysplasia is an inherited disorder characterized by ectodermal dysplasia associated with aplasia or hypoplasia of the sweat glands, hypothermia, alopecia, anodontia, conical teeth and facial abnormalities. Also refer to the explanation of Q. No. 24.

27. Use of which of the following is most important in managing the dental problems of a child with Down's syndrome?

a. Occlusal sealants
b. Local anesthesia
c. General anesthesia
d. Adequate premedication
e. Full coverage when caries occurs
f. A comprehensive preventive program

Ans f.

Refer to the explanation of Q. No. 22.

28. A 4-year-old child has frequent broken bones and exhibits blue sclera. Which of the following dental conditions is suggested?

a. Cleidocranial dysostosis
b. Amelogenesis imperfecta
c. Osteogenesis imperfecta
d. Enamel hypoplasia secondary to rickets

Ans c.

Osteogenesis imperfecta is also referred to as "blue eyes-broken bones disease" or "brittle bone disease". Four autosomal dominant phenotypes are recognized: Type 1 (mild) has blue sclera and bone fragility Type 2 (prenatal lethal) has dark sclera, severe bone fragility, and bone deformity; Type 3 (deforming) has light sclera, bone fragility, progressive deformity, imperfect dentition and short stature; Type 4 (mild deforming) has light sclera, imperfect dentition and mild short stature.

29. One of the following disorders is a single gene disorder

a. Sickle cell anemia
b. Dental caries
c. Malocclusion
d. Cleidocranial dysplasia

Ans a.

When the genetic information is carried into the next generation by a single mutant or defective gene, it is called monogenic inheritance. Sickle cell anemia and cystic fibrosis are examples of monogenic disorders.

30. Allele is

a. Alternate forms of gene
b. Gene pair
c. 'A' is an allele of a gene
d. All of the above

Ans a.

Alternate forms of genes are called alleles. When the alleles are identical the individual is homozygous for that trait; and when the alleles are different the individual is referred to as heterozygous.

31. Amelogenesis imperfecta is inherited as

a. An autosomal dominant disorder
b. An X-linked dominant disorder
c. Any of the above-mentioned forms
d. Only autosomal dominant form

Ans c.

The inheritance of amelogenesis imperfecta can be autosomal dominant, autosomal recessive, X linked and sporadic.

32. Number of genes present in human chromosomes is approximately

a. 10,000–15,000

b. 20,000–25,000
c. 30,000–50,000
d. 50,000–100,000

Ans c.

The entire genome consists of 3.2 billion nucleotide or base pairs within the DNA. This is distributed among the 23 chromosomes. There are about 35,000–50,000 regulatory or structural genes that control the regulation of genes throughout the lifespan.

33. Which of the following disorder is not an autosomal dominant disorder?

a. Dentinogenesis imperfecta
b. Incontinentia pigmenti
c. Achondroplasia
d. Some forms of amelogenesis imperfecta

Ans b.

Autosomal dominant disorders include dentinogenesis imperfecta (Type I), some forms of amelogenesis imperfecta and achondroplasia.

34. Human genome project was started in the year

a. 1980
b. 1990
c. 2000
d. 1995

Ans b.

The human genome project is a multinational effort between public and private sectors to elucidate the genetic content and architecture of human genome. The term "human" is a misnomer because the project also supports sequencing of genomes of infectious microbes, animal and plant models with beneficial effects.

35. Human genome project includes mapping of

a. Human genes
b. Human and microbial genes
c. Human, microbial and some plant genes
d. Human, microbial, animal and plant genes

Ans d.

Refer to the explanation of Q. No. 34.

36. Human DNA contains approximately __________ base pairs.

a. 1.5 billion

b. 2.5 billion

c. 3.2 billion

d. 5 billion

Ans c.

Refer to the explanation of Q. No. 32.

37. RUNX2 factor is related to

a. Cleidocranial dysostosis

b. Williams syndrome

c. Incontinentia pigmenti

d. Down syndrome

Ans a.

RUNX2 is runt-related transcription factor 2. Cleidocranial dysostosis is caused by mutation of *RUNX2*. The *RUNX2* gene provides instructions for making a protein that is involved in bone and cartilage development and maintenance.

Chapter 44

Antimicrobials and Analgesics Used in Pediatric Dentistry

1. One of the following antibiotics is a macrolide derivative:

a. Amoxicillin
b. Dicloxacillin
c. Erythromycin
d. Clindamycin

Ans c.

The following table classifies antibiotics based on their microbial target and also explains the nature of the drugs.

Based on microbial target
A. Used against gram-positive (aerobic) organisms
Natural penicillins (penicillin G, penicillin V)
Penicillinase-resistant penicillins (oxacillin, dicloxacillin)
Aminopenicillins (ampicillin, amoxicillin)
Macrolides (erythromycin, clarithromycin, azithromycin, roxithromycin)
Glycopetides (vancomycin)
Cephalosporins (cefazolin, cephalexin, cephadroxil)
Lincosamides (clindamycin)
Topicals (bacitracin, mupirocin)
B. Used against gram-negative (aerobic) microorganisms
Aminoglycosides (amikacin, tobramycins, gentamicin)
Extended spectrum penicillins (azlocillin, piperacillin)
Antipseudomonal penicillins (carbenicillin, ticarcillin)
Cephalosporins (ceftazidime)
Sulfonamides (trimethoprim, sulfamethoxazole)
Quinolones (ciprofloxacin, ofloxacin, norfloxacin) broad-spectrum antimicrobials
3rd, 4th generation cephalosporins (cefotaxime, ceftriaxone)
β lactam and β lactamase inhibitor combinations (ampicillin + sulbactam, amoxicillin + clavulanate, ticarcillin + clavulanate) tetracycline, chloramphenicol

C. Used against anaerobic bacteria

Penicillins (penicillin G)

Cephalosporins (cefatetan, cefoxitin)

Lincosamides (clindamycin)

Chloramphenicol

Metronidazole

D. Used against fungus

Polyenes (amphotericin B)

Azoles (fluconazole)

Topical agents (nystatin, clotrimazole, miconazole)

E. Used against viruses

Acyclovir, trifluridine, idoxuridine

Based on the mode of action

A. Inhibition of cell wall synthesis

Penicillins, cephalosporins, glycopeptides, azole

B. Inhibition of protein synthesis

1. Binds to 50s ribosome

Macrolides, chloramphenicol, lincosamides

2. Binds to 30s ribosome

Aminoglycosides, tetracyclines

C. Antimetabolites

Sulfonamides

D. Alteration of cell membrane permeability

Clotrimazole, polyene

E. Inhibition of nucleic acid synthesis

Rifampicin, nucleoside antiviral drugs

F. Topoisomerase inhibitors

Nalidixic acid, quinolones

G. Inhibition of cytochrome sterol

Azoles

Based on the effect on bacterial pathogen

A. Bactericidal agents

Penicillins, cephalosporins, glycopeptides, aminoglycosides, quinolones

B. Bacteriostatic agents

Macrolides, tetracyclines, chloramphenicol, sulfonamides, lincosamides

2. **The mode of action of tetracycline**
   a. Inhibits cell wall synthesis
   b. Inhibits protein synthesis
   c. Inhibits nucleic acid synthesis
   d. Alters cell membrane permeability

Ans b.

Tetracycline inhibits protein synthesis by binding to 30S ribosomes. The table in Q. No. 1 also classifies the antibiotics based on their mode of action.

3. **One of the following is bacteriostatic**
   a. Penicillin
   b. Tetracycline
   c. Cephalosporins
   d. Quinolones

Ans b.

Penicillins, cephalosporins, glycopeptides, aminoglycosides and quinolones are bactericidal agents. Macrolides, tetracyclines, chloramphenicol, sulfonamides and lincosamides are bacteriostatic agents.

4. **The term "antibiotic" was proposed by**
   a. Waksman
   b. Jenner
   c. McCallum
   d. Fleming

Ans a.

Waksman proposed the term "antibiotics".

5. **Dosage of amoxicillin for children should be**
   a. 10–20 mg/kg
   b. 25–50 mg/kg
   c. 50–70 mg/kg
   d. 70–100 mg/kg

Ans b.

Amoxicillin should be given 25–50 mg/kg body weight in three divided doses. It is available as 125 or 250 mg tablets and 125 mg/5 mL or 250 mg/5 mL syrup.

6. **According to the American Academy of Pediatric Dentistry (AAPD), the minimal duration of drug therapy should be**

a. 3 days c. 7 days
b. 5 days d. 10–14 days

Ans c.

The minimal duration of drug therapy should be limited to 7 days and usually can be a course of 10–14 days.

7. **Flagyl suspension is**

a. Metronidazole c. Tinidazole
b. Ciprofloxacin d. Cephadroxil

Ans a.

Metronidazole is given 30–50 mg/kg body weight in children with anaerobic infections. It is available as 200 mg tablets and 200 mg/5 mL suspension. Nausea and metallic taste are the characteristic side effects of the drug.

8. **One of the following is an antifungal drug**

a. Acyclovir c. Metamizol
b. Metronidazole d. Fluconazole

Ans d.

Fluconazole and nystatin are commonly used antifungal drugs. Fluconazole is given 6–12 mg/kg/day and is available as 50 and 100 mg dispersible tablets. It can also be given intravenously. Acyclovir is an antiviral drug given 20 mg/kg/dose, 3–5 times daily.

9. **One of the following is a selective COX-2 inhibitor:**

a. Piroxicam c. Nimesulide
b. Rofecoxib d. Ketorolac

Ans b.

Rofecoxib, celecoxib and valdecoxib are selective COX-2 inhibitors. Nimesulide, nabumetone and meloxicam are preferential COX-2 inhibitors. The following table classifies the various analgesics.

Classification of Analgesics
A. Nonselective COX inhibitors (conventional NSAIDs)
1. Salicylates: Aspirin
2. Pyrzolone derivaties: Phenylbutazone, oxyphenbutazone
3. Indole derivatives: Indomethacin, sulindac
4. Propionic acid derivatives: Ibuprofen, naproxen, ketoprofen, flurbiprofen
5. Anthranilic acid derivatives: Mephenamic acid

6. Aryl acetic acid derivative: Diclofenac

7. Oxicam derivatives: Piroxicam, tenoxicam

8. Pyrrolo-pyrrole derivatives: Ketorolac

B. Preferential COX-2 inhibitors

Nimesulide, meloxicam

C. Selective COX-2 inhibitors

Celecoxib, rofecoxib, valdecoxib

D. Analgesic, antipyretic with poor anti-inflammatory action

1. Para-aminophenol derivative: Paracetamol (acetaminophen)
2. Pyrazolone derivative: Metamizol (dipyrone), propiphenazone
3. Benzoxazine derivatives: Nefopam

10. "q.i.d." indicates

a. Once daily
b. Twice daily
c. Thrice daily
d. Four times a day

Ans d.

"q.i.d." indicates *quarter in die*, which means four times a day. "d", "b.i.d." and "t.i.d." indicates once, twice and thrice a day respectively. The common abbreviations used are summarized in the following table.

Commonly used abbreviations in a prescription

S. No.	Abbreviation	Latin	English
1.	d	Die	A day, daily
2.	b.i.d.	Bis in die	Twice a day
3.	t.i.d.	Ter in die	Thrice a day
4.	q.i.d.	Quarter in die	Four times a day
5.	h.	Hora	Hour
6.	h.s.	Hora somni	At bedtime
7.	stat	Statim	Immediately
8.	p.o.	Per os	Orally
9.	tab.	tabella	Tablet
10.	caps.	capsula	Capsule

11. Calculation of drug dosage based on body weight is

a. Clark's rule
b. Young's rule
c. Dilling's rule
d. Rx rule

Ans a.

$$\text{Individual dose} = \frac{\text{Body weight in kg}}{70 \times \text{Adult dose}}$$

Body weight is most commonly used to calculate the drug dosage. Though formulas based on body surface area can be more accurate, it cannot be used routinely for all patients. Young's rule and Dilling's rule are based on age of the patient and are least reliable. Calculations based on body surface area are supposed to be the most accurate.

12. Children younger than 8 years of age should not be given tetracycline because these agents

a. Cause damage to tendons
b. Do not cross the CSF
c. Are not bactericidal
d. Get deposited in tissue undergoing calcification

Ans d.

Children less than 8 years of age administered with tetracycline can have stains on their permanent teeth as they get deposited in them during the calcification process.

13. All of the following are broad spectrum antibiotics except

a. Amoxicillin
b. Tetracycline
c. Doxycycline
d. Chloramphenicol

Ans a.

The answer is self-explanatory.

Chapter 45

Child Abuse and Neglect

1. **The first documented and reported case of child abuse occurred in**

   a. 1874
   b. 1974
   c. 1894
   d. 1924

Ans a.

The first documented and reported case of child abuse occurred in 1874. A child named Mary Ellen was discovered chained to her bedpost. She was beaten regularly and was found to be severely malnourished. A New York City Church group reported the situation to the police.

2. **The term "battered child syndrome" was coined (in 1962) by**

   a. Caffey
   b. Mary Ellen
   c. Henry Kempe
   d. Needleman

Ans c.

Henry Kempe coined the term "battered child syndrome" in his milestone article in 1962. Caffey and Silverman reported cases of child abuse in their article. Mary Ellen is the name of the first documented child who was reported to be abused. Needleman reported cases of child abuse with orofacial trauma.

3. **Battered child syndrome should be considered in any child exhibiting evidence of**

   a. Fractures of any long bone
   b. Subdural hematomas
   c. Failure to thrive, soft tissue swelling or skin bruising
   d. Any of the above

Ans d.

According to Henry Kempe, battered child syndrome should be considered in any child exhibiting evidence of fractures of any long bone, subdural hematoma, failure to thrive, soft tissue swelling and skin bruising.

4. Which one of the following is/are a form of child abuse and neglect?

a. Munchausen syndrome by proxy
b. Sexual abuse or exploitation
c. Intentional drugging or poisoning
d. All of the above

Ans d.

All the above-mentioned conditions are different forms of child abuse and neglect. Munchausen syndrome by proxy is a form of fabricated illness by the parents. Sexual abuse is a form of child abuse where an adult sexually exploits the child. Intentional drugging or poisoning is a form of child abuse where the child is drugged or poisoned by the caretaker.

5. All of the following is/are true regarding physical abuse except

a. Otherwise known as accidental trauma
b. Defined as injuries inflicted on a person under 18 years of age by a caretaker
c. Graded from mild to moderate and severe forms of abuse
d. Usually recognized by the pattern of injury or its inconsistency with the history related

Ans a.

Physical abuse is defined as nonaccidental trauma. The injuries in physical abuse are graded from mild (a few bruises, welts, or scratches) to moderate (numerous bruises, minor burns or a single fracture) to severe (large burns, CNS injury, abdominal injury, multiple fractures or other life-threatening injuries). A careful history by an alert clinician will reveal inconsistency in the history from parent and the child. Also the type and severity of the injuries may not coincide with the history.

6. All of the following are true regarding failure to thrive except

a. A child is overweight
b. When a child fails to grow and develop because of insufficient caloric intake
c. Usually under 2 years of age
d. Can be shown to thrive once they are removed from the home and placed on unlimited feedings of a normal diet for their age

Ans a.

In failure to thrive, the child is underweight and malnourished.

7. One of the following statements regarding Munchausen syndrome by proxy is false.

a. Children who are victims of parentally fabricated or induced illnesses

b. Involvement of children who are too young (under 6 years of age) to be aware of or able to tell others about this deception

c. Fabricated illnesses which may lead to unnecessary medical treatment

d. Bleeding from various sites, recurrent sepsis from injecting contaminated fluids, chronic diarrhea from laxatives, fevers or skin rashes as their signs and symptoms

e. Fractures of long bones, subdural hematomas and soft tissue swellings or skin bruising are characteristic clinical features

Ans e.

Munchausen syndrome by proxy is a malignant disorder of parenting in which the caretaker (usually the mother) relates a fictitious history, produces false signs and symptoms and fabricates illnesses in the child. It results in extensive medical evaluations, testing and often prolonged hospitalizations. Choice "e" has characteristic features of battered child syndrome.

8. All of the following is/are true regarding health care neglect except

a. When a parent or caretaker ignores the treatment recommendations of a health professional for the management of a treatable illness that a child has and becoming worse is health care neglect

b. Dental neglect is a specific type of health care neglect

c. AAPD defines dental neglect as the failure by a parent or a guardian to seek treatment for visually untreated caries, oral infection and or oral pain or failure of the parent or guardian to follow with treatment once informed that the above conditions exists

d. Continual scapegoat and rejection of a child by parents, caretakers or teachers

Ans d.

Continual scapegoat and rejection of a child by parents, caretakers or teachers is a type of emotional abuse.

9. **Match the following:**

   a. 1-E, 2-A, 3-B, 4-C, 5-D
   b. 1-D, 2-E, 3-A, 4-B, 5-C
   c. 1-B, 2-C, 3-D, 4-E, 5-A
   d. 1-A, 2-B, 3-C, 4-D, 5-E

Ans a.

The below mentioned table describes or defines safety neglect, emotional abuse, emotional neglect, physical neglect and educational abuse.

S. No.	Type of Abuse	S. No.	Description
1	Safety neglect	A	Continual scapegoat and rejection of a child by parents, caretakers or teachers
2	Emotional abuse	B	Includes inadequate nurture or affection, i.e. lack of "mothering", knowingly "permitted" maladaptive behavior such as delinquency or substance abuse
3	Emotional neglect	C	Failure to care for a child according to accepted or appropriate standards
4	Physical neglect	D	When a parent or caretaker knowingly permits chronic truancy, intentionally keeps the child home or fails to enroll the child in school
5	Educational abuse	E	Gross lack of direct or indirect supervision of a child which results in an injury

10. **All of the following statements regarding an abused child are true except**

    a. Trauma to the head and associated areas occurs in approximately 50% of the cases of physical abuse to children
    b. Soft tissue injuries (most frequently bruises) are the most common injuries sustained to the head and face and are the single most common injuries sustained in child abuse

c. Injury to the upper lip and maxillary labial frenum may be a characteristic lesion in the severely abused young child
d. The youngest children (infancy to 2 years) tend to be sexually abused most often

Ans d.

Usually the youngest children (infancy to 2 years) tend to be neglected most often and sexually or emotionally abused least often. On the other hand, older children (12–17 years) are the least neglected but the most sexually and emotionally abused.

11. Most difficult form of child maltreatment to identify and treat is

a. Sexual abuse
b. Physical abuse
c. Emotional abuse
d. Munchausen syndrome by proxy

Ans d.

Munchausen syndrome by proxy is a malignant disorder of parenting in which the parents (usually mother) relate a fictitious history, produce false signs or symptoms and fabricate illnesses in the child that results in extensive medical evaluations, testing and often prolonged hospitalizations. Because health care providers are often dependent on the parental history of the child's illness, it takes some time for the practitioner to realize the inconsistencies and possibly fabricated or exaggerated nature of the complaints. Hence, it is very difficult to identify and treat Munchausen syndrome by proxy. The other names of this condition are factitious disorder by proxy and pediatric condition falsification.

12. The Child Abuse Prevention and Treatment Act was signed into law in United States in

a. 1974
b. 1932
c. 1986
d. 1956

Ans a.

In 1974, the Child Abuse Prevention and Treatment Act was signed into law. It established, a national center on child abuse and neglect for the first time within the federal government.

13. Which of the following is an evidence for sexual abuse?

a. Tearing, bruising or specific inflammation of the mouth, anus, or genitals

b. Venereal disease of the mouth, eyes, anus or genitals in a child under 15
c. Pregnancy and the girl is very evasive in naming her partner
d. Any of the above

Ans d.

The answer is self-explanatory.

14. A child aged 4 years reports with the following findings: undernourished, small for age, symptoms of malnutrition with dirty clothes. This is classified as

a. Physical neglect
b. Emotional abuse
c. Emotional neglect
d. Physical abuse

Ans a.

Refer to the explanation of Q. No. 9.

15. Which of the following characterizes an abuser?

a. Abuser may demonstrate psychotic behavior
b. Abuser may view the child as different or bad
c. When the abuser is confronted with allegations of abuse
d. He or she makes no attempt to explain the injuries
e. Any of the above

Ans d.

The answer is self-explanatory. Child abuse is seldom the result of any single factor. Usually it is due to a combination of emotional and environmental stresses, a predisposition towards maltreatment, a personality type, an occasion when for some reason the child happens to trigger the parent's contempt or resentment.

16. Battered child syndrome was first described by

a. Rosenberg
b. Caffey
c. Silverman
d. Kempe

Ans d.

Henry Kempe coined the term "battered child syndrome" in his milestone article in 1962. Also refer to the explanation of Q. No. 2.

17. Rejecting, ignoring, terrorizing, isolating and corrupting are all various forms of

a. Physical abuse
b. Emotional abuse
c. Health care neglect
d. Physical neglect

Ans b.

Emotional abuse can be defined as systematic tearing down of another human being. Types of emotional abuse are rejecting, ignoring, terrorizing, isolating and corrupting.

18. Munchausen syndrome was first described by

a. Rosenberg
b. Caffey
c. Richard Asher
d. Silverman

Ans c.

Munchausen syndrome was first described by Dr Richard Asher in 1951.

19. PANDA is

a. An awareness program related to prevention of child abuse
b. A child protective agency
c. A law, related to child abuse in North American legal system
e. A child who was abused in the 18th century and the first reported victim of abuse

Ans a.

Prevent Abuse and Neglect through Dental Awareness (PANDA) is a program to educate professionals and dental auxiliaries about their role and responsibility in recognizing, reporting and preventing child abuse and neglect.

20. Shaken baby syndrome was first reported by

a. Asher
b. Caffey and Silverman
c. Guthkelch
d. Kempe

Ans c.

This syndrome was first reported by Guthkelch in 1971.

21. Persistent and unexplained metabolic acidosis may be a sign of

a. Intentional drugging or poisoning
b. Physical abuse with cigarette burns
c. Munchausen syndrome by proxy
d. Failure to thrive

Ans a.

Intentional drugging or poisoning is a less common, yet potentially life-threatening form of child abuse. It can occur for many different reasons, and involve a variety of toxic substances and have no classic clinical presentation. Case reports by Saladino in 1991, Woolf in 1992 suggest that persistent, unexplained metabolic acidosis may be the only sign of poisoning.

22. Which type of child neglect is diagnosed based on the weight for age?

a. Emotional neglect
b. Healthcare neglect
c. Failure to thrive
d. Dental neglect

Ans c.

Failure to thrive in infants and children results from inadequate nutrition to maintain physical growth and development. It is best defined as inadequate physical growth diagnosed by observation of growth over time using a standard growth chart. Failure to thrive is often multifactorial, involving some combination of organic disease, subtle neurological or behavioral problems, dysfunctional parenting behaviors and parent–child interaction difficulties.

23. Failure to thrive is diagnosed when a child's weight for age is below

a. Fifth percentile
b. Second percentile
c. Third percentile
d. Fourth percentile

Ans a.

Failure to thrive in infants and children results from inadequate nutrition to maintain physical growth and development. It is a condition commonly seen by primary care physicians and is usually diagnosed when a child's weight for age is below the fifth percentile or crosses two major percentile lines.

Chapter 46

Pediatric Dentistry: Practice Management

1. Children who were accommodated in a relatively more pleasant environment exhibited lowest anxiety levels. Conversely those children who were treated in a standard operatory exhibited highest anxiety levels.

a. Both the statements are true
b. Both the statements are false
c. First statement is true and the second is false
d. First statement is false and the second is true

Ans a.

Swallow, Jones and Morgan in 1975 studied the effect of environment on child behavior and reaction to dentistry. They found that the environment plays a major role in child behavior.

2. All of the following are advantages of exclusive pediatric practice except

a. Preventive dentistry can be dealt in extensively
b. A particular age group comes under this practice which is unique (upto 19 years)
c. Once the child is happy with the pediatric dentist, they do not prefer to be taken to another dentist
d. Children come with single tooth problems commonly

Ans d.

Children tend to come with multiple decayed teeth or in a caries free state. Children with only single tooth decayed are very uncommon.

3. The number of exclusive pediatric practices in India may range from

a. 15–35 in number across India
b. 1–5 in number across India

c. 60–100 in number across India

d. 100–200 in number across India

Ans a.

Across the country the number of pediatric dentistry clinics which cater exclusively to children may range in between 15–35 in number as of 2011 in India.

Chapter 47

Developmental Disturbances

1. Radiographic examination of a child revealed several missing primary and permanent teeth. The history indicated practically no perspiration during hot, summer months. These facts would lead to a preliminary diagnosis of

a. Achondroplasia
b. Ectodermal dysplasia
c. Osteogenesis imperfecta
d. Cleidocranial dysostosis

Ans b.

Ectodermal dysplasias are described as heritable conditions in which there are abnormalities of two or more ectodermal structures such as the hair, teeth, nails, sweat glands, craniofacial structures, digits and other parts of the body. Oligodontia and defective enamel are the most commonly seen dental anomalies.

2. The absence of pulp chamber is suggestive of

a. Dentinogenesis imperfecta
b. Amelogenesis imperfecta
c. Cleidocranial dysostosis
d. All of the above

Ans a.

Dentition in cases of dentinogenesis imperfecta looks gray or brown colored with extensive wear. Radiographic examination would generally show a normal complement of teeth, but extensive deposits of secondary dentin with almost obliterated pulp chambers and canal.

3. Ectopic or delayed eruption in the anterior segment of the arch is caused by

a. Presence of supernumerary teeth
b. Migration of teeth
c. Premature loss of primary teeth

d. Discrepancy between size of teeth and size of arch
e. Unfavorable sequence of eruption
f. All of the above

Ans f.

The answer is self-explanatory.

4. Dentinogenesis imperfecta differs from amelogenesis imperfecta in that the former is

a. A hereditary disturbance
b. The result of excess fluoride ingestion
c. Characterized by a brown color of the enamel
d. The result of faulty enamel matrix formation
e. Characterized by calcification of the pulp chambers and the root canals of the teeth

Ans e.

Refer to the explanation of Q. No. 2.

5. Cleidocranial dysostosis is of interest to the dentist because of

a. Premature loss of teeth
b. Concomitant micrognathia
c. High incidence of clefts
d. Associated high caries index
e. Multiple supernumerary and unerupted teeth

Ans e.

Dental abnormalities seen in cleidocranial dysplasia may include delayed loss of the primary teeth, delayed appearance of the permanent teeth, unusually shaped, peg-like teeth, malocclusion and multiple supernumerary teeth. It is sometimes accompanied by cysts in the oral cavity.

6. A condition characterized by dull orange-brown teeth, absence of pulp canals and shortened roots would most likely be

a. Hemosiderosis
b. Congenital porphyria
c. Osteogenesis imperfecta
d. Hereditary ectodermal dysplasia
e. Hereditary dentinogenesis imperfecta

Ans e.

Refer to the explanation of Q. No. 10.

7. A 10-year-old patient shows a discrepancy in the midlines of maxillary and mandibular dentitions in occlusion. This may be the result of a

a. Severe closed bite condition
b. Class II, Division 1 malocclusion
c. Deviation of the mandible on closure
d. Lateral drift maxillary or mandibular anterior teeth
e. Either (c) or (d)

Ans e.

Deviation of mandible from rest position to closure might be due to premature contacts or occlusal interferences. Lateral drift of anterior teeth can also cause a discrepancy in the midline of both the arches.

8. Fused or geminated teeth occur during which of the following stages of tooth development?

a. Apposition
b. Calcification
c. Eruption
d. Initiation

Ans d.

The answer is self-explanatory.

9. Premature exfoliation of a primary canine may indicate

a. An arch length excess
b. An arch length deficiency
c. A skeletal malocclusion
d. None of the above

Ans b.

Refer to the explanation of Q. No. 27, Chapter 6.

10. At which stage of development of a tooth does dentinogenesis imperfecta occur?

a. Initiation
b. Proliferation
c. Histodifferentiation
d. Morphodifferentiation
e. Apposition

Ans c.

The answer is self-explanatory.

11. The mechanism of tooth eruption is best explained on the basis of

a. Hormonal stimulation
b. Primary tooth exfoliation
c. Programmed cell death at the base of the crypt
d. Osteoclastic activity at the base of the crypt
e. Proliferation of cells at the base of the crypt

Ans e.

The answer is self-explanatory.

12. A 5-year-old child prematurely lost a primary mandibular second molar. The subsequent arch length loss noted at age 6½ years was caused by

a. Growth
b. Muscle imbalance
c. Forces of eruption
d. Forces of occlusion

Ans c.

When the permanent first molars erupt at 6 years, they drift mesially into the primary second molar space causing a reduction in the arch length.

13. After eruption of a permanent tooth, the time required for apical closure of its root is approximately

a. ½–1½ years
b. 2½–3½ years
c. 4½–5½ years
d. None of the above

Ans b.

In primary teeth, root completion occurs 1 year after tooth eruption.

14. The most common microorganism associated with a periapical infection, which results in an alveolar abscess, is

a. Staphylococcus
b. *Streptococcus viridans*
c. Pneumococci
d. *Staphylococcus salivarius*

Ans b.

The *Streptococcus viridans* group of microorganisms produce significant amounts of hyaluronidase and fibrinolysins which act to break down or dissolve hyaluronic acid and fibrin.

15. While making an access opening in an abscessed tooth, the discomfort can be lessened if the tooth is stabilized by the dentist's finger. A splint of impression compound can also stabilize the tooth.

a. Both the statements are false
b. Both the statements are true
c. First statement is true and the second is false
d. First statement is false and the second is true

Ans b.

When the tooth is stabilized, the pressure exerted in the apical direction by the handpiece and the bur is reduced. This reduces the pain and discomfort.

16. In Ludwig's angina all of the following spaces are involved except

a. Submental space
b. Submandibular space
c. Sublingual space
d. Pterygoid space

Ans d.

Cellulitis from an infected mandibular tooth can spread to the floor of the mouth along fascial planes, nerves and vessels. If the infection involves the submandibular, sublingual and submental spaces, it is called *Ludwig's angina*. In this condition, the tongue and floor of the mouth is elevated to the extent that the patient's airway gets obstructed and swallowing becomes impossible.

17. Which of the following is the spreading factor that causes the infection to spread into the tissue spaces in Ludwig's angina?

a. Collagenase
b. Hyaluronic acid
c. Hyaluronidase
d. Polysachharidase

Ans c.

Hyaluronidase breaks down the intercellular cementing substance (hyaluronic acid). Similarly, fibrinolysin breaks down the fibrin. This leads to a rapid spread of the infection.

18. Continued budding of the primary or permanent tooth germ as a result of an abnormal proliferation of cells of the tooth germ results in

a. Dentigerous cyst
b. Odontoma
c. Anodontia
d. Odontogenic keratocyst

Ans b.

The question explains the etiology of odontoma.

19. Treatment for odontoma is usually

a. Observation
b. Surgical excision
c. Allowing it to erupt
d. Orthodontic extrusion

Ans b.

Odontomas are usually removed surgically before they interfere with the eruption of adjacent teeth.

20. All of the following statements are true about fusion except

a. They follow a familial tendency
b. Union of two independently developing primary or permanent teeth
c. When there is fusion in primary teeth, congenital absence of the corresponding permanent teeth is never seen
d. Fused teeth have separate pulp chambers and separate pulp canals

Ans c.

A frequent finding in fusion of primary teeth is the congenital absence of one of the corresponding permanent teeth.

21. All of the following about gemination are true except

a. It represents an attempted division of a single tooth germ by invagination
b. It does not follow a hereditary pattern
c. It appears clinically as a bifid crown on a single root
d. It is seen in both primary and permanent teeth

Ans b.

Gemination follows a hereditary pattern of occurrence, seen in both primary and permanent teeth but more frequently in primary teeth.

22. Dens in dente is most often seen in

a. Permanent maxillary central incisors
b. Permanent maxillary lateral incisors
c. Primary maxillary lateral incisors
d. Primary mandibular lateral incisors

Ans b.

This condition should be suspected whenever deep lingual pits are observed in maxillary permanent lateral incisors.

23. Which of the following regarding dens in dente is true?

a. This condition should be suspected whenever deep lingual pits are observed in maxillary permanent lateral incisors
b. This condition can occur in primary and permanent teeth
c. Prophylactic application of a sealant or restoration is indicated
d. If the condition is detected before the complete eruption of the tooth, the removal of gingival tissue to facilitate cavity preparation and restoration may be indicated
e. All of the above

Ans e.

The answer is self-explanatory.

24. All of the following are true regarding cherubism except

a. It is otherwise known as familial fibrous dysplasia
b. Numerous sharp, well-defined multilocular areas of bone destruction and thinning of cortical plate are usually evident in radiograph
c. It is characterized by delayed exfoliation of primary teeth
d. It has an autosomal dominant pattern of inheritance

Ans c.

In *cherubism*, teeth are frequently exfoliated prematurely as a result of loss of support or root resorption or in permanent teeth as a result of interference with the development of roots. Spontaneous loss of teeth may occur or the child may pick the teeth out of the soft tissue.

25. Which of the following about acrodynia is true?

a. Exposure of young children to minute amounts of mercury is responsible for this condition
b. Otherwise known as pink disease
c. Ointments and medicaments are the usual sources of mercury and dental amalgam restorations do not cause this condition
d. Clinical features include fever, anorexia, desquamation of soles and palms, sweating, tachycardia, gastrointestinal disturbance, hypotonia, oral ulcerations, excessive salivation and early exfoliation of primary teeth
e. All of the above

Ans e.

The answer is self-explanatory.

26. Micrognathia can be a result of

a. Intrauterine injury and deficient nutrition
b. Birth injury
c. Infections of temporomandibular joint
d. All of the above

Ans d.

Forceps delivery can interfere with the growth of the condyle thereby resulting in micrognathia. Similarly, intrauterine injury, deficient nutrition and infections of TMJ can also affect the growth of the condyle resulting in smaller jaws.

27. Which of the following regarding vitamin D-resistant rickets is true?

a. Also known as familial hypophosphatemia
b. Inherited usually as an X-linked dominant trait
c. Absent or abnormal lamina dura is seen in radiographs
d. Dental manifestations include apical radiolucencies, abscesses and fistulas associated with pulp exposures in primary and permanent teeth
e. All of the above

Ans e.

The answer is self-explanatory.

28. All of the following conditions are associated with early exfoliation of teeth except

a. Acrodynia

b. Progeria
c. Juvenile diabetes
d. Hypopituitarism

Ans d.

Premature exfoliation of teeth is seen in acrodynia, progeria and juvenile diabetes. But in hypopituitarism, there is delayed exfoliation of teeth.

29. All of the following conditions are associated with early exfoliation of teeth except

a. Cherubism
b. Hypophosphatasia
c. Histiocytosis X
d. Hypothyroidism

Ans d.

Premature exfoliation of teeth is seen in cherubism, hypophosphatasia and histiocytosis X. But in hypothyroidism there is delayed exfoliation of teeth.

Refer to the explanation of Q. No. 11, Chapter 6.

30. Which of the following is true regarding lead poisoning?

a. The fetus of a lead-poisoned mother can be affected because lead readily crosses the placenta during pregnancy
b. Pica is a common sign of plumbism in children
c. It can result in pitting hypoplasia
d. All of the above

Ans d.

The answer is self-explanatory. Tasting or mouthing of strange objects is normal in children up to the age of 2 years. Persistence of this habit beyond the age of 2 years is termed pica and it may be a manifestation of parental neglect or lack of affection. The child may develop the habit of eating non edible substances such as sand, clay, paint and wall plaster. These children are prone to lead poisoning and often complain of chronic abdominal pain and pallor.

31. Which of the following is not inherited as an autosomal dominant trait?

a. Dentinogenesis imperfecta
b. Cherubism
c. Vitamin D-resistant rickets (familial hypophosphatemia)
d. Hemophilia

Ans c.

Vitamin D-resistant rickets is inherited as an X-linked dominant trait.

32. Dentinogenesis imperfecta without osteogenesis imperfecta is otherwise called
   a. Type I dentinogenesis imperfecta
   b. Type II dentinogenesis imperfecta
   c. Hereditary opalascent dentin
   d. Both (b) and (c)

Ans d.

Type I dentinogenesis imperfecta is associated with osteogenesis imperfecta.

Type III dentinogenesis imperfecta is otherwise called brandywine type.

33. Which of the following is true regarding dentinogenesis imperfecta?
   a. They affect both primary and permanent teeth
   b. The pulp chamber is small or entirely absent and the pulp canals are small and ribbon like
   c. Stainless steel crowns may be considered as a means of preventing gross abrasion
   d. Multiple root fractures are present particularly in older patients
   e. All of the above

Ans e.

All of the above-mentioned statements are true regarding dentinogenesis imperfecta.

34. All of the following are true regarding amelogenesis imperfecta except
   a. It can be of hypocalcified, hypomaturation and hypoplastic type
   b. Taurodontism is sometimes associated with amelogenesis imperfecta
   c. Jacket crowns can be made for young patients
   d. It affects both primary and permanent teeth
   e. It is inherited as an autosomal dominant trait only

Ans e.

Amelogenesis imperfecta can be inherited as an autosomal dominant as well as an X-linked type.

35. In shell teeth, pulp chambers and canals are so enlarged that little more than a shell of enamel and dentin remain. In dentinogenesis

imperfecta, the pulp chamber is small or entirely absent, and the pulp canals are small and ribbon like.

a. Both the statements are false
b. Both the statements are true
c. First statement is true and the second is false
d. First statement is false and the second is true

Ans b.

The answer is self-explanatory.

36. Large pulp chambers are characteristic of all of the following conditions except

a. Shell teeth
b. Dentin dysplasia or dentin aplasia
c. Dentinogenesis imperfecta
d. Taurodontism

Ans c.

In dentinogenesis imperfecta, the pulp chamber is small or entirely absent and the pulp canals are small and ribbon like.

37. The congenital absence of primary teeth is relatively rare. When a number of primary teeth fail to develop, other ectodermal deficiencies are usually evident.

a. Both the statements are false
b. Both the statements are true
c. First statement is true and the second is false
d. First statement is false and the second is true

Ans b.

The answer is self-explanatory. Other deficiencies affecting nails, sweat glands and hair may be seen.

38. Which of the following is/are true regarding erythroblastosis fetalis?

a. It results from the transplacental passage of maternal antibody active against red blood cell antigens of the infant
b. Because of persistent jaundice during the neonatal period, the primary teeth may have a characteristic blue green color or brown color
c. The staining of dentin which occurs after birth is due to the perfusion of bilirubin and biliverdin into the dentin
d. All of the above

Ans d.

In *erythroblastosis fetalis*, there is massive destruction of the red blood cells by the antigen–antibody reaction. All the above-mentioned statements are true regarding erythroblastosis fetalis.

39. A child aged 4 years presents with the following symptoms: hypersensitivity to light, passage of red-colored urine, blisters on hands and face and purplish brown primary teeth. The most probable diagnosis is

a. Erythroblastosis fetalis
b. Porphyria
c. Tetracycline toxicity
d. Cystic fibrosis

Ans b.

Children with congenital erythropoietic porphyria pass red-colored urine, are hypersensitive to light and develop subepidermal bullous lesions when their skin is exposed to sunlight. Their primary teeth are purplish brown as a result of the deposition of porphyrin in the developing structures.

40. Which of the following is/are true regarding tetracycline discoloration?

a. Discoloration is because of chelating properties of tetracycline which forms a tetracycline-calcium orthophosphate complex
b. Exposure of affected teeth to light results in a color change from yellow to brown (oxidation)
c. The larger the dose of drug relative to body weight, the deeper the pigmentation
d. All of the above

Ans d.

Duration of exposure is less relevant than the total dose relative to body weight. Tetracycline is deposited in the dentin and to a lesser extent in the enamel that is calcifying at that time. Tetracycline when yellow in color fluoresces

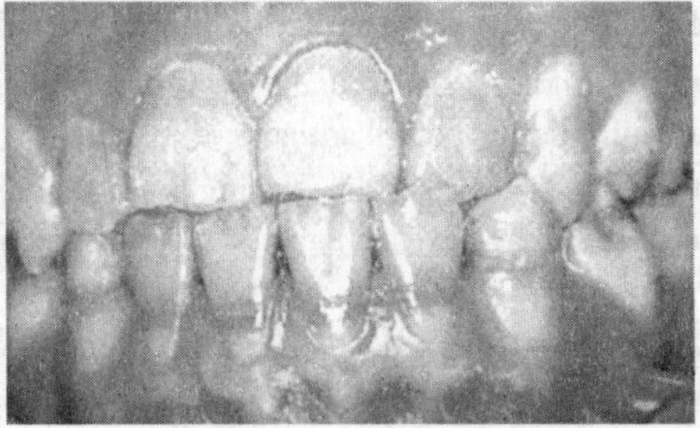

Fig. 47.1 Tetracycline discoloration.

under ultraviolet light (the fluorescence diminishes when it becomes yellow to brown). If administered during pregnancy, crowns of primary teeth show noticeable discoloration. The sensitive period for tetracycline during tooth development is as follows: 4 months in utero to 3 months postpartum for maxillary and mandibular incisors, 5 months in utero to 9 months postpartum for maxillary and mandibular canines, 3 to 5 months postpartum to 7th year of life for permanent maxillary, mandibular incisors and canines. Maxillary lateral incisors are an exception because they begin to calcify at 10–12 months postpartum. Bleaching with superoxol is a method of managing tetracycline discoloration.

41. Which of the following papillae usually show inflammatory and atrophic changes on the dorsum of the tongue?

a. Fungiform papillae
b. Foliate papillae
c. Circumvallate papillae
d. Filiform papillae

Ans a.

Inflammatory and atrophic changes occurring on the dorsum of the tongue usually involve the vascularized fungiform papilla.

42. Which of the following papillae are vascularized?

a. Fungiform papillae and circumvallate papillae
b. Circumvallate papillae and filiform papillae
c. Filiform papillae and foliate papillae
d. Foliate papillae and fungiform papillae

Ans a.

Large circumvallate papillae, 10–15 in number, may be found on the posterior border of the dorsum. These papillae have blood supply and they hold numerous taste buds. Fungiform papillae may be distributed over the entire dorsum of the tongue; however, they are present in greater numbers at the tip and towards the lateral margins of the tongue.

43. The papillae associated with taste sensation are

a. Fungiform papillae
b. Foliate papillae
c. Circumvallate papillae
d. Filiform papillae

Ans b.

Foliate papillae are arranged in folds along the lateral margins of the tongue; the taste sensation is associated with these papillae.

44. The most numerous papillae of the tongue are

a. Fungiform papillae
b. Foliate papillae
c. Circumvallate papillae
d. Filiform papillae

Ans d.

The most numerous papillae are the *filiform papillae,* which are thin and hair like and evenly distributed over the dorsal surface. The *filiform papillae* are without a vascular core and their continuous growth is slight.

45. All of the following conditions are associated with macroglossia except

a. Cretinism
b. Down syndrome
c. Angioneurotic edema
d. Ectodermal dysplasia

Ans d.

Macroglossia refers to a larger than normal size of the tongue. This can be congenital or acquired. Congenital macroglossia caused by an overdevelopment of the lingual musculature or vascular tissues becomes increasingly apparent as the child develops.

46. Which of the following patients can have a fissured tongue?

a. Down syndrome
b. Cretinism
c. Vitamin B complex deficiency
d. Any of the above

Ans d.

The answer is self-explanatory.

47. Which of the following pairs regarding the papillary distribution is incorrect?

a. Circumvallate papillae—posterior border of the dorsum
b. Fungiform papillae—tips and lateral borders predominantly (also entire dorsum)
c. Filiform papillae—even distribution over the dorsum
d. Foliate papillae—middle of the tongue

Ans d.

Refer to the explanations of Q. No. 42, 43 & 44.

48. Scarlet fever is associated with

a. Strawberry tongue
b. Coated tongue
c. Fissured tongue
d. Black hairy tongue

Ans a.

An enlargement of the fungiform papillae extending above the level of the white desquamating filiform papillae gives the appearance of an unripe strawberry. This condition has been observed in cases of scarlet fever and Kawasaki disease in young children.

49. Strawberry tongue is because of

a. Enlargement of filiform papillae
b. Enlargement of fungiform papillae
c. Enlargement of foliate papillae
d. Enlargement of circumvallate papillae

Ans b.

Refer to the explanation of Q. No. 41.

50. Which of the following tongue anomaly is associated with *Candida albicans*?

a. Median rhomboid glossitis
b. Black hairy tongue
c. Strawberry tongue
d. Benign migratory glossitis

Ans a.

Median rhomboid glossitis is an oval, rhomboid or diamond shaped reddish patch on the dorsal surface of the tongue immediately anterior to the circumvallate papillae.

51. Which of the following tongue anomaly is associated with oral and systemic intake of antibiotics?

a. Median rhomboid glossitis
b. Black hairy tongue
c. Strawberry tongue
d. Benign migratory glossitis

Ans b.

Black hairy tongue is rarely seen in children but occurs in young adults and has been related to the oral and systemic intake of antibiotics, smoking and excessive ingestion of dark drinks such as coffee and tea. Accumulations of keratin on the filiform papillae in the middle third of the tongue become elongated into hair-like processes, sometimes as long as 2.5 cm (1 inch).

52. Eruption hematoma or eruption cyst is most frequently seen in

a. Primary incisor region
b. Primary first molar region
c. Primary second molar region
d. Primary canine region

Ans c.

Eruption hematoma or cyst — A bluish purple elevated area of tissue develops a few weeks before the eruption of a primary or permanent tooth. This blood-filled cyst is most frequently seen in the second primary molar or first permanent molar regions.

53. Eruption sequestrum is usually seen in children during the eruption of

a. First permanent molar
b. Second permanent molar
c. First primary molar
d. Second primary molar

Ans a.

A tiny spicule of nonviable bone overlying the crown of an erupting permanent molar just before or immediately after the emergence of the tips of the cusps through the oral mucosa is known as the *eruption sequestrum.*

54. Natal teeth are

a. Teeth that erupt during the first 30 days after birth
b. Teeth present at birth
c. Teeth that erupt during the first 6 months
d. Teeth that erupt 30 days after birth

Ans b.

Natal teeth are teeth which are present at birth and neonatal teeth are the ones which erupt into the oral cavity within the first 30 days after birth.

55. Riga-Fede disease is characterized by

a. Natal teeth with tongue ulcerations
b. Natal teeth with eruption hematoma
c. Natal teeth and eruption cyst
d. Natal teeth and Epstein pearls

Ans a.

The sharp incisal edges of erupted natal or neonatal teeth may cause laceration of the lingual surface of the tongue. This clinical entity is called Riga-Fede disease.

56. Most often the natal teeth are

a. Supernumerary primary incisors
b. Prematurely erupted primary teeth
c. Nothing but dental lamina cyst of newborn
d. None of the above

Ans b.

Zhu and King have reported that 85% of the natal or neonatal teeth are prematurely erupted mandibular primary incisors and only small percentages are supernumerary teeth.

57. Which of the following is/are true about Down syndrome?

a. First primary teeth may not appear until 2 years of age
b. Primary dentition may not be complete until 4–5 years of age
c. The eruption of teeth often follows an abnormal sequence and some primary teeth may be retained until 14–15 years of age
d. All of the above

Ans d.

The answer is self-explanatory.

58. Down syndrome is

a. Trisomy 13
b. Trisomy 18
c. Trisomy 21
d. Trisomy 15

Ans c.

Refer to the following table:

S. No.	Trisomy	Name of the syndrome
1.	13	Patau syndrome
2.	18	Edward syndrome
3.	21	Down syndrome

59. Marie–Sainton syndrome is

a. Achondroplasia
b. Ectodermal dysplasia
c. Cleidocranial dysplasia
d. Hypopituiatarism

Ans c.

Marie-Sainton syndrome is otherwise called *cleidocranial dysplasia* or osteodentin dysplasia or mutational dysostosis.

60. All of the following are true regarding cleidocranial dysostosis except

a. Absence of clavicles or remnants of clavicles as evidenced by presence of sternal and acromial ends
b. Large fontanelles
c. Large frontal sinus
d. Complete primary dentition at 15 years of age resulting from delayed resorption of the deciduous teeth followed by delayed eruption of permanent teeth is not uncommon

Ans c.

The diagnosis of cleidocranial dysplasia is by the absence of clavicles, as evidenced by the presence of the sternal and acromial ends. The fontanelles are usually large and radiographs of the head show open sutures even late in the child's life. The sinuses, particularly the frontal sinus, is usually small. Sometimes all the primary teeth are retained till 15 years of age.

61. Multiple supernumerary teeth is characteristic of

a. Cleidocranial dysostosis
b. Ectodermal dysplasia
c. Dwarfism
d. Hyperthyroidism

Ans a.

Some children have few supernumerary teeth in the anterior region of the mouth. Others may have a large number of extra teeth throughout the mouth.

62. Which of the following conditions are usually diagnosed at birth?

a. Hypothyroidism
b. Hypopituitarism
c. Achondroplastic dwarfism
d. All of the above

Ans d.

Congenital hypothyroidism is the result of an absence or underdevelopment of the thyroid glands and insufficient levels of thyroid hormone. It is routinely diagnosed and corrected at birth because of mandatory blood screening of newborn infants. Hypopituitarism is also diagnosed at birth because of mandatory blood screening of newborn infants. *Achondroplastic dwarfism* is also diagnosed at birth based on the growth of the extremities.

63. The union of two teeth by the cementum of the root is

a. Fusion
b. Ankylosis
c. Germination
d. Concrescence

Ans d.

Concrescence is a twinning anomaly and as it occurs after root development, it is not considered to be a developmental anomaly. Etiology is thought to be trauma or adjacent tooth malposition.

Bibliography

1. Andlaw RJ, Rock WP. A Manual of Paediatric Dentistry (4th edn). Edinburgh, Churchill Livingstone, 1998.
2. Braham RL, Morris ME. Textbook of Pediatric Dentistry (2nd edn). New Delhi, CBS Publishers, 1990.
3. Wright GZ. Behavior Management in Dentistry for Children. Philadelphia, Saunders, 1975.
4. Ash MM, Nelson SJ. Wheelers Dental Anatomy, Physiology and Occlusion (8th edn). Philadelphia, Saunders, 2003.
5. Bhaskar SN. Orban's Oral Histology and Embryology (11th edn). St Louis, Mosby, 1991.
6. Crider AB, Goethals GA, Kavanaugh RD et al. Psychology (3rd edn). Scott, Foresman and Company, 1983.
7. Mathewson RJ, Primosch RE. Fundamentals of Pediatric Dentistry (3rd edn). Chicago, Quintessence, 1995.
8. Finn SB. Clinical Pedodontics (4th edn). Philadelphia, Saunders, 1991.
9. Graber TM. Orthodontics: Principles and Practice (3rd edn). Philadelphia, Saunders, 1992.
10. Pinkham JR et al. Pediatric Dentistry: Infancy through Adolescence (4th edn). New Delhi, Elsevier, 2005.
11. McDonald RE, Avery DR, Dean JA. Dentistry for the Child and Adolescent (8th edn). St Louis, Mosby, 2004.
12. Stephen HYW. Pediatric Dentistry: Total Patient Care. Philadelphia, Lea and Febiger, 1988.
13. Stewart RE, Barber TK, Troutman KC et al. Pediatric Dentistry: Scientific Foundations and Clinical Practice. St Louis, Mosby, 1982.
14. Proffit WR, Fields HW. Contemporary Orthodontics (2nd edn). St Louis, Mosby, 1993.
15. Question papers of National Board Dental Examinations (from 1979-1996): Used as a resource for some of the questions.

Bibliography